GARUM AND SALSAMENTA

STUDIES IN ANCIENT MEDICINE

EDITED BY

JOHN SCARBOROUGH

VOLUME 3

GARUM AND SALSAMENTA

Production and Commerce in Materia Medica

By

Robert I. Curtis

E.J. BRILL
LEIDEN • NEW YORK • KØBENHAVN • KÖLN
1991

The paper in this book meets the guidelines for permanence and durability of the Committee on Production Guidelines for Book Longevity of the Council on Library Resources.

Library of Congress Cataloging-in-Publication Data

Curtis, Robert I. (Robert Irvin), 1943-
Garum and salsamenta: production and commerce in materia medica / by Robert I. Curtis.
p. cm.—(Studies in ancient medicine, ISSN 0925-1421; v. 3)
Includes bibliography references and index.
ISBN 90-04-09423-7 (cloth: alk. paper)
1. Fish, Salted—Therapeutic use—History. I. Title. II. Series.
[DNLM: 1. Fish Products—history. 2. History of Medicine, Ancient. 3. Materia Medica—history. 4. Medicine, Traditional. WZ 51 C978g]
RS160.7C87 1991
615'.36—dc20
DNLM/DLC
for Library of Congress 91-16000
CIP

ISSN 0925-1421
ISBN 90 04 09423 7

PRINTED IN THE NETHERLANDS

D M

OPTIMI

PATRIS FRATRISQUE

ET

MATRI UXORIQUE FILIAEQUE

OPTIMAE

CONTENTS

ABBREVIATIONS

Abbreviations of journals follow those listed in *L'Année Philologique*. In general, abbreviations of ancient authors conform to those listed in the *Oxford Classical Dictionary*, 2nd ed. (Oxford 1970); for papyri and ostraca I have followed those listed in *Checklist of Editions of Greek Papyri and Ostraca*. Supplement No. 4 of *Bulletin of the American Society of Papyrologists*. John F. Oates, Roger S. Bagnall, William H. Willis, and K. A. Worp, eds. 3rd ed. (1985). For abbreviations of other sources cited, attention is drawn to the following list.

ANRW	*Aufstieg und Niedergang der römischen Welt*. H. Temporini and Wolfgang Haase, eds. (Berlin 1972–).
BT	*The Babylonian Talmud*. Rabbi Dr. Isidore Epstein, ed. 18 vols. (London 1961).
CGL	*Corpus Glosssariorum Latinorum*. G. Loewe and G. Goetz, eds. (Leipzig 1888–1923).
CIL	*Corpus Inscriptionum Latinarum*. T. Mommsen et al., eds. 16 vols. (Berlin 1893–).
CMG	*Corpus Medicorum Graecorum*.
CML	*Corpus Medicorum Latinorum*.
Dar.-Sag.	*Dictionnaire des antiquités grecques et romaines*. C. Daremberg and E. Saglio, eds. 10 vols. (Paris 1877–1918).
Ditt. *Syll.*[3]	*Sylloge Inscriptionum Graecarum*. W. Dittenberger, ed. 3rd ed. 4 vols. (Leipzig 1915–24).
Ermerins	F. Z. Ermerins, *Anecdota Medica Graeca* (Leiden 1840).
ESAR	*An Economic Survey of Ancient Rome*. Tenney Frank, ed. 6 vols. (Baltimore 1933–40).
FGrH	*Die Fragmente der griechischen Historiker*. F. Jacoby, ed. (Berlin 1923–).
FHG	*Fragmenta Historicorum Graecorum*. K. Müller, ed., 4 vols. (Paris 1841–51).
IG	*Inscriptiones Graecae* (Berlin 1873–).
IGRR	*Inscriptiones Graecae Ad Res Romanas Pertinentes*. René Cagnat et al., eds. 4 vols. (Paris 1911–27).
ILS	*Inscriptiones Latinae Selectae*. H. Dessau, ed. 3 vols. (Berlin 1892–1916).
Migne, *PG*	*Patrologiae Cursus Completus. Series Graeca*. J. P. Migne, ed. 161 vols. (Paris 1857–86).
Migne, *PL*	*Patrologiae Cursus Completus. Series Latina*. J. P. Migne, ed. 221 vols. (Paris 1844–65).
MGH	*Monumenta Germaniae Historica* (Hannover 1824–)
Not. dign.	*Notitia Dignitatum accedunt Notitia Urbis Constantinopolitanae et Laterculi Provinciarum*. Otto Seeck, ed. (Berlin 1876).
NSc	*Notizie degli Scavi di Antichità*. (Rome 1876–)
OGIS	*Orientis Graecae Inscriptiones Selectae*. W. Dittenberger, ed. 2 vols. (Leipzig 1903–05).
RE	*Realencyclopädie der classischen Altertumswissenschaft*. A. Pauly, G. Wissowa, and W. Kroll, eds. (Berlin 1894–1974).
SEG	*Supplementum Epigraphicum Graecum* (Leiden 1923–).
SEHRE[2]	M. I. Rostovtzeff, *The Social and Economic History of the Roman Empire*. 2nd ed. rev. by P. M. Fraser. 2 vols. (Oxford 1957).
SEHHW	M. I. Rostovtzeff, *The Social and Economic History of the Hellenistic World*. 3 vols. (Oxford 1941).

PLATES

FIGURES

ACKNOWLEDGMENTS

Acknowledging assistance, advice, and encouragement is the most pleasurable of tasks for an author and at the same time the most difficult. One wants to express the utmost appreciation to each and every person who has contributed, but for a work which has taken several years to complete one runs the risk of inadvertently omitting someone deserving of inclusion. For all of those, named and unnamed, who have helped along the way I extend my heartfelt gratitude and hope that the finished product will meet with their approval. The author has been saved from many errors of fact and of judgment by the timely and judicious suggestions of these friends and colleagues. Any errors that remain are the responsibility of the author, who has greatly appreciated but not always followed their advice.

This book traces its roots back to my early days of graduate school when Wilhelmina F. Jashemski, teacher, scholar, and dear friend, first suggested the topic to me. Focusing first on the industry at Pompeii alone, then on its manifestation in the Western Roman Empire, the study has grown to its present form which investigates the role of fermented fish products in all of Graeco-Roman society. These food products and items of materia medica formed an important element in long-distance trade. In regard to the study of their medicinal role, I am particularly indebted for the assistance, freely given, of John Scarborough, whose expertise on ancient medicine has been of inestimable value. His encouragement and advice in the completion of this project are particularly appreciated. Over this long period Anna Marguerite McCann in many enjoyable conversations concerning her work at Cosa as well as about my own research has proven a source of encouragement and inspiration.

Over the past ten years parts of the present work have appeared in different form as articles in various journals and books. Although I specifically indicate in the notes where this material is used, I wish here as well to thank the editors of these journals and publishers who have granted permission for me to incorporate this material into the present work: *American Journal of Archaeology, Classical Journal, Phoenix, Ancient Society, The Journal of the History of Medicine and Allied Sciences, The International Journal of Nautical Archaeology and Underwater Exploration,* and Aristide D. Caratzas Publisher, New Rochelle, New York. I would also like to extend my appreciation to those individuals and publishers who have granted me permission to use photographs and drawings, in some cases providing me with copies of them from their own collections. These include Charles K. Williams, II and Nancy Bookidis of the American School of Classical Studies in Athens, for

Plate Nos. 1a and 8; Anna Marguerite McCann, Guest Investigator for Woods Hole Oceanographic Institution, for Plate Nos. 2 and 5; Piet Stuart of the Rijksmuseum van Oudheden in Leiden, The Netherlands, for Plate No. 6; and Bernard Liou and the Centre Camille Jullian of Aix-en-Provence, for Plate No. 7b. For permission to base my Figure No. 1 on line drawings appearing in their book, *Amphorae and the Roman Economy*, I am indebted to D. P. S. Peacock and D. F. Williams. D. Fletcher, Director of Servicio de Investigación Prehistórica in Valencia, Spain, not only gave permission to use photographs and drawings from *La factoría pesquera de Punta de l'Arenal y otros restos romanos de Jávea (Alicante)* by Gabriela Martin and Maria Dolores Serres but also provided the book *gratis* when the illustrations and photographs themselves were not available. These latter appear as Figure No. 3 and Plate No. 3. Similarly, I wish to thank the Presses Universitaires de France for permission to use photographs for Figure Nos. 2 and 4 and for Plate Nos. 4a and 4b, taken from M. Ponsich and M. Tarradell, *Garum et industries antiques de salaison dans la Méditerranée occidentale*.

The spirit of cooperation I have experienced from many individuals, both in this country and abroad, who have corresponded with me on particular points covered by this book, who have shared with me copies of their published materials, and who have discussed the works of others in related fields, has been particularly gratifying. In this group I wish to acknowledge the contributions of David S. Reese, Elizabeth Lyding Will, Elizabeth Reitz, Genaro Chic Garcia, Gregorio de Frutos Reyes, Aurelio Padilla Monge, Baruch Rosen, Stéfanie Martin-Kilcher, and Liliane Bodson. For assistance in providing translations of works in languages with which I am not proficient, I wish to extend my thanks to John Toohey (Russian) and to my colleague Jared Klein (Hebrew). Over the past seventeen years my visits to Pompeii and Herculaneum have always been pleasurable and productive. I should particularly like to express my thanks to three previous Soprintendenti di Antichità in Campania, the late Alfonso De Franciscis, Fausto Zevi, and Giuseppina Cerulli Irelli, and to Stefano De Caro, former Direttore degli Scavi di Pompei, for permission to work in the Campanian cities and to photograph material *in situ* and in storage. These individuals greatly facilitated and immeasurably assisted my work in Italy.

The preparation of my manuscript for transformation into camera-ready copy has seemed a task of mammoth proportions, but which has been rendered a more pleasurable and far easier one through the assistance of many skilled and knowledgeable individuals at the University of Georgia. Ms. JoAnn Pulliam and Mary Ricks, departmental secretaries, typed several drafts of the manuscript. Mr. Christopher Anderson, of the Computer Department of the university bookstore, offered valuable assistance and advice in matters of computer technology. Ms. Virginia Vaughn, of the Instructional Resources Center, skillfully prepared the plans, maps, and other drawings. I would particularly like to express my gratitude to the following individuals who provided timely and substantial financial assistance toward the cost of publication of this book: Joe L. Key, Vice President for Research, C. Michael Moriarty, Associate Vice President for Research, John J. Kozak, Dean of Franklin College of Arts and Sciences, and Richard A. LaFleur, Head, Department of Classics.

Finally, I would like to express my deepest appreciation to my wife, Susan, who has over these many years shown the patience of Job during periods when she may have felt that her efforts had much in common with those of Sisyphus. As a professional librarian, she has been of direct help in facilitating my access to many sources and in tracking down some old and obscure citations. More importantly, she has been my greatest support, serving at the same time as my sharpest critic and strongest and most persistent encourager. In significant ways this book could not have been completed without her.

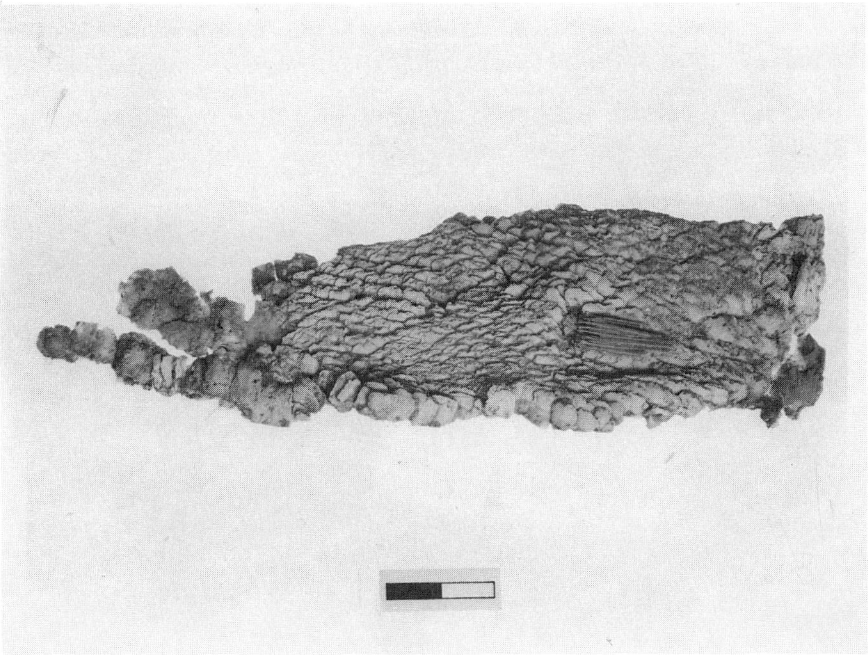

Plate 1a.

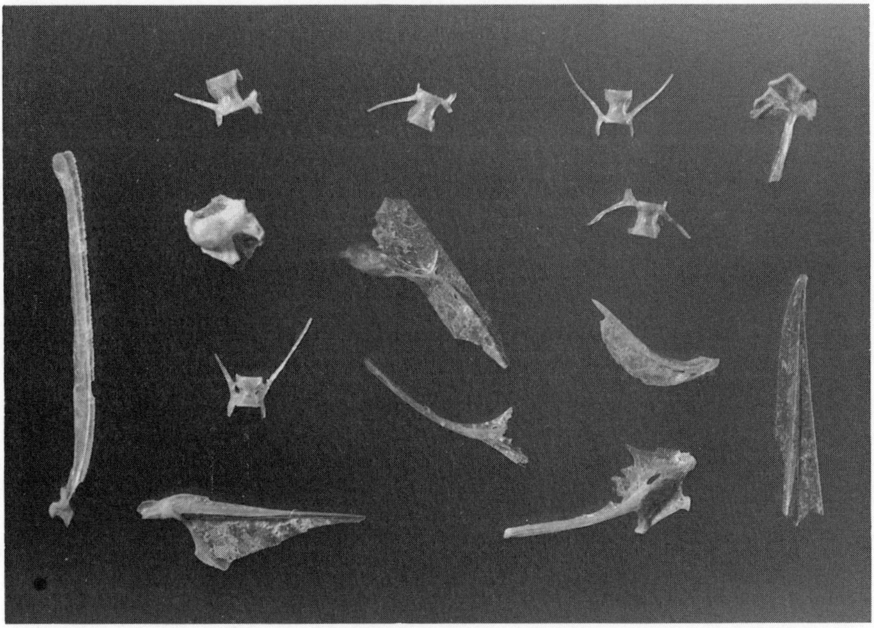

Plate 1b.

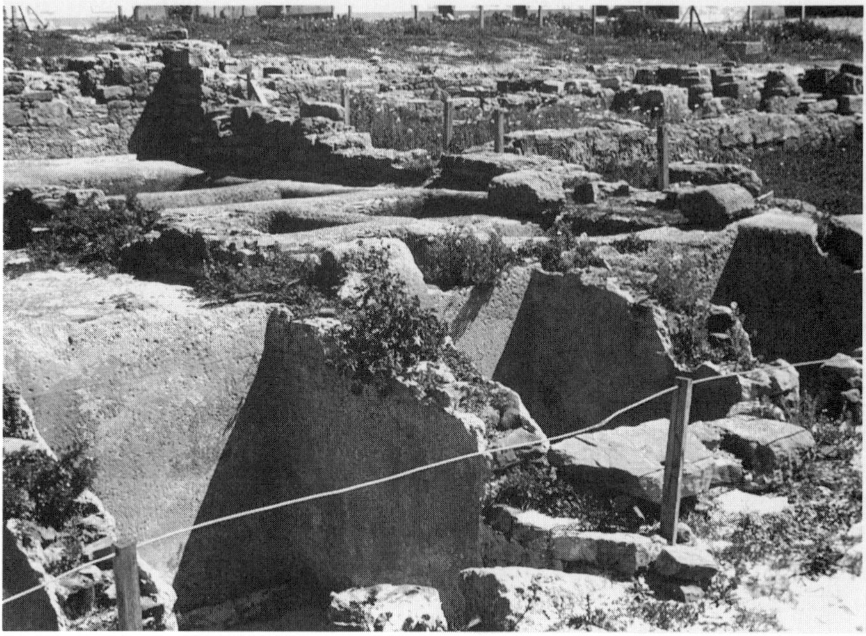

Plate 2.

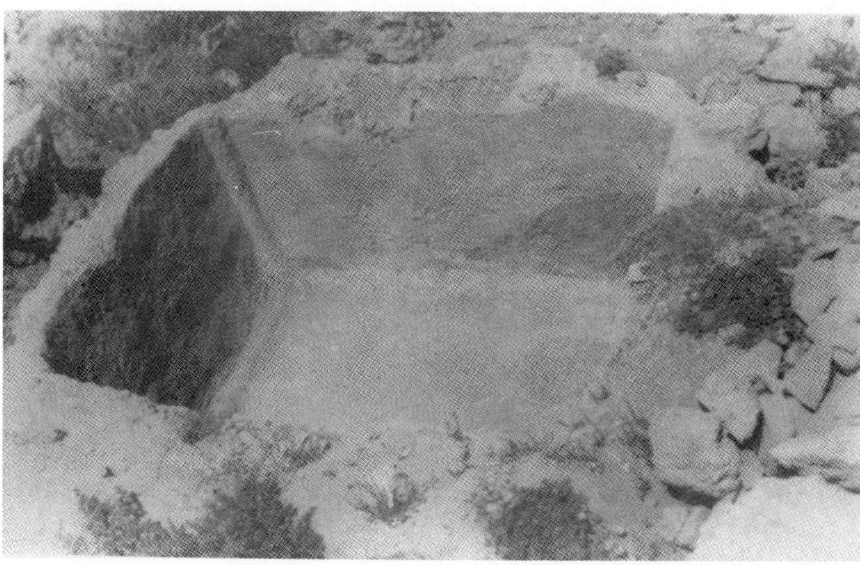

Plate 3.

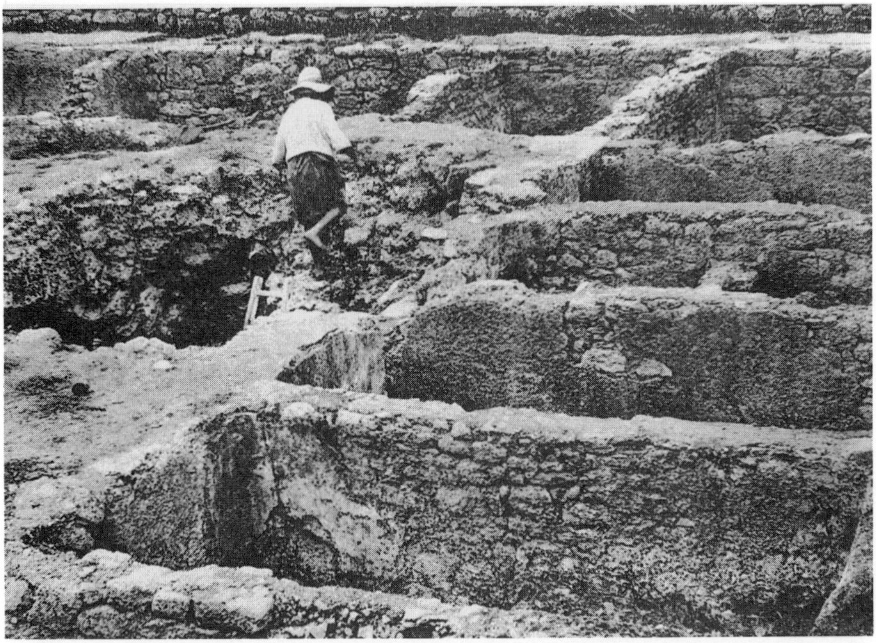

Plate 4a.

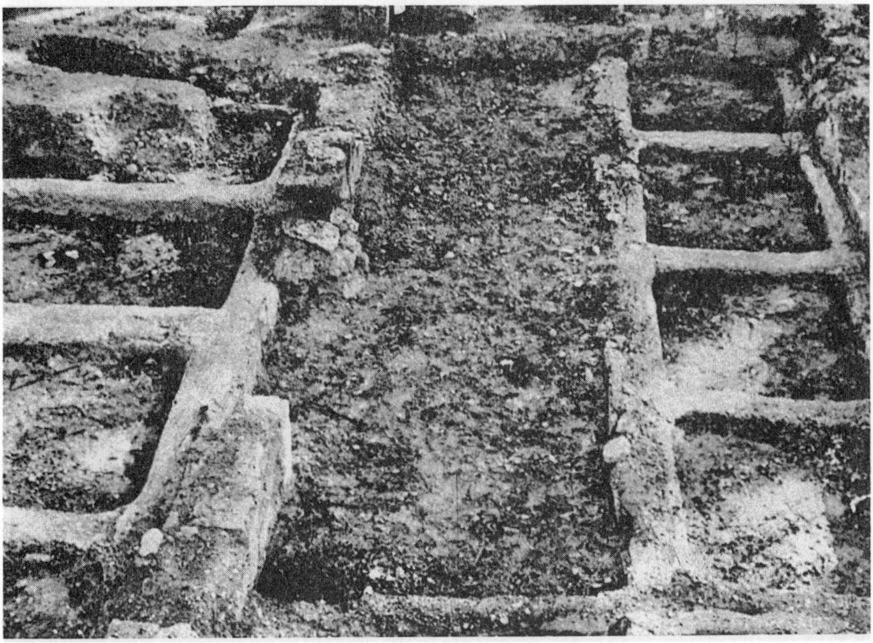

Plate 4b.

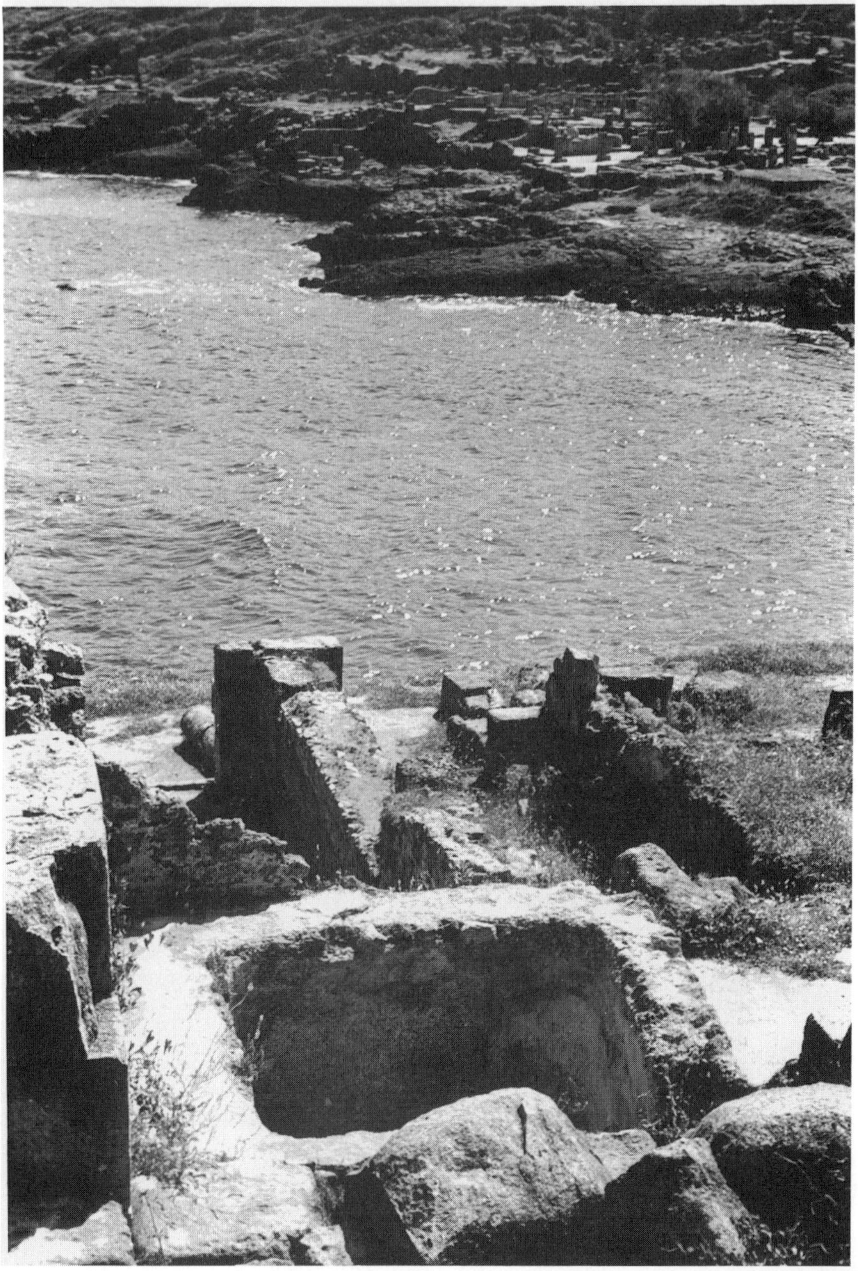

Plate 5.

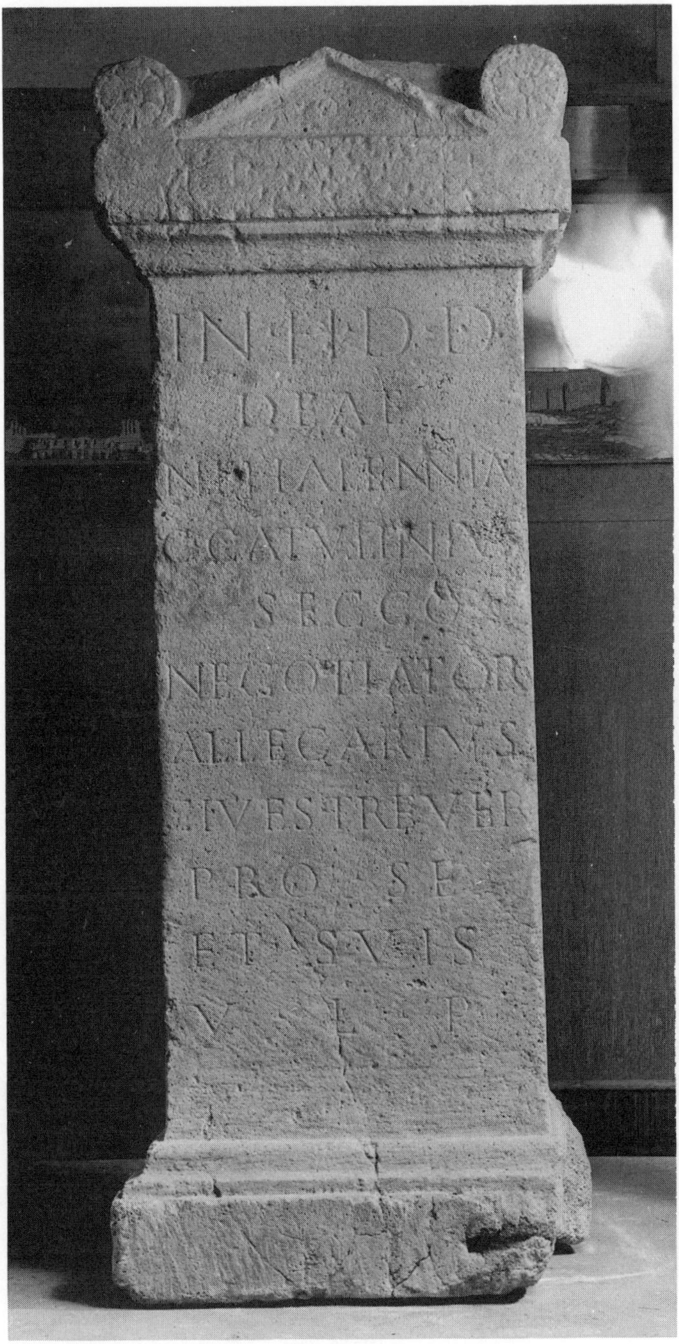

Plate 6.

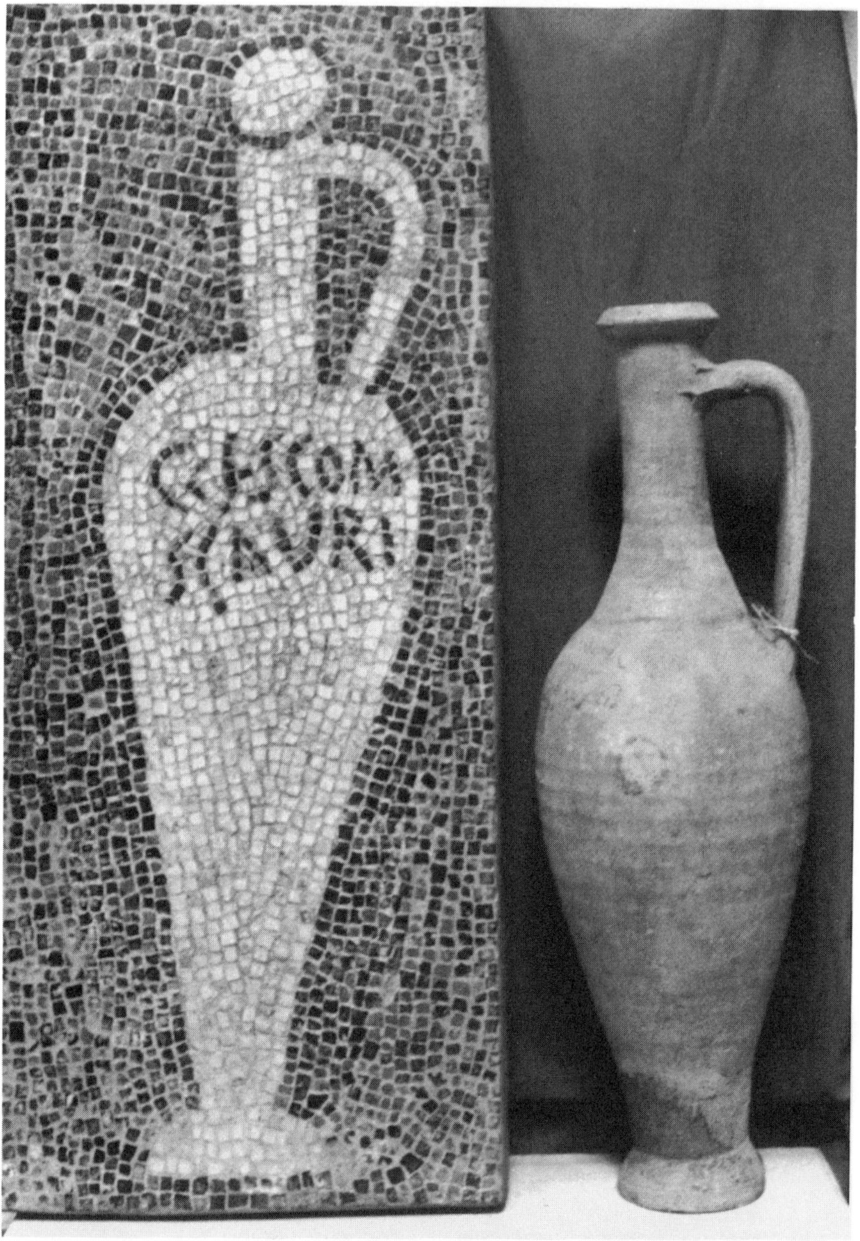

Plate 7a.

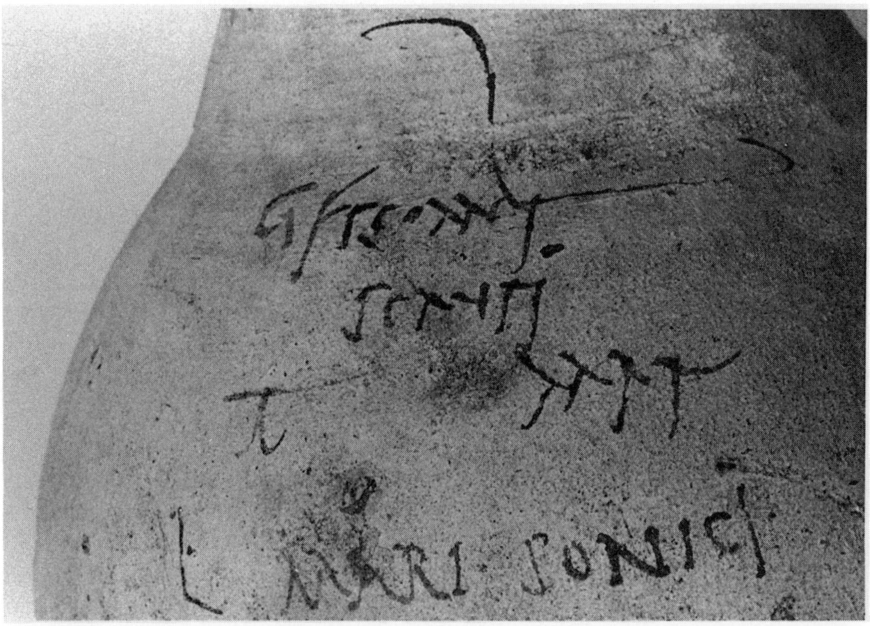

Plate 7b.

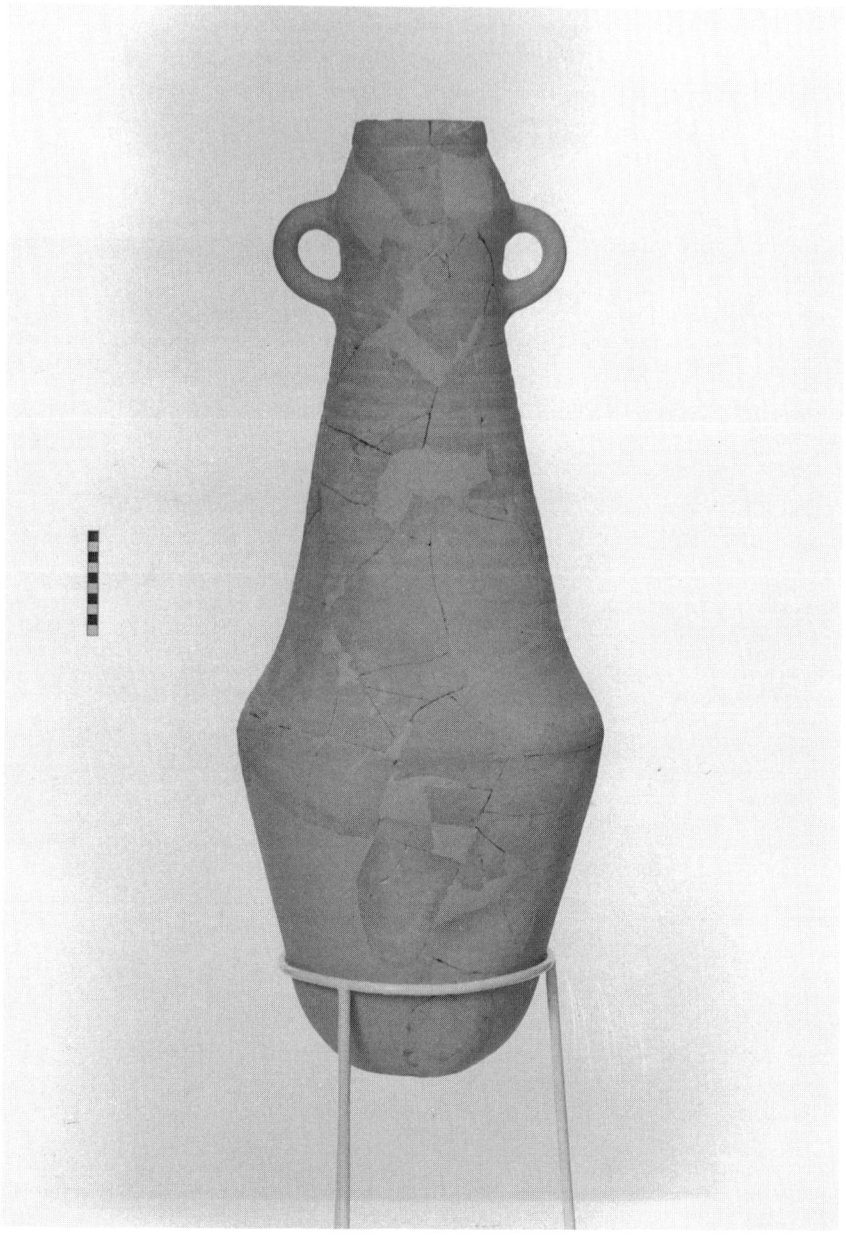

Plate 8.

CHAPTER ONE

INTRODUCTION

Galen, in Book I of *Concerning the Properties of Foods,* states that a dish of lentils seasoned with garum would create a "very pleasant and exceedingly useful medicine and food for not a few suffering from chronic diarrhea."[1] This dual purpose for fish sauces and other salted fish products, that is as a food and medicine, established for them an important place in Greek and Roman life. Galen could also have added here, as he strongly suggests in his discussion of salted foods in Book III of the same work, that preserved fish products were also important items of trade. Writing from Rome as his vantage point, he provides evidence of the far-flung trade in salt-fish, conjuring up in the mind of the reader the image of merchant ships arriving at the port of Rome laden with salt-fish products of both East and West. The best salt-fish (τάριχος) of which he is personally cognizant, he says, was called "Gaderic" by earlier physicians but now goes under the name "sarda." In the same category he includes salted mullet from Pontus. The second place he assigns to salted coracinus, pelamys, and Saxitana.[2] Galen's top choices, therefore, included salted tunny from the Western Mediterranean salteries of Gades in Spain and of the island of Sardinia and mullet from the factories of the Black Sea. His second choices were the coracinus, probably from Egypt or the Black Sea, the pelamys, a young tunny common to the seas of both East and West but especially in the Black

---

[1] Galen *De alimentorum facultatibus* 1.1.42–43: τευτλοφακῆν γοῦν ἡμεῖς τε δίδομεν ἐνίοτε καὶ πρὸ ἡμῶν ὁ Ταραντῖνος Ἡρακλείδης ἐδίδου πολλοῖς πολλάκις οὐ μόνον ὑγιαίνουσιν ἀμέμπτως, ἀλλὰ καὶ πάσχουσί τι. πρῶτον μὲν οὖν ἐμβάλλομεν αὐτῇ πολλὰ τεῦτλα, δεύτερον δὲ κατὰ τὴν ἄρτυσιν ἢ ἁλῶν βραχεῖ πλέον ἢ γάρου γλυκέος˙ ὑπακτικωτέρα γὰρ οὕτως. εἴ γε μὴν πτίσας τὴν φακῆν ἑψήσας τε δίς, ὡς ἀποχέαι τὸ πρότερον ὕδωρ, εἶτ᾽ ὀλίγον μὲν ἁλῶν ἢ γάρου μίξαις, ἐπεμβάλοις δέ τι βραχὺ τῶν ἐφεκτικῶν γαστρός ἄχρι τοῦ μὴ λυπῆσαι τὴν γεῦσιν, ἥδιστόν τε καὶ ὠφελιμώτατον ἐργάσῃ φάρμακόν θ᾽ ἅμα καὶ σιτίον οὐκ ὀλίγοις τῶν διαρροίαις χρονίαις ἐνοχλουμένων. οὐκ ὀλίγοις δ᾽ εἶπον, ἅπασι φυλαξάμενος εἰπεῖν, ὅτι κἀνταῦθα διορισμῶν ἐστι χρεία, καθ᾽ οὓς αἱ διαθέσεις εὑρεθήσονται τῶν διαρροιζομένων χρονίως. References to Galen's *De alim. fac.* come from *Corpus Medicorum Graecorum* V,4,2. G. Helmreich, ed. (Leipzig 1923). All further citations to the *Corpus Medicorum Graecorum* will use the abbreviation CMG. References to the Galenic corpus for works not covered by CMG will be to *Claudii Galeni Opera Omnia*. Carl Gottlob Kühn, ed. 20 vols. (Leipzig 1821–33). Notation will include volume number, page number, and the abbreviation K.

[2] Galen *De alim. fac.* 3.40.1–6. See especially para. 6: πρόδηλον δ᾽ ἐκ τούτων, ὅσα μὲν σκληρὰ καὶ νευρώδη καὶ οἱονεὶ δερματώδη τε καὶ βυρσώδη γίγνεται ταριχευθέντα, δύσπεπτα πάντ᾽ εἶναι˙ τὰ δ᾽ ἐναντίως διατιθέμενα λεπτομερῆ μὲν αὐτὰ γίγνεται, λεπτύνει δ᾽ ἐσθιόμενα τοὺς παχεῖς καὶ κολλώδεις χυμούς. ἄριστα δ᾽ ἐστὶ τῶν εἰς ἐμὴν πεῖραν ἐλθόντων τά τε Γαδειρικὰ πρὸς τῶν ἔμπροσθεν ἰατρῶν ὀνομαζόμενα ταρίχη, σάρδας δ᾽ αὐτὰς καλοῦσιν οἱ νῦν, οἵ τ᾽ ἐκ τοῦ Πόντου κομιζόμενοι μύλλοι. δευτέραν δ᾽ ἐπ᾽ αὐτοῖς ἔχουσι τάξιν οἵ τε κορακῖνοι καὶ αἱ πηλαμύδες καὶ τὰ Σαξιτανὰ καλούμενα.

Sea, and the Saxitana, the Spanish mackerel, named for Sexi, a town in Baetica.[3]

Galen was not the first physician to include preserved fish products in his discussion of dietetics and therapeutics. Salt-fish received attention in the Hippocratic corpus, compiled in the fifth and fourth centuries B.C., but fish sauce does not appear in extant medical literature before its inclusion in Book II of the *De materia medica* by Dioscorides, who flourished in the first century A.D.[4] The Greeks, however, consumed both these products and participated in their commerce as early as the fifth century B.C., and probably earlier. Galen provides proof that the Romans six hundred years later were doing the same thing but on a far greater scale. The present work, therefore, purports to concentrate on the three interrelated aspects of salted fish products which made them so important a part of ancient life: food, medicine, and object of trade.

Few items of materia medica lend themselves so well to a study of their trade. Spices coming from the East, amber from Northern Europe and Scandinavia, and silphium from North Africa are the most important ones which come to mind.[5] Silphium, however, seems the closest parallel to salt-fish products as commercial materia medica. It was a plant which could be used as a food by humans and domestic animals or as a condiment on food; it also served as a pharmaceutical in human and veterinary medicine. Its period of greatest commercial importance ranged from the late seventh century B.C. until around 200 B.C. when overuse rendered it practically extinct. Our knowledge of its history as an item of trade, however, is limited only to mentions of it in literary sources; archaeological evidence is nonexistent, except for scattered numismatic images. Three sharp distinctions, however, set salted fish products off into a unique category different from all other items of materia medica. Preserved fish are part of animal materia medica, not vegetable which forms the vast majority of this material. Second, the history of trade in salt-fish extends over many centuries, from

[3] D'Arcy Thompson, *A Glossary of Greek Fishes* (London 1947), pp. 122–25 (coracinus), 161–62 (mullus), 197–99 (pelamys), 226 (Saxitana), with full ancient references; for the sarda, see Alfred C. Andrews, "The 'Sardinian Fish' of the Greeks and Roman," *AJPh* 70 (1949): 171–85.

[4] *Regimen* II. For *Regimen* I have consulted *Hippocrates*. Vol. 4. W. H. S. Jones, ed. Loeb Classical Library (London and Cambridge, Mass. 1959). Dioscorides *De mat. med.* 2.32: γάρος δὲ πᾶς ὁ ἐκ τῶν ταριχευτικῶν ἰχθύων καὶ κρεῶν καταντλούμενος νομὰς ἐφιστᾷ καὶ κυνόδηκτα ἰᾶται. ἐνίεται δὲ καὶ ἐπὶ δυσεντερικῶν καὶ ἰσχιαδικῶν, ἐφ' ὧν μὲν ἵνα τὰ εἱλκωμένα ἐπισπάσῃ, ἐφ' ὧν δὲ ἵνα τὰ ἀνέλκωτα ἐρεθίσῃ. For Dioscorides' work I have used *Pedanii Dioscoridis Anazarbei De Materia Medica Libri Quinque*. Max Wellmann, ed. (Berlin 1907).

[5] On the drug trade of antiquity, see especially John Scarborough, "Roman Pharmacy and the Eastern Drug Trade: Some Problems as Illustrated by the Example of Aloe," *Pharmacy in History* 24,4 (1982): 135–43; Vivian Nutton, "The Drug Trade in Antiquity," *Journal of The Royal Society of Medicine* 78,2 (Feb. 1985): 138–45; Lionel Casson, "Cinnamon and Cassia in the Ancient World," in *Ancient Trade and Society* (Detroit 1984), pp. 225–46; Manfred G. Raschke, "New Studies in Roman Commerce with the East," in *ANRW* II,9.2 (1978), esp. pp. 650–76 (spice trade); John M. Riddle, "Amber in Ancient Pharmacy," *Pharmacy in History* 15,1 (1973): 3–17; and Chalmers L. Gemmill, "Silphium,"*BHM* 40,4 (July–Aug. 1966): 295–313.

perhaps as early as the seventh century B.C. to well into the Byzantine period. Its heyday apparently fell between the second century B.C. and the fourth century A.D. Evidence, both literary and archaeological, are particularly abundant for the first three centuries of the Roman Empire. And finally, ancient salt-fish products have their modern counterparts, which, though not so much used now medicinally, still fulfill for certain parts of the world similar and essential alimentary functions as well as form an important item of trade. Salt-fish products, then, evidence for which derives from extensive medical and non-medical literary sources and from abundant and widespread archaeological material, offer a unique opportunity to study in detail trade in an important item of materia medica.

Even though preserved fish products played a major role in Graeco-Roman society for many centuries, little serious study has been devoted to them by modern scholars. In part at least, this is probably because the mere mention of garum, for example, frequently evokes the image created by ancient comedy writers and particularly Roman satirists. This portrait usually takes the form of an expensive, malodorous product derived from the fermentation of fish. "Putrid" is a favorite adjective used to describe it.[6] Influenced by these pejorative descriptions modern historians usually have concluded, with Ugo Paoli, that "Our stomachs would probably revolt at a dish prepared with garum."[7] Garum, frequently perceived to be an expensive item and so not in widespread use among the general population, and salt-fish, perhaps seen as too mundane a topic for discussion, have had scant appeal to most modern social and economic historians. Numerous references in non-medical Greek and Latin sources to preserved fish products, augmented by archaeological evidence for their role in commerce and daily life, however, provide a clear picture of their popularity in classical antiquity. The frequent mention of salt-fish and fish sauce in ancient medical literature on dietetics and therapeutics, therefore, should elicit no surprise. Interestingly, what we know from ancient literary sources concerning the production and commerce of preserved fish products is in no small way owed to information supplied by Greek and Roman medical writers. Yet salted fish products have likewise elicited little interest among modern historians of ancient medicine.

Lack of modern interest in medicinal aspects of salt-fish products probably derives from the fact that animal substances as a whole in materia

---

[6] Cf. Plato Comicus fr. 198 (=*The Fragments of Attic Comedy*. John M. Edmonds, ed. 4 vols. [Leiden 1957–61], 1: 552): σαπρὸν γάρον.Where a fragment can be found in the collection of Edmonds, I have indicated so. See also Artemidorus *Onirocriticon* 1.66 (=*Onirocriticon Libri V*. Roger A. Pack, ed. [Leipzig 1963], p. 72): ἔστι γὰρ οὐδὲν ἄλλο ὁ γάρος ἢ σηπεδών; Pliny *HN* 31.93 (=*C. Plinii Secundi Naturalis Historiae Libri XXXVII*. Carl Mayhoff, ed., 6 vols. [Leipzig 1897–1909]): *putrescentium* (see Appendix I-2). Martial (3.77.5) criticizes a certain Baeticus for eating onions floating *putri allece*. See also Manilius *Astronomica* 5.673 (=*M. Manilii Astronomicon*. A. E. Houseman, ed. 5 vols. [Cambridge 1937]): *putris*. See Appendix I-3.

[7] Ugo Paoli, *Rome, Its People, Life and Customs*. R. D. McNaughton, transl. (Florence 1940; rpt. New York 1963), p. 91.

medica received less attention from ancient writers, such as Dioscorides, Pliny, and Galen, than herbals, spices, and other plant materials. The Hippocratic corpus stressed regimen, including diet, over pharmaceutical remedies, but even here animal products received less attention than vegetables.[8] The latter were, of course, far more plentiful and readily available for the most part. Nevertheless, use of animal substances did persist. Internally, various concoctions, some of simple design, others quite complicated, took the form of foods, medicinal solids, and potions; externally, as ashes, powders, salves, and poultices. Recipes frequently involved fish, though not always salted fish products.[9]

Köhler, who in 1832 published the earliest and still the standard treatment of salted fish products, devotes a mere two pages to the medicinal role of preserved fish; while Zahn, who in his *Real-encyclopädie* article of 1912 on garum devotes almost one-half to therapeutic uses, pays little attention to dietetics and attempts not at all to fit salt-fish products into the overall framework of ancient medicine. The best recent treatment is that of Claude Jardin in 1961, but his discussion is rather brief and no longer wholly accurate.[10]

Greeks and Romans, lacking an effective means of refrigeration, could not easily transport large quantities of fresh fish long distances. Fresh and sometimes live fish were exported from one city to another, but the quantities were small and the prices high.[11] Trade in fresh fish, therefore, primarily involved fishermen selling their catch in local markets, or, at most, conveying them as rapidly as possible to markets located nearby. Most ancient trade in fish consequently involved processed fish products packaged in industrial installations located throughout the Mediterranean and Black Seas.

Scholars, although for many years aware of Roman production and com-

---

[8] Loren C. MacKinney ("Animal Substances in Materia Medica: A Study in the Persistence of the Primitive," *JHM* 1 [1946]: 149–70) notes that of Dioscorides' five books *De materia medica* only one-half of Book II concerns animal substances; Pliny devotes only 5 books to them from a total of 18 on materia medica; and Galen includes only 2 books from 11 devoted to simples. Book II of the Hippocratic treatise *Regimen* includes much on animal products in diet.

[9] MacKinney, "Animal Substances," pp. 149–70; and Léon Moulé, "La Zoothérapie au temps de Dioscoride et de Pline," in *1er Congrés de l'Histoire de l'Art de Guérir, Anvers, 7–12 août 1920* (Anvers 1921); pp. 458–61. William Radcliff (*Fishing from the Earliest Times* [London 1921; rpt. Chicago 1974], p. 278) states that in Book XXXII alone of Pliny's *Natural History* fish figures in over 342 medicinal remedies.

[10] (?) Köhler, "Τάριχος, ou recherches sur l'histoire et les antiquités des pêcheries de la Russie méridionale," in *Mémoires de l'Académie Impériale de Sciences de St. Petersburg*. 6th sér., tome 1, 1832 [extract]; R. Zahn, s.v. "Garum," *RE* 7 (1912): cols. 841–49; Claude Jardin, "Garum et sauces de poisson de l'antiquité," *RSL* 27 (1961): 70–96.

[11] Citations to live or fresh fish imported to Rome are numerous. For the species of fish and expense, see Thomas Corcoran, "The Roman Fishing Industry of the Late Republic and Early Empire," Ph.D. diss., Northwestern University, 1957, esp. pp. 20–65. For a small fishing boat found at Ostia and equipped with a fish-well for maintaining live fish, see Otello Testaguzza, *Portus. Illustrazione dei porti di Claudio e Traiano e della città di Porto a Fiumicino* (Rome 1970), pp. 132, 143–44.

merce in fish products, have not until recently begun to investigate the full scope of this activity. Following the work of Köhler, several publications on the general topic followed during the remainder of the nineteenth century, all of which had one thing in common: they relied almost exclusively on literary evidence.[12] The twentieth century has seen the appearance of several important works, but these have also included little archaeological evidence, although the amount of material relating to ancient fish processing has accumulated at an ever-increasing volume since the turn of the century. Intensified archaeological excavation in the Mediterranean basin, especially in Spain and Gaul, and rapid growth of the study of amphorae and of underwater archaeology have necessitated a new look at this topic. Much that is of importance to our knowledge of this industry, however, remains buried in scattered archaeological reports, articles, monographs, and books. There has not been an attempt to bring together this diffuse material to see how it relates to the literary evidence and to draw, however tentatively, some general conclusions on this important aspect of ancient medicine and Roman social and economic life. This study seeks to fill that lacuna.

---

[12] Hugo Blümner, *Die gewerbliche Thätigkeit der Völker des klassischen Alterthums* (Leipzig 1869), passim; J. K. Smidth, "Historical Observations on the Conditions of the Fisheries Among the Ancient Greeks and Romans, and on Their Mode of Salting and Pickling Fish," U. S. Congress, Senate, 43rd Congress, 2nd Session. *Miscellaneous Documents*, No. 108 (Washington 1875): 3–20; Joachim Marquardt, *Das Privatleben der Römer* (Leipzig 1882), esp. pp. 416–27; Maurice Besnier, s.v. "Salsamentum," *Dar.-Sag.* 7: 1022–25; Paul Rhode, *Thynnorum Captura Quanti Fuerit Apud Veteres Momenti* (Leipzig 1890), passim; and Georg Eberl, *Die Fischkonserven der Alten* (Stadtamhof 1892), passim. The British physician C. David Badham also participated in this discussion. Although he devotes relatively little space to the medicinal role of fish in antiquity, he does include some revealing parallels drawn between ancient and nineteenth-century fishing and fish preservation techniques. See C. David Badham, *Prose Halieutica or Ancient and Modern Fish Tattle* (London 1854).

CHAPTER TWO

FERMENTED FISH PRODUCTS: ANCIENT AND MODERN

Ancient Processed Fish: The Literary Evidence for Production

The principal commodity produced at Roman salting installations was salted fish, called *salsamentum* (Greek τάριχος, or sometimes τέμαχος).[1] This was a general term, derived from the Latin *sal* (salt) and used to designate any meat, but particularly fish, preserved by various methods of salting. The details of these processes are not easily learned from literary sources. We must lament the loss of many works, such as those of Mnesitheus of Athens and Diocles of Carystus, both of the 4th cent. B.C., Diphilus of Siphnos (fl. early 3rd cent. B.C.), Euthydemus of Athens (fl. ca. 2nd cent. B.C.), Hicesius of Smyrna (fl. ca. 100 B.C.), and Dorion (fl. 1st. cent. A.D.), extant only in excerpts from the works of later writers, for example the *Deipnosophistae* of Athenaeus (fl. 2nd cent. A.D.). Since the focus of these authors, physicians and writers on hygiene, food, and fish, was primarily on fish as food, we cannot be sure that they described the production process at all. Nevertheless, from fragments of their writings and those of others which record the diverse forms in which salted fish products were manufactured, we can gather some idea of these products and the various techniques of production.

The end products received specific names dependent upon the shape or form in which they were processed, saltiness, type of fish, and so forth. Τρίγωνον, τετράγωνον (Pl. 1a), and κύβιον designated salted fish of a particular shape; ἀκρόπαστος (lightly salted), ἡμιτάριχος (half-salted), τέλειος (fully salted), τάριχος τιλτόν (salted with scales), and τάριχος λεπιδωτόν (salted without scales) imply particular methods of production used; ὑπογάστρια (stomach portion) and μελάνδρυα (dorsal slice) denote the particular part of the fish used. The term ὡραῖον may signify a young tunny or a

[1] Salsamentum can, in general, refer to any salted food, but salted fish seems to have been the commodity produced in greatest quantity, and so the one most frequently referred to in the sources. Τέμαχος denoted specifically a slice of salted fish, whereas τάριχος could refer to whole fish as well. The sources rarely distinguish between salted, dried, smoked, or pickled fish. All are subsumed under the terms salsamentum or τάριχος. For this reason, I shall also use these terms unless a distinction is clear or a comment is necessary. In general, one can assume that salted, dried, or smoked fish is meant if the container in which the product is held is a basket; and pickled or salted, if the vessel is an amphora or similar container. For τάριχος see Demetrius J. Georgacas, *Ichthyological Terms for the Sturgeon and Etymology of the International Terms Botargo, Caviar and Congeners* (Athens 1978), pp. 154–61; and Köhler, Τάριχος, esp. pp. 26–37. Besnier ("Salsamentum," *Dar.-Sag.*, pp. 1022–23), Eberl (*Fischkonserven*, pp. 11–30), and Corcoran ("Roman Fishing Industry," passim) draw heavily upon the discussion of Köhler.

fish prepared during a certain season.[2] Some salted fish products received specific names derived from the type of fish used: for example, βωρίδια, from the βωρεύς; κορακίδια, from the κορακῖνος; and τυφλινίδια from the τύφλη. Tunny cut into quarters were called θύννεια or θυννίδες.[3] Latin did not distinguish the various kinds of salted fish to the same extent. Except for the occasional use of Latinized Greek terms, such as cybium, melandryum, trigonum, and horaeum, all salted fish were included under the word salsamenta.[4]

Manufacturers did not waste any part of the fish, but used everything, such as the tail, stomach, neck or head.[5] The innards, gills, and any other parts normally considered refuse also had a use; these were made into fish sauce.[6] The Romans produced four different sauces: garum, liquamen, allec, and muria. Garum was the primary product, while allec (Pl. 1b), the sediment created in making garum, was of secondary importance.[7] The Roman penchant for using the terms liquamen and muria imprecisely renders allusive a firm understanding of these products. The former term, which probably originally designated a sauce distinct from garum, acquired before the fifth century A.D. almost generic value for any fish sauce, while the latter was a word sometimes used to mean garum and at other times to signify the liquid used in making garum or in packing salted fish products in vessels for transport.[8] Greek expressions for fish sauce were not so var-

---

[2] Τρίγωνον (Athen. 3.116c); τετράγωνον (*ibid*. 3.116b); κύβιον (*ibid*. 3.116e, 118a-b); ἀκρόπαστος (Xenocrates *ap*. Orib. 2.58.150; for παστὸς see esp. Georgacas, *Ichthyological Terms*, pp. 161–63); ἡμιτάριχος or ἡμίνηρον (Athen. 3.117a; 118f; cf. Xenocrates *ap*. Orib. 2.58.151); τάριχος τέλειος (Athen. 3.120d); τάριχος τιλτόν and τάριχος λεπιδωτόν (Pollux *Onom*. 6.49; Hesychius s.v. τιλτόν); ὑπογάστριον (Athen. 3.116b; 7.302d; 9.399c); μελάνδρυα (*ibid*. 3.121b; 7.315e); ὡραῖον (*ibid*. 3.116a,e; 120e-f; Pollux *Onom*. 6.48; cf. Pliny *HN* 11.36). ᾿Ωμοτάριχος is a term which may refer either to a lightly salted fish (Eberl, *Fischkonserven*, p. 20) or to the shoulder portion of a tunny (Köhler, Τάριχος, p. 30). See Nicostratus fr. 1 Edmonds, Alexis fr. 15 Edmonds, and Xenocrates *ap*. Orib. 2.58.144. Other terms for salted fish products will be met as the discussion progresses. Xenocrates' work is preserved in Book II of Oribasius' *Medical Collections* (= *Oribasii Collectionum Medicarum Reliquiae*. Johann Reader, ed. 4 vols. *CMG* VI,1,1 [Leipzig 1928–33], pp. 47–57).

[3] Athen. 3.118d (θυννίδες), 116e (θύννεια), and Hesychius s.v. θυννίδες: θύννων τεμάχη, and s.v. θυννάδες˙ Τεμάχη ταρίχου. Cf. below, p. 133, and note 107.

[4] Melandryum: Martial 3.77.7; Varro *Ling*. 5.77; and below note 16; cybium: Pliny *HN* 9.48, 32.151; Martial 5.78.5; Varro *Ling*. 5.77; horaeum: Plaut. *Captivi* 851; Varro *Ling*. 5.77; trigonum: Plaut. *Captivi* 851.

[5] Tail: Persius *Sat*. 5.183 (*cauda thynni*); Pliny *HN* 9.48; Martial 11.31.14. Stomach, neck and head: Pliny *HN* 9.48. See also Manilius *Astron*. 5.656–81 (Appendix I-3).

[6] Pliny *HN* 31.93. For Roman fish sauces see Zahn, "Garum," *RE*, cols. 841–49; Thomas Corcoran, "Roman Fish Sauces," *CJ* 58 (1963): 204–10; Pierre Grimal and Thomas Monod, "Sur la véritable nature du 'Garum'," *REA* 54 (1952): 27–38; Jardin, "Garum," pp. 70–96; and Robert I. Curtis, "In Defense of *Garum*," *CJ* 78 (1983): 232–40.

[7] Pliny *HN* 31.95. The dregs (*faex*) of garum was variously spelled allec (Hor. *Sat*. 2.8.9), hallec (Plaut. *Aul*. fr. 5), allex (Pliny *HN* 31.95), and hallex (Plaut. *Poen*. 1310; Cato *Agr*. 58). The latter form is found most often in painted inscriptions on commercial amphorae.

[8] Liquamen: Caelius Aurelianus *On Chronic Diseases* (*Tardarum passionum*) 2.1.40: *garum, quod appellamus liquamen*; *idem*. 2.3.70: *ex garo . . . quod vulgo liquamen appellant*. For Caelius Aureli-

ied. Greek γάρον gave rise to Latin garum, while ἅλμη has its nearest equivalent in Latin muria.[9] The Roman sauces allec and liquamen, however, lack corresponding Greek terms. When the words ἅλιξ and λικουάμεν do appear, and they do so only rarely, they seem to be merely transliterations of the Latin.[10] The author of the *Geoponica*, a Byzantine agricultural manual, uses the word αἱμάτιον (bloody) to refer to a product prepared from the tunny and reputed to have been the best garum (τὸ κάλλιον γάρος).[11] The names of mixed fish sauces (ὀξύγαρον, οἰνόγαρον, ὑδρόγαρον, and ἐλαιόγαρον or γαρέλαιον) appear almost exclusively in literary sources in contexts which tell us little about their production or commerce.[12]

---

anus, see *Caelius Aurelianus. On Acute Diseases and On Chronic Diseases*. I. E. Drabkin, ed. (Chicago 1950), pp. 590, 610. Muria: Columella *Rust*. 12.55.4: *et tanquam salsamentum in muria sua permanet*; Pliny *HN* 31.83: *muria salsamentorum*; Martial 13.103, entitled *amphora muriae: Antipolitani, fateor, sum filia thynni/ essem si scombri, non tibi missa forem*; Isidore *Orig*. 20.3.20 (Appendix I-6); and *Geoponica* 20.46.5 (Appendix I-8). Pseudo-Acron, the fifth-century A.D. scholiast to Horace, comments on the word muria found in Horace *Sat*. 2.4.65: *Muriam antiqui dicebant liquamen et Syrorum lingua sic dicitur*; and on garum in *Sat*. 2.8.46: *Hoc liquamen de suco piscis fit*. See *PseudoAcronis Scholia in Horatium Vetustiora*. Otto Keller, ed. (Leipzig 1904), pp. 167, 201.

9 Greek sources give variously ὁ γάρος (Aeschylus *ap*. Athen. 2.67c; Artemidorus *On*. 1.66; Suidas s.v. γάρος), τὸ γάρος (Galen *De compositione medicamentorum secundum locos* 12.622K); τὸ γάρον (Strabo 3.4.6), and τὸ γάριον (Arrian *Epic. diss*. 2.20.29). The papyrological sources frequently use ὁ γάρος or τὸ γάρον, but the other forms do appear. See Francis T. Gignac, *A Grammar of the Greek Papyri of the Roman and Byzantine Periods*. Vol. II: *Morphology* (Milan 1981), pp. 98–99. The derivation of the word garum remains obscure. Pliny (*HN* 31.93) says that *Hoc* [garum] *olim conficiebatur ex pisce quem Graeci garon vocabant*. Isidore (*Orig*. 20.3.19), apparently using Pliny as a source, explains that *Garum est liquor piscium salsus qui conficiebatur ex pisce quem Graeci* γάρον *vocabant; et quamvis nunc ex infinito genere piscium fiat, nomen tamen pristinum retinet a quo initium sumsit*. D'Arcy Thompson's objection (*Greek Fishes*, p. 43) notwithstanding, there is little reason to reject Pliny's derivation. For muria and ἅλμη compare *muria salsamentorum* of Pliny *HN* 31.83 with ἅλμη τῶν ταριχηρῶν ἰχθύων of Oribasius *Synopsis ad Eustathium* 2.2; 9.61.5–6 (= *Oribasii. Synopsis ad Eustathium*. Johannes Raeder, ed. *CMG* VI,3 [Leipzig 1926], pp. 29, 312); Leo Medicus Σύνοψις ἰατρικῆς (*Synopsis of Medicine*) 2.8 (= *Anecdota Medica Graeca*. F. Z. Ermerins, ed. [Leiden 1840], p. 97); Aetius 2.151 (= *Aetii Amidenis Libri Medicinales I-IV*. Alexander Olivieri, ed. *CMG* VIII,1 [Leipzig 1935], pp. 207–08); and Galen *De simplicium medicamentorum temperamentis ac facultatibus* 12.377K. Cf. Columella *Rust*. 12.55.4 (Appendix I-1); Quintilian *IO* 8.2.3: *duratos muria pisces*; Hesychius s.v. ἅλμη· ὁ τῶν ἰχθύων ζωμός; and Herodotus 2.77: ἰχθύων δὲ τοὺς μὲν πρὸς ἥλιον αὐήναντες ὠμοὺς σιτέονται, τοὺς δὲ ἐξ ἅλμης τεταριχευμένους.

10 *Geoponica* 20.46.1–3. See also Paul of Aegina 3.59.11 (= *Paulus Aegineta*. I. L. Heiberg, ed. *CMG* IX,1 [Leipzig 1921], p. 274); *P.Got*. 17_{20}. The Greek word ἅλιξ or ἄλιξ does not occur before the time of Dioscorides (*De mat. med*. 4.148). Cf. *CGL* III. 257; Charisius *Ars gram*. 1.11: ὁ ἄλληξ ἰχθὺς ταριχευόμενος. The Latin liquamen does not appear in literature before Columella (*Rust*. 9.14.3) in the first century A.D., and exists in Greek form only in the *Geoponica*.

11 *Geoponica* 20.46.6. Zahn ("Garum," *RE*, col. 843) equates γάρον αἱμάτιον with γάρος μέλαν (Aetius 3.83), and says that both refer to the Spanish fish sauce garum sociorum.

12 I have excluded discussion of mixed garums since, although found frequently in literature, only three examples occur in papyrological sources (*P.Bas*. 16: γαρέλεον; *UPZ* 89.14: ἐξάλμη; and *P.Vindob. G*. 29567: οἰνόγαρος) and are almost completely absent from archaeological evidence. For *P.Vindob. G*. 29567, see P. J. Sijpesteijn, "Vierzehn Wiener Papyri," *Aegyptus* 61(1981): 82–83; cf. also below, p. 146 and note 179. Peter Remark, (*De Amphorarum Inscriptionibus Latinis Quaestiones Selectae* [Tübingen 1912], p. 27) suggests that *CIL* IV.5728, which reads

One last item deserves mention because of its almost total absence from the ancient evidence. Diphilus of Siphnos is the only ancient author to mention salted fish eggs, a product which we usually call caviar.[13] The reason for this silence is unknown, but may arise from the lack of any widespread commerce in the product. Most fish roe probably went into the vats along with other fish innards to be made into fish sauce.

Among Latin sources only Manilius and Columella provide information on Roman salting methods. Manilius, in *Astronomica* 5.656–81, although primarily giving a brief and somewhat ambiguous description of the production of fish sauce, alludes to what must have been a general practice in Roman salting installations. He describes how fishermen processed their tunny catch on the shore. They cut the tunny into pieces, designating each one for a specific purpose. Evidently, no part of the fish was wasted. But Manilius confines his discussion to fish sauce and we are left wondering about the other salted fish products. Columella throws some light on the question when he describes two methods for salting pork, the second of which, he implies, was similar to that for salting fish:[14]

CICER/HAL[lex], refers to a mixture of allec and chick peas. The label, or *titulus pictus*, however, probably only indicates that the amphora had been used first for peas and subsequently for fish sauce, or vice versa. Cf. Pliny *HN* 18.308. For mixed fish sauces see Zahn, "Garum," *RE*, cols. 842–46. For purposes of this study I have also intentionally omitted discussion of certain other products which, according to some scholars, may be related to fish sauce but whose identification as such is based almost exclusively on the type of container used to transport them. These include limphatum (*CIL* IV.5615–20; XV.4736), laccatum (*CIL* IV.5640–43; XV.4733–34), largarinum (*CIL* XV.4741), and something known only as CoD (*CIL* IV.5629–38, 9609, 10730; XV.4732). For limphatum, see Heinrich Dressel's commentary to *CIL* XV.4736, and Jean Andreau, *Les affaires de Monsieur Jucundus*. Collection de l'École Française de Rome, no. 19 (Rome 1974), p. 231, note 5 and bibliography cited therein. For laccatum, see Fausto Zevi, "Appunti sulle anfore romane," *ArchClass* 18 (1966): 243, who follows Remark, *De Amphorarum Inscriptionibus*, p. 24; but cf. M. H. Callender, *Roman Amphorae* (London 1965), p. 38, and Pio Ciprotti, "Brevi note su alcuni scritte pompeiane," in *Neue Forschungen in Pompeji*. Bernard Andreae and Hemut Kyrieleis, eds. (Rechlinghausen 1975), p. 274. For largarinum, see Callender, *Roman Amphorae*, p. 40. For CoD, see Albert Grenier, "Le matériel de la navigation les amphores," *Manuel d'archéologie gallo-romaine*. Vol. 2 (Paris 1934), pp. 618–20; but cf. Callender, *Roman Amphorae*, p. 37, and Oskar Bohn, "Pinselschriften auf Amphoren aus Augst und Windisch," *Anzeiger für schweizerische Altertumskunde* 28 (1926): 204. For a recent discussion of the suggestion that COD may refer to co(r)d(ula), a young tunny, see Bernard Liou, "Inscriptions peintes sur amphores: Fos (suite), Marseille, Toulon, Port-la-Nautique, Arles, Saint-Blaise, Saint-Martin-de-Crau, Mâcon, Calvi," *Archaeonautica* 7 (1987): 66–69.

[13] Diphilus *ap*. Athen. 3.121c: τὰ μέντοι τῶν ἰχθύων καὶ τῶν ταρίχων ᾠὰ πάντα δύσπεπτα, δύσφθαρτα, μᾶλλον δὲ τὰ τῶν λιπαρωτέρων καὶ μειζόνων. See also Köhler, Τάριχος, pp. 69–72; Otto Keller, *Die antike Tierwelt*. 2 vols. (Leipzig 1913), 2: 338; and Georgacas, *Ichthyological Terms*, pp. 148–49, 167–78, 189–237, 243–54.

[14] Columella *Rust*. 12.55.4 (Appendix I-1). It is interesting to compare this with the present-day process of salting whole fish in Southern India. The fish are gutted and stacked in large concrete vats with a fish-to-salt ratio of 3:1. The "pickle" produced from this process is used to pack cured fish in barrels for export to Sri Lanka. Fish cured in this manner remain edible for a year or more. See I. M. Mackie, R. Hardy, and G. Hobbs, *Fermented Fish Products*, FAO Fisheries Reports, No. 100 (Rome 1971), p. 10. For a more detailed discussion, see below pp. 15–19.

> And there is another salting method which can even be used in hot places at every season of the year. When the pigs have been prohibited from water for a day, on the next day they are slaughtered and are deprived of hair either with boiling water or with a small flame made from slender pieces of wood, for in each way the hairs are removed. The flesh is cut up into pieces of a pound each. Parched salt, but moderately broken as we have said above, is laid down in large containers. The small pieces of meat are thickly arranged, and salt is placed on alternately. But when the throat of the jars has been reached, the remaining part is filled with salt and with weights placed on top is pressed down into the containers. And this flesh is always preserved, just as salt-fish is preserved in its own liquid.

It seems from this that fish were salted in a container filled with alternating layers of fish and salt. When these had filled the vessel, a final layer of salt was added and the entire mass pressed down by weights. The process apparently produced a salty liquid which was placed with the salsamenta into vessels used to transport the product commercially.

The shape of salsamenta is not hard to visualize. Some came in cubes, squares, and triangles; others perhaps in irregular shapes. The appearance of salted fish, however, is more difficult to imagine. Those salted with scales were no doubt coarse looking and rougher to the touch than those salted without scales. Apparently some salt-fish were dry with a hard consistency, others soft and moist. The former kind was probably heavily salted for a long period of time and appeared rather tight and stretched (ἐπιτεταμένος), while the latter describes more lightly processed fish. The particular species or portion of fish might also account for this general differentiation. Lean fish produced a harder product, while fatty fish pieces resulted in a soft salt-fish which spoiled more easily.[15] Pliny says that melandrya were shaped like oak-wood, and his contemporary Xenocrates asserts that they had the form of darkened roots.[16] Köhler vouches for the accuracy of these descriptions by pointing out that in his day salted sturgeon, called *balyk*, produced at the mouth of the Don and Volga Rivers and at Kerch had a similar appearance.[17] The taste of preserved fish was appar-

---

[15] Xenocrates *ap*. Orib. 2.58.133–35: Περὶ ἰχθύων ταριχηρῶν κητωδῶν. Οἱ δὲ τάριχοι κοινῶς μέν εἰσιν εὔστομοι, κακόχυλοι δὲ καὶ κακοστόμαχοι, λεπτυντικοί τε καὶ ταρακτικοὶ κοιλίας. ταρίχων δ' οἱ μὲν σκληρόσαρκοι, οἱ δὲ φύσει ὑγροπαγεῖς καὶ οἱ ἁπαλοί, οἱ δὲ μέσως· καὶ οἱ μὲν σαρκώδεις, οἱ δ' ἐμπίμελοι· καὶ οἱ μὲν παλαιοί, οἱ δὲ μέσοι, οἱ δὲ πρόσφατοι· ὧν οἱ παλαιοὶ ἐπιτεταμὲνοι, οἱ δὲ νεαλεῖς ὑποβεβηκότες, οἱ δὲ μεσοχρόνιοι σύμμετροι· καὶ οἱ μὲν ἄγαν πίονες ἐπιπολαστικοί, ⟨οἱ δ'⟩ ἧττον ἐκείνων θρεπτικώτεροι· τῶν δ' ἄλλων οἱ σκληρόσαρκοι δύσφθαρτοι, οἱ ἁπαλώτεροι φθείρονται ῥᾳδίως. For pieces of processed fish found in Corinth, see below, p. 115.

[16] Pliny *HN* 9.48: *melandrya vocantur, quercus assulis similia*. Xenocrates *ap*. Orib. 2.58.146: Τὰ δὲ λοιπὰ μέρη, μελάνδρυα διὰ τὴν ἐμφέρειαν πρὸς τὰς μελαινούσας τῆς δρυὸς ῥίζας, παρορμητικὰ ὀρέξεων νάπους παραπλοκῇ, τοῦ δ' ὑπογαστρίου δυσφθαρτότερα, τῷ πιμελῆς ἀπηλλάχθαι. See also Varro *Ling*. 5.77. Paulus, in his commentary on Festus *De verborum significatu*, p. 76M (Lindsay, ed., p. 67), says that *melandrya* was the common word for *elacatena*, a kind of salted fish: *elacatena, genus salsamenti, quod appellatur vulgo melandrea*. For ἠλακατῆνες see Thompson, *Greek Fishes*, p. 75.

[17] Köhler, Τάριχος, p. 32.

ently quite salty since at times it had to be soaked to reduce its sharpness.[18]

Ancient writers offer little toward our understanding of the salting process. Were different pieces, such as trigona and cybia, salted in separate containers, or in the same vessel and separated at a later time? How long did the salting process take? Were the different species of fish mixed together or always separated? What was the relationship in the salting process between salsamentum and fish sauce? This last question can be partially answered, since on the subject of garum production the sources are more numerous and detailed.

Manilius, who flourished during the reign of Tiberius, and Pliny the Elder, who died in A.D. 79, are the earliest writers known to have described the process of garum production. Pliny's remarks offer little information beyond the ingredients used, that is, viscera and other fleshy parts of fish combined with salt.[19] Manilius, on the other hand, presents a good description of fish sauce production by tunny fishermen.[20] The basic ingredients consisted of fish and salt. Manilius describes two preparations, one with many small fish and the other with pieces of large ones. Although he offers no description of the facilities used in making garum from tunny, he does specify wine dolia and vats (*lacus et Bacchi dolia*) as receptacles for preparing the sauce from small whole fish. Manilius does not specifically name the products being prepared, but their identification as fish sauce is assured through the phrases he uses to describe the process. He alludes, somewhat pejoratively, to the general process of mixing the salt and fish: "here flowed the expensive liquid and expelled the flower of the blood; and when salt has been added, it regulates the taste of the mouth. There the entire mass of putrid confusion is mixed together" (*Astron.* 5.670–74). These lines recall similar characterizations by his younger contemporaries Pliny the Elder, who refers to garum as "that liquid of putrifying matter" (*illa putrescentium sanies*), and Seneca, who calls the same sauce "the expensive liquid of bad fish" (*pretiosa malorum piscium sanies*).[21]

Three other texts describe the process. Those attributed to Gargilius Martialis (fl. 3rd cent. A.D.) and Rufius Festus (fl. late 4th cent. A.D.) must be treated with caution, since both may date much later than the author to whom they are attributed. The extant manuscript of Gargilius Martialis

---

[18] Cf. Plautus *Poen.* 240–44: *Soror, cogita, amabo, item nos perhiberi*
quam si salsa muriatica esse autumantur
sine omni lepore et sine suavitate:
nisi multa aqua usque et diu macerantur,
olent, salsa sunt, tangere ut non velis.

[19] Pliny *HN* 31.93–95 (Appendix I-2).

[20] Manilius *Astron.* 5.656–81 (Appendix I-3). Cf. Firmicus Maternus *Mathesis* 8.17.5: *In extremis partibus Piscium in laeva parte consurgit Belua quae a Graecis Cetus vocatur. Quicumque hoc sidere oriente nati fuerint, erunt piscatores sed magnorum piscium. Hi enim focas canes marinos xifias thynnos corcodillos capient. Habebunt etiam officia quae ex salibus sunt vel ex salsamentis et a liquamine, et haec mercabuntur.*

[21] Pliny *HN* 31.93; Seneca *Ep.* 95.25: *illud sociorum garum, pretiosam malorum piscium saniem, non credis urere salsa tabe praecordia?*

may contain medieval intrusions,[22] while the garum recipe attributed to Rufius Festus is more obviously of medieval date.[23] Although the texts may date much later than the respective authors, as will be presently shown, the processes described therein vary little from those common to the first three centuries of the Roman Empire.

The recipe of Ps-Rufius Festus employed a rather quick method of preparing garum.[24] Fish mixed with salt and wine formed the primary ingredients. Artificial heat reduced the mixture, which was then strained into a glass flask. The length of time for heating the sauce was unimportant; what mattered was that the volume be reduced by two-thirds. The recipe of Ps-Gargilius Martialis, on the other hand, took considerably longer to prepare.[25] He describes a method by which layers of herbs and spices, fish, and salt are placed alternatingly upon each other up to the capacity of a "solid well-pitched container." This mixture was allowed to ferment in the sun for twenty-seven days. After the seventh day, however, the material required stirring two or three times daily. At the end of the period the garum was strained and collected in a vessel.

The best and most complete description of garum production comes from the *Geoponica*, a tenth-century Greek agricultural manual which may derive from a sixth-century A.D. Latin treatise. In the chapter entitled "Preparation of Garums," the author describes two methods of preparing garum: a slow way, warming by solar heat in a baker's kneading trough for up to three months; and a fast method, heating the material in a small container using an artificial source:[26]

> 1. The so-called liquamen is made in this manner: the intestines of fish are thrown into a vessel and salted. Small fish, either the best smelt, or small mullet, or sprats, or wolffish, or whatever is deemed to be small, are all salted together and, shaken frequently, are fermented in the sun.

---

[22] The controversy surrounding the date centers on the inclusion in the recipe of the aringus, or herring, a fish otherwise unknown before the Medieval period. Valentine Rose ("Aringus, der Hering," *Hermes* 8 [1874]: 224–27) believes that its absence from classical literature is purely accidental. Cf. Antoine Thomas, "Latin *sclareia*," *RPh*, 2d ser. 31 (1907): 199. See Robert I. Curtis, "*Negotiatores Allecarii* and the Herring," *Phoenix* 38 (1984): 147–58.

[23] Only a single manuscript of the *Breviarium rerum gestarum populi Romani* preserves a recipe for garum. Entitled *Confectio gari*, the recipe appears at the head of the tenth-century A.D. manuscript *Codex Parisinus P* and was written in the same hand as the text itself. Since it exists in only one manuscript and bears no direct relationship to the subject matter of the *Breviarium*, this recipe should not be considered part of the work by Rufius Festus. C. Wagener, in the Teubner edition of 1886, and J. W. Eadie, in *The Breviarium of Festus. A Critical Edition with Historical Commentary* (London 1967), omit any mention of the garum recipe included by Wendel Förster in the Teubner edition of 1874, page 23.

[24] Ps-Rufius Festus *Brev.* (Förster, p. 23) (Appendix I-4).

[25] Ps-Gargilius Martialis 62 (= Rose, "Aringus, der Hering," pp. 226–27) (Appendix I-5).

[26] *Geoponica* 20.46.1–6 (Appendix I-8). The work probably contains material dating earlier than the sixth century. See E. Oder, s.v. "Geoponica," *RE* 7 (1912), cols. 1221–25; and Eugen Fehrle, *Studien zu den griechischen Geoponikern* (Leipzig 1920), esp. pp. 49–50. For the text I have used *Geoponica sivi Cassiani Bassi Scholastici De Re Rustica Ecologae*. Heinrich Beckh, ed. (Leipzig 1895), pp. 528–29.

2. After it has been reduced in the heat, garum is obtained from it in this way: a large, strong basket is placed into the vessel of the aforementioned fish, and the garum streams into the basket. In this way the so-called liquamen is strained through the basket when it is taken up. The remaining refuse is alex.

3. The Bithynians prepare it in this manner: It is best if you take small or large sprats, but if not, wolffish, or horse-mackerel, or mackerel, or even alica, and a mixture of all, and throw these into a baker's kneading trough, in which they are accustomed to knead meal. Tossing into the modius of fish two Italian sextarii of salt, mix up thoroughly in order to strengthen it with salt. After leaving it alone for one night throw it into a vessel and place it without a lid in the sun for two or three months, agitating it with a shaft at intervals. Next take it, cover it, and store it away.

4. Some add to one sextarius of fish, two sextarii of old wine.

5. Next, if you wish to use the garum immediately, that is to say not ferment it in the sun, but to boil it, you do it this way. When the brine has been tested, so that an egg having been thrown in floats (if it sinks, it is not sufficiently salty), and throwing the fish into the brine in a newly-made earthenware pot and adding in some oregano, you place it on a sufficient fire until it is boiled, that is until it begins to reduce a little. Some throw in boiled-down must. Next, throwing the cooled liquid into a filter you toss it a second and third time through the filter until it turns out clear. After having covered it, store it away.

6. The best garum, the so-called haimation, is made in this way: the intestines of tunny along with the gills, juice and blood are taken and sufficient salt is sprinkled on. After having left it alone in the vessel for two months at most, pierce the vessel and the garum, called haimation, is withdrawn.

It is apparent from the preceding discussion that the basic preparation process of fish sauce remained unchanged throughout antiquity, although some variations in detail do appear among the sketchy descriptions of Pliny and Manilius and the more complete ones of Ps-Gargilius Martialis, Ps-Rufius Festus and the author of the *Geoponica*. Using any one of these recipes, a commercial producer, a villa owner, or even a town dweller could make whatever amount of garum he desired. The size of the container was unimportant. A variety of vessels are named by the authors recording production processes. The largest containers mentioned include the dolium and *lacus Bacchi* of Manilius and the kneading trough recorded in the *Geoponica*. But even these are of unknown capacity. Only Ps-Gargilius Martialis suggests a certain size vessel, and even then he is not specific, suggesting a container of "three or four modii." The primary concern was not the size of the vessel, but the proportion of salt and fish. The author of the *Geoponica* (20.46.3) suggests a mixture of one modius of fish for two sextarii of salt, that is, a fish-to-salt ratio of 8:1. When producers employed fish and muria the ratio was unimportant so long as the brine was salty enough to float an egg.[27]

[27] No extant recipe designates the amount of brine necessary; only its salinity was important. As will become clear later, the amount was probably only enough to keep the fish covered and protected from exposure to air. Cf. *BT. Shabbath* 108b (Epstein, p. 527), where a mixture of two parts salt and one part water was declared sufficient to float an egg and was used to make fish sauce.

A producer of garum could choose among a variety of alternatives in preparing his product. He could make a simple sauce composed only of salt and fish as ingredients, or he might include wine or one or more herbs and spices.[28] The greatest variety, however, lay in the choice of seafood. Pliny states that garum was made from an infinite variety of fish, but the mackerel (*scomber*) was by far the most popular.[29] Indeed, he says that this fish served no other useful purpose. Other desirable fish, large and small, include the tunny, murry, sprat, mullet, smelt, and coracinus.[30] Most of the fish used to produce fish sauce were pelagic. This is not surprising, since the Romans did not use river fish to any large extent in their diet.[31] They also used marine animals, such as oysters, sea urchins, sea anemones and various shellfish, to produce fish sauce.[32]

The appearance of ancient sauces is unknown, although the carmelized residue of what was probably garum has been found in a Roman saltery at Plomarc'h in Western Gaul and the bones of small fish found in dolia in Pompeii may be the desiccative remains of allec (Pl. 1b). From this and from numerous epigraphical and literary references one can postulate that ancient garum was a clear liquid; allec, the residue, was no doubt a mushy, paste-like substance containing fish bones and other undissolved fish material. Exactly what liquamen was remains unclear. When viewed as a product distinct from garum, its appearance most likely resembled that of garum, but as a liquid it was probably weaker in salinity and color. Muria, the solution resulting from salting fish, was probably similar to that of liquamen.[33]

What conclusions may be drawn from this survey of the literary sources for the production of garum? First, the production of garum and of salsamentum are closely related and can be different parts of the same process. Manilius' description of tunny processing included both products and Columella's description of salting pork (and fish) closely parallels Ps-Gargilius Martialis' recipe for garum production. Second, the basic ingredients con-

---

[28] Garum and wine only: *Geoponica* 20.46.4; Ps-Rufius Festus *Brev.* (Förster, p. 23); garum with herbs and spices: *Geoponica* 20.46.5; Ps-Gargilius Martialis 62 (= Rose, "Aringus, der Hering," pp. 226–27).

[29] Pliny *HN* 31.94–95. See also Isidore *Orig.* 20.3.19 (Appendix I-6). The scomber: Pliny *HN* 31.94; Martial 3.50.9; 13.102,103; Strabo 3.4.6; *Geoponica* 20.46.3.

[30] The *apua*, a generic word referring to all small fry, appears in Pliny *HN* 31.95 as the name of a specific fish. See also Alciphron 1.21 and Isidore *Orig.* 12.6.40 and 20.3.20 for small fish used in garum production. Pliny (*HN* 9.66) reports that Apicius made an allec from only the livers of red mullet.

[31] André, *L'alimentation*², p. 107. The silurus, a river fish, was used to prepare fish sauce. See Caelius Aurelianus *On Chronic Diseases* 2.1.40 (Drabkin, p. 590); Oribasius *Ad Eunapium* 4.116.19; and Rufus of Ephesus 64.47. See *Oeuvres de Rufus d'Éphèse*. Ch. Daremberg and Ch. Émile Ruelle, eds. (Paris 1879; rpt. Amsterdam 1963), p. 338.

[32] Pliny *HN* 31.95.

[33] Liquamen was probably equivalent to one of the modern-day leached or lixiviated fish sauces. See below pp. 17–19 (muria), 20–21 (liquamen).

sisted of salt or a strong brine plus fish, primarily sea fish or shellfish, but especially the mackerel, tunny, and various small fish. Optional ingredients included wine, herbs and spices. Third, garum could be made in any amount desired, as long as the prescribed ratio of salt to fish was maintained or the brine was of sufficient salinity. The type or size of vessel was unimportant, although for the most part extant sources speak of rather small containers. Fourth, garum production required a period of maturation, two to three months if allowed to age in the sun, but a shorter, unspecified time if cooked. Fifth, garum production frequently called for straining as the last step to acquire a clear product. This procedure finds specific mention in the first century A.D. in Pompeii on a container which bears an inscription identifying its contents as "the best strained liquamen."[34] Sixth, the rather bizarre production process and odor of fish sauce did not escape the notice of several ancient authors who generally spoke of these characteristics in pejorative terms.[35] Finally, a comparison of production methods described by authors of the first century A.D. with those recorded by writers of the third, fourth and sixth centuries indicates that production methods of garum changed little over the centuries.[36] This remained true even up to the present day.

Modern Processed Fish: Production and Nutritive Value

Modern technology has devised new methods of fish preservation unavailable to the ancients, such as freezing or dehydration through vacuum or freeze drying, and has invented new containers for storage and long-distance transportation, such as vacuum-packed cans. Nevertheless, natural drying and smoking continue to be used. The first method involves exposure to the sun and wind and creates a shrunken, tough product susceptible to infestation by various insects. Smoking, even at elevated temperatures, produces a dried product subject to spoilage and the growth of molds. The palatability of both products is heavily dependent upon the freshness of the fish at the time of processing. More frequently, however,

---

[34] *CIL* IV.7110: *liquamen/ optimum/ saccatum*. Cf. Apicius *De re coq*. 7.6.14: *allec collatus*.

[35] For the odor of garum, see Martial 6.93.6 and Pliny *HN* 31.90; for muria, cf. Horace *Sat*. 2.4.63–66; and implied for allec, Martial 11.27. The odor and production method of fish sauce gave rise to a rather stereotyped description. Cf. Curtis, "Defense," pp. 232–40. Garum, however, was no more malodorous than the Vietnamese fish sauce *nuoc-mam*, since the amount of salt used in its production inhibited putrid fermentation and prevented, for the most part, any rancid smells (see below pp. 23–24). In effect, garum smelled no worse than Limberger cheese. See A. Balil Illana, "Un estudio sobre el 'garum'," *AEA* 26 (1953): 184. The close association between the odor of fish sauce and that of cheese is of ancient standing. See below, p. 189 and note 18. Nevertheless, garum could go bad. The cookbook attributed to Apicius contains a recommended means of improving fish sauce, "if it should have a bad odor." See Apicius *De re coq*. 1.7: *liquamen si odorem malum fecerit*.

[36] Cf. the garum recipe recorded in the Carolingian manuscript from the abbey of Echternach (Appendix I-7).

to insure longer keeping quality, salting precedes both drying and smoking.[37] The smoking of Atlantic mackerel (*Scomber scombrus*), a fatty fish, for example, involves a combination of all three processes.[38] Salting, then, is a basic step in fish preservation and is itself a primary process leading to a variety of products.

Salting is the most important method of preservation practiced in those areas where climatic conditions, lack of storage facilities, and poor transportation resources militate against the accumulation of large quantities of fresh fish, such as in Southeast Asia and the Philippines. In areas where these factors are not significant and modern processing equipment is available, the preservative nature of salting is secondary to the flavor or texture it can impart to the finished product. Salt retards or, at least, controls the decomposition of fish which commences soon after removal from water and death. In general, the term used to describe the process whereby organic substances break down into simpler compounds in the presence of salt and enzymes is fermentation.[39] The term "fermented fish product" is, however, misleading, since all fish processed with salt ferment after a period of time. Some biochemists prefer more precision and so speak of two distinct processes: bacterially fermented products and products created by enzyme hydrolysis. The latter term, reserved for non-microbial action, further subdivides into processes using added enzymes or naturally occurring enzymes. Where only indigenous enzymes play a role, the process is called autolysis.[40] The term autolysis, therefore, best corresponds to the ancient salting process and to many modern ones as well.

The principal ingredients necessary for fermentation are dry salt and fish. To speed up the process a very salty water can be used; this is called "brining." From this simple beginning many variables can, and often do,

---

[37] The combination of salting, then drying is probably the most widespread method of fish preservation. In the 1970s salted, then dried fish made up about 77% of all processed fish in Malaysia. S. Y. Yu, C. L. Siaw, and A. Z. Idrus, "The Application of Technology to the Processing of Dry-salted Fish in Peninsular Malaysia: Comparison of Sun-dried and Oven-dried Fish," *Journal of Food Technology* 17,2 (April 1982): 211. See also A. G. Van Veen, "Fermented and Dried Seafood Products in Southeast Asia," in *Fish as Food*. Georg Borgström, ed. 4 vols. (New York 1965), 3: 242–43; C. L. Cutting, "The Influence of Drying, Salting and Smoking on the Nutritive Value of Fish," in *Fish in Nutrition*. Eirik Heen and Rudolf Kreuzer, eds. (London 1962), pp. 169, 173–75; and *idem*, "Smoking," in *Fish as Food*. Georg Borgström, ed. 4 vols. (New York 1965), 3: 90–91.

[38] A. K. M. Aminullah Bhuiyan, R. G. Ackman, and S. P. Lall, "Effects of Smoking on Protein Quality of Atlantic Mackerel (*Scomber scombrus*)," *Journal of Food Processing and Preservation* 10,2 (1986): 116; and A. K. M. Aminullah Bhuiyan, W. M. N. Ratmayake, and R. G. Ackman, "Effect of Smoking on the Proximate Composition of Atlantic Mackerel (*Scomber scombrus*)," *Journal of Food Science* 51,2 (March–April 1986): 327.

[39] I. M. Mackie et al., *Fermented Fish Products*, p. 1; and C. G. Beddows, "Fermented Fish and Fish Products," in *Microbiology of Fermented Foods*. Brian J. B. Wood, ed. 2 vols. (London 1985), 2: 1–2.

[40] J. D. Owens and L. S. Mendoza, "Enzymically Hydrolysed and Bacterially Fermented Fishery Products," *Journal of Food Technology* 20,3 (June 1985): 273–74.

come into play to produce almost innumerable end products.[41] Since fish tissue deteriorates rapidly following death, the length of time elapsing between catch and initiation of processing can strongly influence the taste and keeping quality of the fish.[42] Other variables include the species of fish, where it was caught, its age, fat content, size, and whether it is processed whole or eviscerated. The purity and quantity of salt or the salinity of the brine play a major role, as does the process itself. For example, the length of time given to salting and subsequent ripening, the ambient temperature of the fish-salt mass, and the use of additives, such as sugar or pineapple, to speed up the process or to inculcate a desired taste or to create a certain appearance, all affect the end product. The decision to dry and/or smoke following fermentation also determines the ultimate outcome.[43]

Salt exerts a strong osmotic effect on fish tissue, producing a pickle. If the fish remains in contact with the pickle for only a short time and the amount of salt used is small, a relatively soft salt-fish results. If the amount of salt and the period of contact time is increased and the pickle is occasionally drained off, the result is fish paste. Over a long period of time and if the amount of salt used is great, the proteolytic enzymes (from the muscle and gastro-intestinal tract if retained) produce almost complete degradation of fish material, creating fish sauce. All of these products, salt-fish, fish paste, and fish sauce, therefore, form part of the same process.

The production of salt-fish normally requires the removal of the gastro-intestinal tract from the fish before mixing with salt or brine. This eliminates the most active enzymes leading to autolysis. Mildly cured fish are those treated with only a little salt or with high concentrations of salt but for only a short period of time, followed perhaps by drying and/or smoking; they keep little better than fresh fish.[44] Hard cures have as their goal long-term preservation and involve increased concentrations of salt for ex-

---

[41] In Southeast Asia alone there are around 60 different types of fermented fish products. See K. Amano, "The Influence of Fermentation on the Nutritive Value of Fish with Special Reference to Fermented Fish Products of Southeast Asia," in *Fish in Nutrition*. Eirik Heen and Rudolf Kreuzer, eds. (London 1962), p. 180. H. L. Wang and C. W. Hesseltine (*Indigenous Fermented Food of Non-western Origin*. Mycologia Memoirs, No. 11 [Berlin 1986], pp. 335–40) identify 68 different products of Southeast Asia, Korea, and Japan.

[42] This rapid deterioration of fish tissue is caused by the same process which in the presence of salt induces preservation; that is, the attack of proteolytic enzymes on fish muscle proteins. See Gunther Siebert, "Enzymes of Marine Fish Muscle and Their Role in Fish Spoilage," in *Fish in Nutrition*. Eirik Heen and Rudolf Kreuzer, eds. (London 1962), pp. 80–82; and Alberto Pedrosa-Menabrito and Joe M. Regenstein, "Shelf-life Extension of Fresh Fish—A Review. Part I—Spoilage of Fish," *Journal of Food Quality* 1,2 (1988): 117–27.

[43] See, for example, Van Veen, "Fermented and Dried Seafood Products," 3: 233, 243–44; Cutting, "Influence," pp. 172–73; and Mackie et al., *Fermented Fish Products*, pp. 2, 8, 15.

[44] *Pedah siam* from Thailand is a salt-fish product from a *scomber* species, whole but with entrails removed and salted in a fish-to-salt ratio of 3:1 for one day. It is then packed in crates which allow the brine to drain out. The result is a fish product which is fatty and partly dried, having only a slight fish odor and brown color. Packed, it can keep for months; removed from

tended periods of time. A minimum of 10% salt concentration is needed to inhibit the growth of bacteria and molds.[45] Hard curing creates a very salty product which keeps well in hot regions, such as in Southeast Asia; in western countries, where modern technology is more readily available and where taste preferences require that hard cured products be desalted in fresh water or oil before eating, mild cures tend to be more popular.[46]

Three general methods are employed to salt fish: dry salting, which forms its own brine, brining with a prepared salt solution, and a combination of the first two. As osmosis draws water out of fish tissue and replaces it with salt, the overall weight of the fish decreases. As time goes on, the salt concentration in the outer layers of fish tissue equalizes with that in the surrounding brine. The whole process slows down, salt passing from the brine into the outer fish tissues to the same degree as the inner tissues absorb salt from the outer layers. Finally, as the fish continues to absorb salt, its weight increases slightly. The fish meat is now dense and contracted. A strong flavor of salt replaces both the odor and taste of raw fish.[47]

The technology within which this process occurs can be seen in the processing of herring and anchovies practiced today in Europe and Russia. Although individual processes vary considerably from one country to another dependent upon climate, species and size of fish, season of the year, use of barrels or vats, and so on, the principles are basically identical.[48] The bottom of the vat receives a layer of salt. A layer of fish, sometimes washed, at least partially eviscerated, and occasionally rubbed with salt, is then laid down. This is topped by a second layer of salt, then more fish laid down at right angles to the previous fish layer, and so on.[49] When the top of the vat is reached, a final layer of salt is added and the whole covered in some manner. Stone or concrete weights press down the fish so that they are submerged by the pickle which begins to form within twenty-four hours.

---

the crates, it spoils within a few weeks. See Beddows, "Fermented Fish and Fish Products," pp. 28–29; Van Veen, "Fermented and Dried Seafood Products," pp. 238–41; and Mackie et al, *Fermented Fish Products*, pp. 9–10.

[45] N. A. Voskresensky, "Salting of Herring," in *Fish as Food*. Georg Borgström, ed. 4 vols. (New York 1965), 3: 114–16; Cutting, "Smoking," p. 88; and *idem*, "Influence," p. 162.

[46] Cutting, "Influence," p. 162; and Henri Cheftel, "The Processing of the Anchovy: *Engraulis encrasicholus* Linnaeus," in *Fish as Food*. Georg Borgström, ed. 4 vols. (New York 1965), 3: 219. Mild cures are, nevertheless, produced in hot climates, but their shortcomings are obvious. In Malaysia, for example, fish processors construct concrete vats under sheds to ward off the hot sun and rain. They place fish into the vats in alternating layers with rock salt and apply weights which press down the mass. After only 1–5 days the processors remove the fish and dry them on bamboo platforms. In the hot Malaysian climate these products spoil easily and are infested with flies. S. Y. Yu et al, "Application of Technology," pp. 211–12.

[47] Voskresensky, "Salting of Herring," pp. 111–15.

[48] *Ibid.*, pp. 121–28; Cheftel, "Processing of the Anchovy," pp. 215–25.

[49] In salting small herring in Russia, Japan, and elsewhere, sometimes about 15–20 cm. of saturated brine are added to the first layer of ca. 0.5–1.0 cm. of solid salt. For large fish layering with dry salt only is practiced. See Voskresensky, "Salting of Herring," pp. 126–28. At least some of the fish viscera is retained, ostensibly for development of the proper flavor. See Mackie et al., *Fermented Fish Products*, p. 14.

The weights expel air bubbles and the brine covering the mass prevents the oxidation of unsaturated fatty acids which accelerates spoilage. The pressure of weights also increases the penetration of salt into the fish tissue.[50] The period of ripening depends upon the degree of salt penetration desired and can range from only a few days to several months.[51] Vat salting is the best way to accommodate catches of migratory fish where large quantities are involved. The major problem encountered is an unevenness of the product because the height of the vat and the pressure exerted by weights can create different degrees of salinity at different levels in the same vat. To allow for this, oftentimes the top layers receive almost double the amount of salt as the bottom layers.[52]

Brining, at an optimum strength of about 70%, is a more rapid method to cure fish than is dry-salting alone. The lower the salt concentration and the fatter the fish, the longer the period of brining required to ensure long-term keeping quality. The major problem encountered here is that as the fish absorbs salt from the brine and gives up water from within its tissues, the brine becomes diluted. Salt must, therefore, be added from time to time and the solution stirred frequently to ensure that the added salt does not merely settle to the bottom. Brining, for this reason, is usually reserved for curing small fish. The production of *surstrømming*, a Scandinavian salt-fish made from non-fatty herring, for example, involves brining whole, eviscerated fish for a short period of time in a solution of low salt concentration. The prepared product is packed in its own brine for shipment.[53]

Fish sauces today are produced in only a few places in the Western Mediterranean and in Greece and Turkey, but in very small quantities in relation to the total fish catch.[54] They are, however, extensively produced in the Far East, where a strong salt taste is not so objectionable and where the hot climate and poor storage facilities necessitate fish products with longer

---

[50] Cheftel, "Processing of the Anchovy," p. 220; Beatriz E. Filsinger, "Effect of Pressure on the Salting and Ripening Process of Anchovies (*Engraulis anchoita*)," *Journal of Food Science* 52,4 (July–Aug. 1987): 919–27; Cutting, "Influence," p. 174; and Pedrosa-Menabrito and Regenstein, "Spoilage of Fish," pp. 124–25.

[51] Small herring in Russia are mildly cured, ripening for only 10–14 days, larger ones for at least 25. Mediterranean anchovies, however, ripen for up to 6–8 months. Herring: Voskresensky, "Salting of Herring," pp. 126–27; anchovies: Cheftel, "Processing of the Anchovy," p. 221; and Beatriz E. Filsinger, C. A. Barassi, H. M. Lupin, and R. E. Trucco, "An Objective Index for the Evaluation of the Ripening of Salted Anchovy," *Journal of Food Technology* 17,2 (1982): 193–94.

[52] Voskresensky, "Salting of Herring," pp. 109, 127. Cf. *P.Oxy.* XXXIII. 2680 (2nd-3rd cent. A.D.), where the writer of the letter notes that the jar of salt-fish (ταρείχιον) had sunk in and needed topping off. He adds that the ones on the bottom were better than the one on top.

[53] Brining: Cutting, "Smoking," pp. 88–90; *surstrømming*: Beddows, "Fermented Fish and Fish Products," p. 30.

[54] *Pissala* (France): P. Creac'h, "Un actuel 'garum' français: le pissala. Le pêche du Nonnat et de la Pontine," *Pêches Maritimes* (Institut Scientifique et Technique des Pêches Maritimes, Paris) 17 (1952): 57–60; *garos* (Greece and Turkey): Georgacas, *Ichthyological Terms*, pp. 192–98. *Pissala* is a product made from small fish (anchovies, etc.) in a short fermentation period; *garos*, from the livers only of the *Scomber colias*. See also Mackie et al., *Fermented Fish Products*, p. 12.

keeping quality. Among the most noted are *nuoc-mam* (Vietnam), *nam-pla* (Thailand), *budu* (Malaysia), and *patis* (Philippines). In general, they are all clear, filtered liquids made in salt concentrations greater than 20% with whole, uneviscerated, usually pelagic fish which undergo a slow process of enzyme hydrolysis extending over long periods of time.[55] Although details of the methods of production for each type vary to greater or lesser extent from one country to another and even between one region of a country and another, for example in fish-to-salt ratio, type and size of fish, and length of ripening, the principles, as is the case with salt-fish, remain the same.

Fish sauce can be made in any amount desired. The home process for Philippine *patis*, for example, involves the mixing of small fish, normally the inexpensive kinds caught year round, such as anchovies and herring fry, with salt derived from the evaporation of sea water.[56] The mixture, in a fish-to-salt ratio of 2.5–3.0:1, undergoes fermentation in earthen or glass jars covered with some sort of lid. The mass is stirred occasionally during the ripening period which lasts until the fish have been almost totally digested. The clear *patis* is then drawn off, leaving a thickish residue of undigested fish tissue. This residue is the fish paste *bagoong*, used in ways similar to *patis*.

The commercial processing of fish sauce involves huge quantities of fish, both large and small, and is performed in wooden or concrete vats housed in sheds to protect the product from sun and rain. The fish-to-salt ratio can vary, but rarely falls below 5:1. The ratio for commercial *patis*, for example, is the same as that for the home preparation, from 4:1 to 3:1; that for Vietnamese *nuoc-mam*, 3:1 to 6:5; Malaysian *budu*, 5:1 to 3:1; and Thai *nam-pla*, 5:1 to 1:1. Indonesian *ketjap-ikan*, however, is produced at a ratio of 6:1; Cambodian *nuoc-mam-gau-ca*, made with only the livers of fish, is prepared in a ratio of 10:1.[57] The best sauces keep for several years, the ones with lower salt concentrations for a considerably shorter period of time.[58]

Uneviscerated fish are placed in vats in alternating layers with salt;

---

[55] In 1961, fish sauce production formed the single largest portion of the fisheries industry in Thailand, Cambodia, and Vietnam. See Prasert Saisithi, Bung-orn Kasemsarn, J. Liston, and Alexander M. Dollar, "Microbiology and Chemistry of Fermented Fish," *Journal of Food Science* 31 (1966): 105. See also Mackie et al., *Fermented Fish Products*, p. 3. For a list of different fish sauces, see Wang and Hesseltine, *Indigenous Fermented Food*, pp. 335–40, and Beddows, "Fermented Fish and Fish Products," p. 5.

[56] Keith H. Steinkraus et al., *Handbook of Indigenous Fermented Foods* (New York), p. 506. For the household production of Vietnamese *nuoc-mam*, see *ibid.*, pp. 516–17.

[57] *Ibid.*, pp. 505–26; Amano, "Influence," p. 183; Beddows, "Fermented Fish and Fish Products," p. 5; Saisithi et al., "Microbiology," p. 105; Eli V. Crisan and Anne Sands, "Microflora of Four Fermented Fish Sauces," *Applied Microbiology* 29,1 (Jan. 1975): 106–07; and Florian M. Orejana and John Liston, "Agents of Proteolysis and Its Inhibition in Patis (Fish Sauce) Fermentation," *Journal of Food Science* 47,1 (Jan.-Feb. 1982): 198. The *garos* of Greece is made from the livers only of the *Scomber colias* in a fish-to-salt ratio of 9:1. See Mackie et al., *Fermented Fish Products*, p. 12.

[58] The best Malaysian *budu*, for example, keeps up to two years; the lowest quality, for less than a week. See Steinkraus et al., *Handbook*, p. 522.

sometimes a concentrated brine is used.[59] When the top of the vat has been reached, the whole is pressed down by weights. After a few days the first bloody liquid (called *nuoc-boi* in Vietnam) is drawn off, to be added back later. With more salt and possibly the first extract now added and the vat sealed, ripening begins, during which the mass is occasionally stirred with paddles. The ripening period, at ambient temperatures of about 30° C, varies according to the type and size of fish, and can extend up to eighteen months. Elevated temperatures, but only up to about 45° C, and the use of pure salt can hasten autolysis. Conversely, salt with impurities, such as magnesium and calcium, can hinder salt penetration and so retard autolysis since they have a hardening effect on fish tissue.[60] When fully matured, the sauce is transferred to settling tanks where a clear first-quality sauce, called in Vietnamese *nuoc-nhut,* is filtered and separated from the thick residue of undigested fish material (*nuoc-xat*). The liquid sauce is then either bottled for shipment or else aged, sometimes up to four years.[61] The residue can be leached or lixiviated with a boiling salty brine to produce a sauce of lower quality. A poorer quality sauce arises from each successive leaching. Since the sauces from second and subsequent washings have a lower salt concentration, they have a poorer keeping quality and can go bad. Additives, such as higher quality sauce, caramel, and molasses, can improve both keeping quality and color. The color of the best sauces varies somewhat, from the clear, straw-yellow to amber of *patis* to the brown color of *nuoc-mam* and *nam-pla*. The taste is rather distinctive, unlike fish altogether. It can best be described as ranging from the salty, almost cheese-like flavor of *patis,* to the salty, strong cheese-like taste of *nuoc-mam,* to the "meaty" odor and flavor of *nam-pla*. The odors, particularly of lesser quality types, can be quite strong. The best ones actually exude an appetite-stimulating aroma.[62]

[59] Layers (*nuoc-mam*): Van Veen, "Fermented and Dried Seafood Products," p. 231; Beddows, "Fermented Fish and Fish Products," p. 6; brine (*nam-pla*): Crisan and Sands, "Microflora," p. 106. For flow charts showing graphically the process of making fish sauces, see Steinkraus et al., *Handbook*, p. 505 (*patis*); and Owens and Mendoza, "Enzymically Hydrolysed and Bacterially Fermented Fishery Products," p. 276 (*nuoc-mam*).

[60] William S. Hamm and John A. Clague, *Temperature and Salt Purity Effects on the Manufacture of Fish Paste and Sauce*. Fish and Wildlife Service Research Report 24 (Washington, D.C. 1950), pp. 3–5. The experiments concentrated on Manila salt used to produce Philippine *patis*. See also Mackie et al., *Fermented Fish Products*, pp. 18–19.

[61] *Nam-pla* ripens from 10–12 months, followed by further aging in the sun in earthenware containers for up to an additional three months. See Saisithi et al., "Microbiology," p. 105. Mackie et al. (*Fermented Fish Products*, p. 7) say that the better qualities age for up to two or three years. *Ounago*, a Japanese sauce made from shrimp, is aged four years; *kaomi*, a similar shrimp sauce, for two years. See Crisan and Sands, "Microflora," pp. 106–07.

[62] Methyl ketones probably produce the cheese-like flavors of fish sauce, while amines, such as pyridine, putrescine, and cadavarine, account for the full range of fish odors. If concentrations of amines are high in comparison to those of amino acids, the odor can be quite strong indicating a spoiled product. The colors result perhaps from the interaction of amines with carbonyl compounds. The aldehydes produced by autoxidation also react with amines in a Maitland-type reaction. The role of bacteria in the development of odor and taste is unknown, but seems minimal. See Van Veen, "Fermented and Dried Seafood products," p. 231; Bed-

Fish paste, primarily a by-product in the preparation of fish sauce, is itself an important food item. *Bagoong*, the residue of *patis* production, for example, is a staple of the Filipino diet. Frequently producers do not permit complete autolysis of the fish mass so that *bagoong*, not *patis*, is the desired end product. *Bagoong* is a thick, pasty, grayish, partially hydrolyzed mash of undissolved fish or shrimp, ripened only 2–3 months. The flavor is salty; the odor of the best quality, cheese-like. The Vietnamese equivalent is *mam;* that of Indonesia, *trassi;* and of Cambodia, *prahoc.*[63] The ancient equivalent is apparently allec, which Pliny (*HN* 31.95) states is the residue of garum production and a product which can be made for its own sake as well.

Fish, in general, are a good source of protein in the human diet, both in terms of protein quality and quantity. In 1982, for example, it accounted for 14% of the world's animal protein requirement and nearly 5% of total protein needs.[64] In addition, fish and fish oil are high in unsaturated fats, potentially useful in the control of cholesterol levels in blood. Where bones are also eaten, as with small fish such as anchovies, fish can provide calcium and phosphorus. Fish also supply some important B-vitamins and certain minerals, such as iron and copper.

Processed fish is an excellent supplement to anyone subsisting on a low-protein, high-cereal diet typical of people living in Southeast Asia. The high salt content, however, prevents it from being a major portion of the diet, but the cheaper fish sauces, used especially as condiments, are particularly helpful for the poorer populations.[65] Fresh fish are usually not readily affordable to the very poor of Southeast Asia. For instance, the Filipino poor eat the fish paste *bagoong* three times per day, in addition to the sauce *patis*, which on boiled rice is a staple. In rural areas *patis* is also eaten with vegetables. Both paste and sauce are priced within reach.[66] In Vietnam,

---

dows, "Fermented Fish and Fish Products," pp. 6, 13–20; Steinkraus et al., *Handbook*, pp. 505–06, 516–17; Mackie et al., *Fermented Fish Products*, pp. 3–4, 14–15, 20–22; Crisan and Sands, "Microflora," p. 106; and Orejana and Liston, "Agents of Proteolysis," pp. 199–203. See also Roger I. Brooks and G. A. Reineccius, "Identification of Neutral and Basic Flavor Compounds in Fermented Fish Sauce," Abstract, *Papers of The American Chemical Society* 172 (1976): AGFD 158, who conclude that among basic and neutral volatile compounds, such as dimethylamine, trimethylamine, and 2–methyl pyrazine, lactones predominated as flavor constituents.

[63] Steinkraus et al., *Handbook*, pp. 488–500; Mackie et al., *Fermented Fish Products*, pp. 7–9; Van Veen, "Fermented and Dried Seafood Products," pp. 234–38, and Beddows, "Fermented Fish and Fish Products," pp. 23–28.

[64] Pedrosa-Menabrito and Regenstein, "Spoilage of Fish," p. 117. The proportion of protein in an individual fish varies with species, but for marine fish it is usually 9–26%. The quality of fish protein is comparable to that of meat, milk, and eggs. See B. C. Guha, "The Role of Fish in Human Nutrition," in *Fish in Nutrition*. Eirik Heen and Rudolf Kreuzer, eds. (London 1962), pp. 40–41; Mackie et al., *Fermented Fish Products*, p. 27. In Malaysia, 49% of the total animal protein consumed and 12% of the total protein intake come from fish. See Yu et al., "Application of Technology," p. 211.

[65] Owens and Mendoza, "Enzymically Hydrolysed and Bacterially Fermented Fishery Products," p. 282; Amano, "Influence," p. 180; and Beddows, "Fermented Fish and Fish Products," p. 4.

[66] The retail price of *bagoong* in 1977 was about $0.34 per bottle of 200 grams; for *patis*, the price was $0.37–$0.39 per 750 ml. bottle. See Steinkraus et al., *Handbook*, pp. 489, 493, 498, 505,

likewise, the poorer classes consume almost four times the *nuoc-mam* of the wealthy, but usually of the lower grades. This is also in addition to other processed fish products which approach 20 grams daily.[67]

The nutritional importance of modern fermented fish products, as also for their ancient counterparts, derives from the biochemical and microbiological processes occurring during the salting and ripening stages. Little experimentation has been done on the nutritional value of salt-fish, so the amount of information is less than that for the fish sauces which have received greater attention. It is clear, however, that salt-fish provides a more concentrated source by weight of protein than fresh fish, since processing removes most of the moisture from fish tissue and replaces it with salt.[68] Although protein loss in processing can vary, brining of fatty Atlantic mackerel caught in the fall, for instance, results in a loss of only 5% protein, while protein quality and retention of polyunsaturated fatty acid content is only a little affected, even when hot smoking follows salting.[69] In salting, however, particularly if the liquid formed is drained off, as in "kench" curing, some water soluble nutrients, such as minerals and B-vitamins, are lost. Salt-fish, therefore, is an excellent source of concentrated protein, but is not a particularly good source of B-vitamins.[70]

The production of fish sauce involves entirely enzymic proteolysis, primarily from enzymes of the digestive tract (pyloric caeca). In the best products there is little or no bacteria involvement, except in so far as what appears between catch and the initial stages of processing. The quality of the final product depends upon the extent to which the growth of microorganisms are controlled. The better quality sauces do not constitute a health hazard, since a salt concentration of 5:1 or greater and a relatively low pH value of 5.0 to 6.5 common in fish sauces are not conducive to the growth of aerobic bacteria. This prevents putrefaction and reduces the

515. In January of 1990, I could purchase locally a 750 ml. bottle of imported *patis* for $1.79. Owens and Mendoza ("Enzymically Hydrolysed and Bacterially Fermented Fishery Products," p. 282) report that in the 1970s annually the Philippines produced 12.5 million liters of fish sauce and paste from over 100,000 tons of fish.

[67] Van Veen, "Fermented and Dried Seafood Products," p. 232; Steinkraus et al. (*Handbook*, p. 516) give the figures as 15 ml. per day for the wealthy; 30 ml. for the middle class; and 60 ml. for the poor. Amano ("Influence," p. 180) estimates that a daily consumption of 40 grams of Vietnamese fish sauce can account for 7.5% of an individual's total nitrogen intake.

[68] Pelagic fish, such as herring, sardines, and sprats, often used in fermented fish products, have protein contents of 15–20% and an oil content as high as 25%. See Mackie et al., *Fermented Fish Products*, p. 15. The quality of the proteins and their hydrolytic products, such as amino acids, does not substantially degrade during processing, at least where the product is of high quality. See *ibid.*, p. 27.

[69] Aminullah Bhuiyan et al., "Effect of Smoking on Proximate Composition," p. 328. Protein quality and polyunsaturated fatty acid content even increased in leaner mackerel caught in the spring. See also Aminullah Bhuiyan et al., "Effects of Smoking on Protein Quality," pp. 15–24; and Cutting, "Influence," p. 168, esp. Table III, pp. 164–67 and Table IV, p. 169.

[70] Salted herring, for instance, has only about one-half the percentage of B-vitamins as fresh herring. See Olaf R. Braekkan, "B-vitamins in Some Fish Products," in *Fish in Nutrition*. Eirik Heen and Rudolf Kreuzer, eds. (London 1962), p. 144.

chances of botulism poisoning.[71] Enzymes, such as trypsin of the pyloric caeca and to a lesser extent pepsin found in the stomach, attack fish tissues at the same time as salt by osmosis removes moisture.[72] Since the proteolytic activity of these enzymes varies with fish species, and in some species varies with the season of the year, but generally is low, the process can take a considerable length of time. Eventually the fish loses its shape and begins to liquify as protein dissolves in the liquid formed. The proteins slowly decompose into amino-nitrogen compounds, especially peptides, amino acids, and nitrogenous bases, such as ammonia, trimethylamine, urea, and creatin. *Nuoc-mam*, for example, has a good concentration of eight of the nine essential amino acids, but not a significant amount of B-vitamins.[73] Since enzymic hydrolysis is not total, an insoluble residue remains. This fish material is also high in protein and is used as a condiment or as an additive for highly seasoned food, for example Philippine *bagoong*; in Vietnam, however, the *nuoc-xat* is used as a fertilizer.[74] Progressively greater bacterial spoilage of the product lowers the ratio of amino acids to amines and creates a stronger smelling sauce of poorer quality. Fish sauce of lower quality produced by leaching likewise results in a smaller amount of amino acid nitrogen and so a product of less nutritional value.[75]

Although it seems clear from the above discussion that the consumption of fresh and processed fish, particularly as fermented sauces, can contribute to a healthful diet, recent studies give cause for some concern. In dietary studies of Japanese in Japan and Japanese immigrants to Hawaii, a strong connection appeared between the incidences of stomach cancer and frequency of consumption of dried and salted fish and pickled vegetables.[76] The relative risks were higher in those of the lower socio-economic scale among whom the consumption of these products was greater. The risk for

---

[71] Orejana and Liston, "Agents of Proteolysis," pp. 198–209. On botulism see Owens and Mendoza, "Enzymically Hydrolysed and Bacterially Fermented Fishery Products," pp. 283–86. See also Mackie et al., *Fermented Fish Products*, pp. 15, 19–20.

[72] The action of trypsin-like enzymes is not consistent. Initially low, it increases rapidly, then falls off after a few months. This characteristic may be related to the increase of amino acids in solution. See Orejana and Liston, "Agents of Proteolysis," pp. 199–203. Cathepsin, the enzyme in fish muscle, likewise plays an important, but secondary role. See *ibid.*, p. 201, and Mackie et al., *Fermented Fish Products*, p. 16.

[73] It is low in histidine. Steinkraus et al., *Handbook*, pp. 505–24; Mackie et al., *Fermented Fish Products*, pp. 15–20; and E. Hess, "Fishery Products of Indochina," in *The Technology of Herring Utilization*. M. Jul and M. Kondrup, eds. (Bergen 1953), pp. 131–44. Steinkraus et al. (*Handbook*, p. 520) list the following values per 100 grams of high quality *nuoc-mam*: Kcal., 268; water, 46 grams; protein, 17.5 grams; fat, 12 grams; carbohydrates, 20.8 grams; ash, 3.4 grams; thiamine, 0.09 milligrams; and riboflavin, 0.86 milligrams.

[74] Orejana and Liston, "Agents of Proteolysis," pp. 198–203; Steinkraus et al., *Handbook*, pp. 488–89, 517.

[75] Mackie, *Fermented Fish Products*, pp. 20, 27.

[76] Tokuro Sato et al. "Studies of the Causation of Gastric Cancer: 2. The Relation Between Gastric Cancer Mortality Rate and Salted Food Intake in Several Places in Japan," *Bulletin of the Institute of Public Health* (Tokyo, Japan) 8 (1959): 187–98; William Haenszel et al., "Stomach Cancer Among Japanese in Hawaii," *Journal of the National Cancer Institute* 49 (1972): 969–88, esp. Table 5, p. 977; William Haenszel et al., "Stomach Cancer in Japan," *Journal of the National*

users of both dried and salted fish was two to three times higher than for non-users when the frequency of use reached six or more times per month. A similar result was also found for pickled vegetables when two or more were consumed twenty-one or more times each month. The elevated risk was not found for fresh vegetables or raw fish; and, indeed, it seems that diets high in sources of vitamin C showed a negative relationship with incidences of gastric cancer.[77] The connection between salted fish and stomach cancer has also been observed for inhabitants of Norway and Newfoundland.[78] The fact that this was not the case for a study of smoked fish ingestion in Iceland, nor have extensive studies been made of populations in Southeast Asia, indicates that further study is needed.[79]

Although the exact biochemical processes leading to this perceived link between gastric cancer and diets high in salted foods are yet to be determined, the latest work has concentrated on the role of carcinogenic nitrosamines formed from dietary precursors, such as nitrates, nitrites, and secondary amines.[80] Nitrates, found frequently in nature, such as in water and vegetables, easily reduce to nitrites in the presence of certain bacteria. This is particularly true in the mouth where oral microorganisms react with saliva which is heavy in nitrate.[81] Nitrites, therefore, occur naturally in the human stomach. Secondary amines, such as dimethylamine and trimethylamine, are found in significant quantities in salt-fish and fish sauce, and may be increased by cooking.[82] It seems, then, that a diet rich in processed fish, even though not eaten with great frequency, may cause significant chemical changes in the stomach when the secondary amines of the fish react with the nitrites naturally occurring there. These chemical changes

Cancer Institute 56 (1976): 265–274; and Laurence N. Kolonel et al., "Association of Diet and Place of Birth with Stomach Cancer Incidence in Hawaii Japanese and Caucasians," *The American Journal of Clinical Nutrition* 34 (1981): 2478–85. The Japanese consume a wide variety of fermented fish products in great amounts, until recently perhaps more so than any other country. See Mackie et al., *Fermented Fish Products*, pp. 2, 10–12.

[77] Kolonel et al., "Association of Diet and Place of Birth," pp. 2478–85.

[78] Erik Bjelke, "Epidemiologic Studies of Cancer of the Stomach, Colon, and Rectum; With Special Emphasis on the Role of Diet," *Scandinavian Journal of Gastroenterology* 9, Suppl. 31 (1974): esp. pp. 47–48, 158–63. The inclusion of vitamin C in the diet of Norwegians also produced a negative correlation with stomach cancer.

[79] For Iceland, see *ibid.*, p. 160. I have been unable to find any studies on the relationship between salt-fish and stomach cancer in the Philippines, Vietnam, and Thailand.

[80] Haenszel et al., "Stomach Cancer Among Japanese in Hawaii," pp. 985–86.; Kolonel et al., "Association of Diet and Place of Birth," pp. 2483–84.

[81] William Lijinsky and Samuel S. Epstein, "Nitrosamines as Environmental Carcinogens," *Nature* 225 (Jan. 3, 1970): 21; Jonathan W. White, Jr., "Relative Significance of Dietary Sources of Nitrate and Nitrite," *Journal of Agricultural and Food Chemistry* 23 (1975): 886–91.

[82] Even raw fish, particularly fish roe, contain some secondary amines which also increase in cooking. Lijinsky and Epstein, "Nitrosamines as Environmental Carcinogens," pp. 22–23; Kolonel et al., "Association of Diet and Place of Birth," pp. 2483–84; Morizo Ishidate et al., "Secondary Amines, Nitrites and Nitrosamines in Japanese Foods," in *Topics in Chemical Carcinogenesis*. Waro Nakahara, Shozo Takayama, Takashi Sugimura, and Shigeyoshi Odashima, eds. (Baltimore 1972), pp. 313–21; and Brooks and Reineccius, "Identification of Neutral and Basic Flavor Compounds," AGFD 158.

produce nitrosamines, known cancer-causing agents. Since several studies suggest that ascorbic acid blocks the formation of nitrosamines, diets rich in vitamin C potentially may serve to offset the deleterious effects of salt-fish products.[83]

In summary, one can draw certain conclusions on the health value of modern fermented fish products. The best quality products are high in protein and provide several important vitamins, especially of the B group, and some minerals, such as calcium, phosphorus, iron, and copper. Lower quality products, those partially spoiled and so high in amines or excessively leached and so possessing less amino acid nitrogen, are not as nutritious but do contribute something to a healthful diet. In terms of life expectancy, the price of a diet high in products so obviously beneficial in many ways, however, may be steep. In countries, such as those in Southeast Asia and until recently in Japan, where consumption of salty foods (cured meat, fermented fish, and pickled vegetables) is high in comparison to fresh fish, vegetables, and fruit incidences of stomach cancer are significant.

---

[83] Kolonel, "Association of Diet and Place of Birth," pp. 2483–84.

ERRATUM

The first line of footnote 2 in Chapter 7, page 160, should read:

[2] Several *tituli* which arguably could have been included as fish sauce labels have been ex- ...

CHAPTER THREE

SALTED FISH PRODUCTS IN ANCIENT MEDICINE

Human Medicine

Although the Greeks knew and used salted fish products as early as the fifth century B.C., and probably earlier, the appearance of garum in extant medical literature does not antedate the reference to it by Dioscorides in Book II of his *De materia medica,* in which it plays a therapeutic role to which I shall return later.[1] Τάριχος, on the other hand, receives prominent attention in the Hippocratic corpus and in works of later physicians, both Hellenistic and Roman.

Ancient dietetics, as defined in *Regimen* and generally followed by subsequent writers, was an attempt to guide a healthy life and to prevent disease through adherence to diet and exercise, both geared to variations not only of a personal kind, such as temperament, age, and sex of the person, but also of an external character, such as the season of the year, geographic location, and so on.[2] Eating the proper foods was of paramount importance. Lacking a modern biochemistry, the ancients relied on sensual observations based on perceived common sense relationships derived from experience. Thus they categorized foods as heating or cooling, moist or dry, laxative or binding, and the like. These categories, frequently accompanied by lists of representative food items, became traditional and were called upon as needed by most subsequent writers.[3]

---

[1] Dioscorides *De mat. med.* 2.32. Garum: Plato Comicus fr. 198 (Edmonds), Pherecrates fr. 173 (Edmonds), Athenaeus 2.67c; τάριχος: Aristophanes *Eq.* 1247, *Ranae* 558; *Acharn.* 1101; Herodotus 2.77. Instances of dietetic and therapeutic uses of salted fish products can be multiplied by frequently citing medical writers who wrote after Galen, such as Marcellus Empiricus, Ps-Pliny, Leo Medicus, Caelius Aurelianus, Oribasius, Alexander of Tralles, and others, but little of substance would be thereby gained. Since the later sources are mainly derivative and frequently repetitive, I have, therefore, with only a few exceptions limited references to sources written between the fifth century B.C. and the fourth century A.D. No effort, therefore, has been made to be exhaustive. The sources for veterinary medicine, however, wth a few notable exceptions, as extant, generally date to the late third century A.D. and after. Much of the information contained in them, however, no doubt applies as well to the first two centuries A.D. For Post-Galenic medical authorities and the third century "lacuna," see John Scarborough, "The Galenic Question," *Sudhoff's Archiv* 65,1 (1981): esp. 21–24. This chapter appeared earlier in slightly altered form in the *Journal of the History of Medicine and Allied Sciences* 39,4 (Oct. 1984): 430–45. I wish to thank the editor for permission to incorporate this material here.

[2] Ludwig Edelstein, "The Dietetics of Antiquity," in *Ancient Medicine: Selected Papers of Ludwig Edelstein.* Oswei Temkin and C. Lilian Temkin, eds. (Baltimore 1967), pp. 303–16; Jerry Stannard, "Hippocratic Pharmacology," *BHM* 35 (1961): 510–17; E. D. Phillips, *Aspects of Greek Medicine* (New York 1973), pp. 75–92; and Wesley D. Smith, "Erasistratus' Dietetic Medicine," *BHM* 56 (1982): 398–409.

[3] W. D. Smith, "The Development of Classical Dietetic Theory," in *Hippocratica.* Actes du Colloque hippocratique de Paris (4–9 septembre 1978). M. D. Grmek, ed. (Paris 1980), pp. 439–48.

Regimen 2.48 declares that τάριχος is drying and attenuating, at least partially, one may presume, because salted fish was itself dry and appeared thin. Physicians expounded as well upon its degree of nourishment, ease of digestion, wholesomeness, and effect upon the appetite and bowels, but failed to agree on all particulars. Diphilus, for example, states that τάριχος offers little nourishment, is dry, and provocative of the appetite. He adds also that ὠμοτάριχος specifically is difficult to digest. Hicesius declares that young tunny were not easy to digest.[4] *Regimen* 2.56 says, in words no doubt appropriate to fish as well, that salted meats were less nutritious because the brine deprived them of their moisture. Thus they were dry, attenuated, and easily excreted. Most writers agreed that salt-fish was wholesome, promotive of the appetite, and stimulative of the stomach and intestines.

Xenocrates' (fl. ca. A.D. 70) treatise, *Food from Aquatic Animals*, particularly Book IV, which treats large sea fish which have been salted, and Book V, which discusses salted river and lake fish, is the most complete work extant devoted to the dietetic value of specific fish.[5] He says that, in general, salt-fish are palatable, but have bad juices, are attenuating, and disturb the stomach. Differentiating between various kinds of salt-fish, he adds that some have hard flesh, others soft, still others are in between. Some are fleshy, others fatty. The very fat ones float on the stomach; those less so are more nourishing.[6] He then discusses the value of different species which have been salted and praises those from certain geographic regions. The *colias*, or Spanish mackerel, for example, is palatable, and stimulates the appetite. Those caught in Spain are best.[7] The small pelamys, a type of tunny which arises in Lake Maeotis in the Black Sea region, is palatable, easy to digest and to excrete. He goes on to discuss other types of salt-fish, such as horaion, orkynus, and kybion. He does state that some salted tunny are hard to digest.[8] Distinguishing different salted fish based on parts of an individual fish, on species, or on country of origin was a commonplace in ancient dietetics and can be seen in other authors as well. Diphilus praises the τάριχος of Spain, as do Euthydemus and Galen. Τάριχος from the Pontic region finds favor with Euthydemus, Hicesius, Dorion, and Galen. Diphilus and Galen praise Sardinian salt-fish too.[9] In

---

[4] Athen. 3.120e-f (Diphilus); 116e (Hicesius). See also John Scarborough, "Diphilus of Siphnos and Hellenistic Medical Dietetics," *JHM* 25 (1970): 194–201. On the dietetic qualities of various fish cited by Diphilus and Mnesitheus, see Jacques Dumont, "Les critères culturels du choix des poissons dans l'alimentation grecque antique: le cas d'Athénée de Naucratis," in *Anthropozoologica*. 2d spec. no.: *L'animal dans l'alimentation humaine. Les critères de choix*. Liliane Bodson, ed. (Paris 1988), pp. 105–12.

[5] Xenocrates *ap*. Oribasius *Medical Collections* 2.58.133–52.

[6] *Ibid*. 2.58.133–35. These differentiations coincide well with what is known today of hard-cured and mildly-cured fish.

[7] *Ibid*. 2.58.133–35. Diphilus (*ap*. Athen. 3.121a) says that the *colias* was purgative, pungent, and possessed a poorer flavor. He adds, however, that the Spanish variety is best.

[8] Xenocrates *ap*. Oribasius *Medical Collections* 2.58.136–44.

[9] Athen. 3.121a (Diphilus), 3.116c (Euthydemus), 3.116f (Hicesius), 3.118b-c (Dorion); Galen *De alim. fac*. 3.40.5.

doing so, these physicians provide non-medical information important to social and economic historians for locating production centers and for understanding better the commerce of these products.[10]

The value of fermented fish sauces in ancient dietetics is more difficult to document because vis-à-vis τάριχος they receive less attention. *Regimen* 2.56 asserts that stale and putrid things—fish sauce would presumably fall into this category—are more readily excreted than fresh foods because they are nearer to corruption. In general, however, garum seems to fall into the same categories as τάριχος. Celsus says as much when he includes all salted fish and fish sauce among foods which have bad juices, are alien to the stomach, and move the bowels.[11] It is somewhat difficult to explain why fish sauce received so little specific notice in writings on ancient dietetics, but probably the answer lies in its principal use as a condiment. Whereas salt-fish was bulkier and so could serve as a substantive part of the diet, fish sauce, being a strongly saline liquid, was used primarily to flavor other foods, in this capacity substituting for salt. Indeed, Pliny says that the taste of salt was the desirable result in eating garum. Its use as a condiment can be easily documented in Greek and Latin literature from the fifth century B.C. into late antiquity. Apicius, the noted chef of the mid-first century A.D., in his *De re coquinaria*, as extant, for example, records 31 recipes which use salt, but nearly 350 which contain a fish sauce.[12] Garum flavored meat, fowl, fruit, vegetables, and even fish. Ancient writers readily acknowledged that fish sauce aided digestion and promoted the appetite. This would account for its common use, as well as salt-fish, as part of the *gustatio* of a Roman meal.[13] Galen, in his *Properties of Foods*, lists garum at least 32

---

[10] These differentiations are not mere casual statements. Today, different fish products from different regions do have different taste, color, consistency, and so on, because processes can vary greatly (See above esp. pp. 18–23). Differences in taste of fish caught at different times of the year, for instance, may be due to varying enzymic activity and fat content. See Voskresensky, "Salting of Herring," pp. 117–28, and Van Veen, "Fermented and Dried Seafood Products," p. 244.

[11] Celsus *Med.* 2.21 (bad juices), 25 (alien to stomach), 29 (move the bowels).

[12] Apicius *De re coq.*, passim. Cicero (*Att.* 4.8, 14.16; *Fam.* 9.16.7) mentions *tyrotaricha*, a cheese and salt-fish stew, and Apicius (*De re coq.* 4.17) gives a recipe with the same dish. For salsamenta and garum as a food and condiment see Jacques André, *L'Alimentation*², pp. 109–13; and Zahn, "Garum," *RE*, cols. 845–46. Pliny *HN* 31.87: *conditur* (sc. sal) *etiam odoribus additis et pulmentarii vicem implet, excitans aviditatem invitansque in omnibus cibis ita, ut sit pecularis ex eo intellectus inter innumera condimenta, item in mandendo quaesitus garo.* The frequent use of garum in the preparation of food and the association of the term garum with liquamen by the fifth century A.D. (cf. above, p. 7 and note 8) render identification of the liquamen of Apicius' *De re coquinaria* as a fish sauce quite likely. This seems particularly probable since the extant text of Apicius dates to the late fourth or early fifth century A.D. See *Apicius. De Re Coquinaria.* M. E. Milham, ed. (Leipzig 1969), p. v. Cf. Eugenia Salza Prina Ricotti, *L'arte del convito nella Roma antica* (Rome 1985), esp. pp. 223–34.

[13] Apicius *De re coq.* 1.34.1–2 (*oxygarum digestible*), 9.10.12; Alexander of Tralles (Puschmann, II, pp. 257, 261); Horace *Sat.* 2.8.6–9; Martial 3.50; 10.48; cf. Pliny *HN* 20.34; . Both Marcellus Empiricus (*De med.* 20.120) and Leo Medicus (*Synopsis of Medicine* 5.6 [Ermerins, pp. 170–73]) say that fish sauce remedied indigestion. For Alexander of Tralles I have consulted *Alexander von Tralles*. Theodor Puschmann, ed. 2 vols. (Wien 1878–79); for Marcellus Empiricus, see *Mar-*

times as part of food preparation; such as with lentils, lupines, fenugreek, beans, olives, mallows, nuts, lettuce, cabbage, and others. In nearly all cases, its addition frequently in combination with oil or vinegar, was primarily to provide a palatable dish, but often to increase the purgative effect of the recipe as well.[14]

It seems then that the role in ancient dietetics assigned to salted fish products derived from observation and experience. Although *Regimen* 2.48 indicates that the driest τάριχος comes from the driest fish, generally sea fish, it appears that in reality it is the physical appearance of salted fish—dry and stretched—which accounts for its assumed powers of dryness and attenuation.[15] Its saltiness naturally inclined it to be categorized with all salty foods, thus it possessed powers of heat and dryness. Experience indicated that salty foods promoted the appetite and moved the bowels, so also must salted fish. This observation was not totally mistaken, since salt can act as an osmotic cathartic in the intestines. Fish sauce, because of its salt content, when mentioned at all, also fell into the same categories, with the added conclusion that its putrid appearance also accounted for its ease of excretion.[16] Garum's primary role in Graeco-Roman life as a condiment, rather than as a basic food element, relegated it to a nearly insignificant place in the discussion of dietetics. Nevertheless, salt-fish, consumed as a significant element in the diet, and fish sauce, frequently used as a condiment on foods of all kinds, like their modern counterparts in Southeast Asia, added an important protein supplement to the ancient diet.

Ancient therapeutics concerned the treatment of diseases through physical means, such as tepid baths, and through pharmaceutical remedies. A cursory glance at the types of affliction for which salt-fish products formed a remedy shows that their uses arose from their assumed powers, principally those of heat and dryness and of loosening the bowels. A basic tenet of *Regimen* was to ensure a proper balance within the body between hot and cold, dry and moist, and so on. To do this a diet of opposites was prescribed if an imbalance were perceived. So it was also in therapeutics.

---

celli De Medicamentis Liber. Maximilian Niederman, ed. *Corpus Medicorum Latinorum* V (Leipzig 1916). For salt-fish see Athen. 3.120d (τάριχος) and Martial 5.78.5 (*cybium*).

[14] Galen *De alim fac.*, passim.

[15] *Regimen* 2.48 says that the driest τάριχος comes from sea fish, followed by that from rivers, then lake fish. Earlier, the author had declared sea fish which lived in and fed upon muddy water to be heavier than those which lived in rocky places or which moved about. In other words, he listed fish on a scale from lightest (and so driest) to heaviest (thus moistest) based upon their manner or location of life. It seems that τάριχος was judged in similar fashion to be consistent with this conclusion. On fish in the Hippocratic corpus see Janine Bertier, "Les animaux dans la diététique hippocratique," in *Anthropozoologica*, 2d. spec. no., pp. 86–88; in Galen, see Juan Antonio Lopéz Férez, "L'animal dans l'alimentation humaine selon Galien," in *ibid.*, p. 94.

[16] As to its powers of heat and dryness, we need not, however, take Seneca (*Ep.* 95.25) too seriously when he complains that Spanish garum "burns up the stomach with its salted rottenness!" (*illud sociorum garum, pretiosam malorum piscium saniem, non credis urere salsa tabe praecordia?*).

Ulcers, seen as moist, called for something to dry them; constipation demanded something to loosen the bowels.[17]

Garum differs from many medicinal substances of animal origin in several ways. It is first and foremost a foodstuff, functioning importantly as a condiment for many types of foods. Second, it is a drug, since it is often prescribed as a medicine by itself or as part of a mixture.[18] Third, most animal materia medica includes the entire animal (insect, worm, and so on) or its excrement, or, more usually, part of the animal (blood, eyes, brains, shell, fat, and so forth). Although derived from fish or parts of fish, garum is a medicament *sui generis*. One never finds, for instance, a prescription for preparing it which goes "Take such and such a fish, add salt in prescribed proportions, let it stand for a specified period of time, drain the liquid, and apply it to cure this or that." The closest one comes to this is a passage in Pliny's *Natural History* (31.95–97) where, after briefly defining garum, allec, and muria, he goes on to relate certain medical problems for which they are useful. All other medical contexts simply call for garum alone or garum mixed with something. The medicine, therefore, is ostensibly garum, not a specific fish per se; and since it is not formed naturally but must be produced by man, it is so-to-speak a manufactured animal and mineral drug combination. I would hasten to add, however, that its role as a food item—it is, after all, essentially a by-product of salting fish—predominates over its use as a medicine. And fourth, garum, being a liquid, easily combines with other elements, animal and vegetable, in a complicated recipe designed to create or to increase the potency of a desired effect. The use of compound medicines is typical of the polypharmacy which arose in the late Hellenistic period. Besides at times adding its own efficacious powers, garum can play two additional roles. Like honey and wine, it can ensure the proper consistency of the medicinal solution; it can also counteract another part of the mixture. Because of this, it is often difficult to determine which drug in a complex concoction actually provides the relief desired.

Of the therapeutic value of fish sauce, the ancient physicians, in general, are in agreement. In the treatment of internal conditions and diseases fish sauce played an important role in the creation of medicinal foods administered by mouth or of solutions injected as a clyster. The afflictions so remedied involved primarily the digestive tract. Galen, in his treatise *Mixtures and Properties of Simples*, says that "Garum has the considerable capacity of heat and dryness, and on account of this some doctors treat putrefying ulcers with it, and inject it into people with dysentery and sciatica." He adds next that ἅλμη τῶν ταριχηρῶν ἰχθύων had identical powers and so

[17] Phillips, *Aspects*, p. 89.

[18] Garum easily fits Stannard's definition of a drug: "The distinction between drugs and foodstuffs is, I believe, a purely pragmatic one: If an item is administered to a sick person with a curative aim, regardless of its mode of administration and the nature of the complaint, it is *ipso facto*, a drug." Stannard, "Hippocratic Pharmacology," p. 512.

was used for similar purposes.[19] Garum, used in conjunction with other foods, was frequently prescribed as a laxative. Celsus, for example, says that fish sauce and salt-fish move the stomach, and Galen often included fish sauce in compound medicines for the same purpose. Marcellus Empiricus (fl. A.D. 310–410), in a chapter on the use of salts, potions, and pills to loosen the stomach and combat or prevent jaundice, describes a *liquamen catharticum* composed of ginger, rock-parsley, pepper, laser, scammony, and liquamen. Aetius gives several similar recipes involving garum mixed with water (ὑδρόγαρον), wine (οἰνόγαρον), and vinegar (ὀξύγαρον).[20]

In one instance, ironically, garum was included in a mixture designed to treat chronic diarrhea. In *De alimentorum facultatibus* 1.1.43, Galen discusses the use of lentil soup in treating diarrhea. After commenting that Heracleides of Tarentum (fl. ca. 70 B.C.) gave a lentil and beet dish (τευτλοφακῆ) to both healthy and sick people, he says that this food with many beets added and seasoned with salt or "sweet garum" was more evacuant (ὑπακτικωτέρα).[21] Continuing his discussion, he declares that if, after braying lentils and then boiling them twice and pouring off the first liquid, you add salt or garum and something to bind the stomach, but not so much as to ruin the taste, you would simultaneously create a good food and a good medicine. The use of garum, a common purgative, in medicines to combat diarrhea seems contradictory, but is entirely consistent. In the first recipe Galen knew that lentil soup (*lenticula*) with beets bound the stomach, a fact known as well to earlier Latin authors, such as Celsus (ca. A.D. 14–37). Knowing also that beets and fish sauce by themselves were evacuants, he merely comments that their addition, particularly with greater numbers of

---

[19] Galen *De simplicium medicamentorum temperamentis ac facultatibus* 12.377K: Γάρος δυνάμεώς ἐστι θερμῆς ἱκανῶς καὶ ξηρᾶς, καὶ διὰ τοῦτο πρὸς τὰ σηπεδονώδη τῶν ἑλκῶν ἐχρήσαντό τινες αὐτῷ τῶν ἰατρῶν, ἐνιᾶσί τε τοῖς δυσεντερικοῖς τε καὶ ἰσχιαδικοῖς. Ἅλμη τῶν ταριχηρῶν ἰχθύων ὁμοίως τῷ γάρῳ πρός τε τὰς σηπεδόνας ἁρμόζει καὶ πρὸς ἰσχιάδας καὶ δυσεντερίαν ἐνιεμένη, τῇ δὲ δριμύτητι τοὺς μὲν τὸ ἰσχίον ἐνοχλοῦντας χυμοὺς ἐπισπᾶται καὶ διὰ τῶν ἐντέρων ἐκκενοῖ, τὰ δὲ σηπεδονώδη τῶν ἑλκῶν ἐν τῇ δυσεντερίᾳ περικλύζει τε καὶ ξηραίνει. μάλιστα δὲ τῇ τῶν ταριχηρῶν σιλούρων καὶ τῇ τῶν μαινίδων ἅλμῃ πρὸς τὰ τοιαῦτα κέχρηνταί τινες ἰατροὶ, καὶ ἡμεῖς δ' ἐπὶ τῶν ἐν στόματι σηπεδονωδῶν ἑλκῶν ἐχρησάμεθα. See also Dioscorides *De mat. med.* 2.32; Pliny *HN* 31.97; and Oribasius *Syn. ad Eust.* 9.61.5–6; *Ad Eunap.* 2.5.3–4, 4.116.19. To treat paralysis of the anus Caelius Aurelianus (*On Chronic Diseases* 2.1.40 [Drabkin, p. 590]) prescribes a garum enema. Cf. Georges Desse, "Sur un condiment marin," in *Archéologie et Médecine. VIIèmes Rencontres Internationales d'Archéologie et d'Histoire, Antibes, Octobre 1986* (Juan-les-Pins 1987), pp. 479–88.

[20] Celsus *Med.* 2.29; Galen *De alim. fac.* 1.24 (with fenugreek), 2.68 (with raw vegetables), and passim; Marcellus Empiricus *De med.* 30.52; and Aetius 3.83–84, 86–88. For liquamen used to mean any fish sauce, especially garum, see Caelius Aurelianus *On Chronic Diseases* 2.1.40, 3.70 (Drabkin, pp. 590, 610).

[21] Exactly what "sweet garum" (γάρος γλυκύ) was remains unknown, perhaps a sauce mixed with something like honey or passum to cut its saltiness. Celsus (*Med.* 2.30) says that cooked honey binds the stomach. For γλυκύς = passum, see André Tchernia, *Le vin de l'Italie romaine* (Rome 1986), p. 244. If Galen had meant vinegar or oil, formal expressions existed at hand, such as, for example, Galen *De alim. fac.* 1.23.1 (ὀξύγαρον) and 3.26.4 (γαρέλαιον).

the former, would render the lentil soup less binding.[22] The garum here, as he explicitly states, functions primarily to season the dish. Its use would have also strengthened the power of beets to loosen the stomach, but this is not emphasized. The second recipe, lentil soup without beets, also bound the stomach. Boiling the soup twice and pouring off the first liquid concentrated the mashed lentils. Garum again served primarily as a seasoning, but being a liquid its use would also have replaced the moisture lost in pouring off the liquid. The addition of something else to bind the stomach seems a recognition by Galen of garum's power as an evacuant and so serves to offset this possible effect. In summary, both recipes aided those suffering from diarrhea by binding the stomach, the garum in each case would have seasoned the dish, making it more palatable, and in the latter recipe also ensured an acceptable consistency.

Although garum could be made from many different species of fish, a requirement to use fish sauce made from a specific fish for medicinal purposes is unusual and, when it does occur, more often than not the fish demanded is the maena or silurus. Dioscorides recommends a gargle of garum made specifically from the maena to cure sores in the mouth, while Caelius Aurelianus (fl. ca. A.D. 410) prescribes an enema of garum made from the silurus in the treatment of paralysis of the anus.[23] Other internal problems remedied with a dose of garum alone or in combination with something else include thrush, an oral disease of children, catarrh, an inflammation of the mucous membrane of the nose, quinsy, and others whose remedy more readily can be assigned to the realm of superstition than to experience, such as migraine headache, lethargy, depression, and tuberculosis. It should come as no surprise that salted fish products, being

[22] Celsus *Med.* 2.29 (beets and fish sauce move the stomach), 30 (lentil soup with beets binds the stomach).

[23] Maena: Dioscorides *De mat. med.* 2.29; Marcellus Sidetes *Medicina ex piscibus* 101; Pliny *HN* 26.23, 27.127, 31.83, 32.88; Galen *De simplicium medicamentorum temperamentis ac facultatibus* 12.377K; silurus: Dioscorides *De mat. med.* 2.27; Caelius Aurelianus *On Chronic Diseases* 2.1.40 (Drabkin, p. 590); Galen *De simplicium medicamentorum temperamentis ac facultatibus* 12.377K; and Rufus of Ephesus 64.47 (Daremberg and Ruelle, eds., p. 338). For Marcellus Sidetes, I have used *Medicina de piscibus*. F. S. Lehrs, ed. in *Poetae Bucolici et Didactici*. A. Koechly, ed. (Paris 1862), pp. 169–71. Fish were not the only marine life used by ancient physicians for dietetic and therapeutic purposes. Shellfish, such as oysters, sea urchins, and sea anemones, often appear in medical sources. See, for example, Xenocrates *ap.* Oribasius *Medical Collections* 2.58.50–132, and Pliny *HN* 31.95. See also E. Caprotti, "Molluschi e medicine nel I° d.c.," *Conchiglie* 13 (1977): 137–44. Extracts from shellfish are today finding medicinal uses as well, though in ways unforeseen by the ancient Greeks and Romans. See, for example, Jean Théodoridès "Considerations on the Medicinal Use of Marine Invertebrates," in *Oceanography: the Past*. M. Sears and D. Merriman, eds. (New York 1980), p. 734–49. The pharmacology of all types of marine life has in the last few decades been the object of much study. See, for instance, *Drugs and Food from the Sea: Myth and Reality*. Puskar N. Kaul and Carl J. Sindermann, eds. (Norman, Oklahoma 1978); *Food-Drugs from the Sea: Proceedings 1972*. Leonard R. Worthen, ed. (Washington, D.C. 1973); and *Drugs from the Sea*. Transactions of the Drugs from the Sea Symposium, University of Rhode Island, 27–29 August 1967. Hugo D. Freudenthal, ed. (Washington, D.C. 1968).

useful food items common to both rural and urban populations, should become part of folk medicine which pervaded much of Greek and Roman medical writing. One example from Pliny, the ever-practical Roman encyclopedist, will suffice. Pliny, who elsewhere denounces the use of magic, says that garum eaten with snails benefits the stomach, but adds charmingly that it works best if the number of snails eaten was odd![24]

Garum's efficacy extended to external afflictions as well. Although the form was different, the motivation was the same as that for internal remedies. Pliny recommends a liniment of the ash of garlic mixed with oil and garum to cure several skin problems, such as leprous sores, lichen, and freckly eruptions.[25] The external uses, however, on the whole seem more derived from folk medicine than from any real practical success. Garum, for instance, was supposed to treat the bites of dogs and crocodiles; while allec was good against the bite of the sea draco. Garum supposedly cured burns, but Pliny admonishes that one must not mention the word garum when applying it![26]

There were times, on the other hand, when garum had to be avoided. Marcellus Empiricus, for example, contrary to a prescription of Caelius Aurelianus, advises people suffering from catarrh to avoid liquamen, as well as vegetables and salty and fatty foods. Alexander of Tralles (fl. 6th cent. A.D.) states that garum should not be drunk with medicine taken for gout, nor should sufferers of melancholy produced through bilious and acrid blood take food with garum on it.[27] The noted hypochondriac Aelius Aristides (ca. A.D. 117–81), in Book Three of his *Sacred Discourses*, records that Aesclepius warned him in a dream not to eat garum because it "was not safe for the head, and least of all for teeth." This is an interesting prohibition in light of possible good dental effects *nuoc-mam* may have on the Vietnamese today.[28] In the vast majority of cases, however, garum's medicinal powers were fully recognized and recommended. St. Pachomius (ca. A.D.

[24] Thrush: Marcellus Sidetes *Medicina de piscibus* 101; catarrh: Caelius Aurelianus *On Chronic Diseases* 2.2.107 (Drabkin, p. 634); quinsy: Pliny *HN* 32.90; migraine headache: Alexander of Tralles (Puschmann, I, p. 501); tuberculosis: Marcellus Empiricus *De med.* 16.89; magic: Pliny *HN* 30.1–3; snails: *ibid.* 30.44. On folk medicine and learned medicine see John Scarborough, "Adaptation of Folk Medicine in the Formal Materia Medica of Classical Antiquity," in *Folklore and Folk Medicines.* John Scarborough, ed. (Madison, Wisconsin 1987), pp. 21–32; John Riddle, "Folk Tradition and Folk Medicine: Recognition of Drugs in Classical Antiquity," in *ibid.* pp. 33–61; and W. H. S. Jones, "Ancient Roman Folk Medicine," *JHM* 12 (1957): 459–72.

[25] Pliny *HN* 31.97 (burns), 20.55 (skin problems).

[26] Pliny *HN* 31.96 (sea draco), 97 (dog and crocodile); Dioscorides *De mat. med.* 2.32 (dog); Pliny *HN* 31.97 (burns). For the treatment of lumbago (?) see *BT. Gittin* 69b (Epstein, p. 331).

[27] Gout: Alexander of Tralles (Puschmann, II, p. 573); melancholy: *ibid.* (Puschmann, II, p. 601); catarrh: Marcellus Empiricus *De med.* 5.2,18–19, and Caelius Aurelianus *On Chronic Diseases* 2.2.107 (Drabkin, p. 634).

[28] *Nuoc-mam* contains a significant quantity of fluorine, about 100 mg. per liter. See Steinkraus et al., *Handbook*, p. 521. See Aelius Aristides *Sacred Discourses* 3.35. For Aelius Aristides, I have used *Aelii Aristidis Smyrnaei Quae Supersunt Omnia.* Bruno Keil, ed., vol. 2 (Berlin 1898), Chapter xlix, p. 421. Cf. Marcellus Empiricus (*De med.* 12.6) who recommends *muria ex piscibus lacertis veteribus* to alleviate pain in the teeth.

292–346), founder of several monasteries in Egypt, in his "Rules of the Order" (*Regulae*), as found in St. Jerome's Latin translation of the 5th century A.D., proscribes the consumption of garum by monks, but specifically makes an exception when they were sick (*absque loco aegrotantium*). In fact, St. Pachomius was himself served γαρέλαιον when he was ill.[29]

Τάριχος played a small role relative to fish sauce in therapeutics. In most cases where Pliny recommends salt-fish, for instance, the illness is identical to the ones for which garum was a remedy also; for example, abscesses, burns, ulcers, and bites of various animals. Salted fish was highly tauted as a purgative. Among specific fish singled out in particular circumstances, the most frequently mentioned were the silurus, maena, perch, and tunny. Pliny passes along some interesting suggestions; such as the statements that salted silurus was good for the voice, that preserved tunny blood, gall, and liver were useful for removing superfluous hair, and that salsamenta, in general, were beneficial in removing weapons which have pierced the skin.[30]

Veterinary Medicine

The use of salted fish products, especially fish sauce, in veterinary medicine should not be unexpected. Farm animals, such as sheep, cattle, and horses, were particularly valuable to the farmer and, especially the latter,

---

[29] *Regula Sancti Pachomii* 45 (= *S. Eusebii Hieronymi Stridonensis Presbyteri Translatio Latina Regulae Sancti Pachomii* in Migne, *PL*, vol. 23 [Paris 1845], col. 69): *vinum et liquamen absque loco aegrotantium nullus contingat*. For St. Pachomius' prohibition against the consumption of garum, see *Regula* 46: *Si aliquis eorum qui peregre mittuntur, in itinere, vel in nave aegrotaverit, et habuerit necessitatem sivi desiderium comedendi liquamen de piscibus, vel aliarum rerum, quae in monasterio comedere non consueverunt, non manducabit cum fratribus caeteris, sed separatim: et dabitur ei a ministris ad omnem abundantium, ne in ullo frater languidus contristetur*. Migne excises the *non* following *comedere* from the *editio princeps* for no good reason, as *Regula* 54 shows: . . . *non gustabunt liquamen, nec vinum bibent, nec aliud quidpiam, quorum edendi consuetudinem non habent*. Cf. *Praecepta Sancti Pachomii* 20 (= *SS. Patrum Aegyptiorum Opera Omnia* in Migne, *PG*, vol. 40, col. 949): Ἐὰν παρασκευάζωσιν αὐτοῖς φαγεῖν, οὐ μὴ γεύσωνται ἑψημένου γεύματος, οὔτε γάρος, οὔτε οἶνον πώσωσιν. That these *Regulae* accurately reflect St. Pachomius' attitude toward fish sauce the *Vita Prima Graeca*, the earliest existing Greek biography of Pachomius composed ca. A.D. 390, shows conclusively. For St. Pachomius' readiness to suspend rules when brothers were sick, see *Life of Pachomius* 53 (= *The Life of Pachomius* [*Vita Prima Graeca*]. Apostolos N. Athanassakis, transl. and ed. [Missoula, Montana 1975], pp. 77–79). For St. Pachomius being served garum and oil while he himself was sick, see *Life of Pachomius* 64: Καὶ ἐσθίοντος αὐτοῦ μίαν ὅτε ἦν ἀρρωστῶν, ἠνέχθη αὐτῷ γαρέλαιον πεποιημένον· For a recent discussion of St. Pachomius, the sources for his life, and the daily life in Pachomius' monasteries, see Philip Rousseau, *Pachomius. The Making of a Community in Fourth Century Egypt* (Berkeley 1985).

[30] Pliny *HN* 32.45–47 (salsamenta used for bites of snake, crocodile, and mad dog, plus sting of scorpion and weever fish), 79–80 (toothache), 90 (maena used for quinsy; silurus, for voice improvement), 95 (salted cybia is a purgative), 101 (salsamentum with pepper treats jaundice), 105 (ashes of the head of salted pelamys cures chaps and condyloma), 106–07 (salsamentum and, in particular, salted coracinus treat superficial absesses), 108 and 127 (salsamentum reduces carbuncles), 119 (salted silurus heals burns), 125 (salsamenta used to extract weapons), 126 (salted perch and cybia treat creeping ulcers), 127 (salsamentum cures fistulas), and 135 (tunny blood, gall, and liver are good for removing superfluous hair). Cf. Celsus *Med.* 2.29 (garum and salsamentum are laxatives).

to the army. Pliny states that man and horse suffered the same afflictions and that man could learn remedies from other animals.[31] It was only logical that cures used on the farm for man were applied to animals, and vice versa.

As in human medicine, the veterinary problems for which fish sauce was prescribed included primarily those of the digestive tract and of afflictions for which a drying or heating agent was required. Columella recommends that a mare suffering from sudden emaciation should receive four sextarii of garum administered through the nose, but one congius if the animal were large. He adds that this draws off the phlegm through the nostrils and serves as a laxative.[32] Gargilius Martialis advocates the use of the "best muria of salted fish" (*muria salsamenti optima*) mixed with vinegar, water, and a few ground herbs for sick oxen.[33] The inclusion of fish sauce in combination with other vegetable ingredients reflects its similar purpose in human medicine, that is to create a palatable food or potion which also brings about the desired medicinal effect.

The efficacious properties of particular ingredients within a recipe, including those with fish sauce, are not always apparent as it applies to specific diseases. The author of the *Mulomedicina Chironis* (written ca. A.D. 400), for example, recommends a potion of the best wine and a little liquamen mixed with the juice of myrrh and cabbage leaves to cure an excess of blood in beasts of burden.[34] Vegetius (fl. ca. A.D. 385) says that the best liquamen mixed with honey, pulverized nuts, and fifteen figs, all rolled into little balls and soaked in passum, helps to cure asthma or dry cough; while Columella recommends cabbage stems dipped in oil and garum to cure a cow with fever.[35] Other animal diseases supposedly treatable with a fish sauce include spavin, a swollen tongue in oxen, jaundice, tympanites, glaucoma, and "strumous blood."[36]

Since ancient veterinary medicine derived largely from rural experiences, it possessed a strong element of superstition. Some of the uses for which fish sauce was prescribed may have their origin in this rather than in

---

[31] Pliny *HN* 8.97, 166. See also John Scarborough, *Roman Medicine* (Ithaca, New York 1969), p. 171. Genuine concern for the welfare of domestic animals over and above concern for a valuable possession may also explain man's readiness to use healing methods similar to those for himself. See Lilian Bodson, "The Welfare of Livestock and Work Animals in Ancient Greece and Rome," *Medical Heritage* 2 (1986): 244–49.

[32] Columella *Rust.* 6.34. Cf. Celsus *Med.* 2.23.

[33] Gargilius Martialis *Curae Boum* 4. For Gargilius Martialis, see *Curae Boum Ex Corpore Gargili Martialis*, bound with *P. Vegeti Renati Digestorum Artis Mulomedicinae*. E. Lommatzsch, ed. (Leipzig 1903), pp. 307–08. Vegetius' work will be abbreviated *Mulomed.*

[34] *Mulomedicina Chironis* 359 (= *Claudii Hermeri Mulomedicina Chironis*. Eugenius Oder, ed. [Leipzig 1901], p. 110).

[35] Vegetius *Mulomed.* 2.132.4; Columella, *Rust.* 6.9.1.

[36] Columella *Rust.* 6.38.2 (spavin), 6.8.2 (swollen tongue); Vegetius *Mulomed.* 2.22.8, 3.28.10 (glaucoma), 2.91.2 (tympanites); Pelagonius (fl. A.D. 365) *Ars vet.* 1.11 (jaundice), 13.213 (tympanites), 30.428 (glaucoma), 30.455 (scabies); Palladius *De vet. med.* 14.36.4 (strumous blood). For Pelagonius, see *Pelagonii Ars Veterinaria*. Klaus-Dietrich Fischer, ed. (Leipzig 1980); for Palladius, *Palladii De Veterinaria Medicina*. Robert H. Rodgers, ed. (Leipzig 1975).

any organized conscious effort to bring specific efficacious powers to bear on particular diseases. The superstitious aspects are more readily apparent when one considers the circumstances under which the medicine containing the fish sauce was sometimes administered. For a sick animal with a green mucous pouring from its nose, for example, Vegetius (*Mulomed.* 1.10.1) recommends a warm potion of the best oil, the "flower of liquamen" (*liquaminis flos*), and old wine poured through a funnel into the animal's nostrils. This must be done, he urges, on a clear and tranquil day.

The notice of "flower of liquamen" returns our attention once again to the importance of ancient medical sources for understanding Graeco-Roman social and economic life. Columella (*Rust.* 6.38.2–3) suggests that to cure spavin in mules one should use a concoction of oil, egg whites, and "the best garum" (*garum optimum*). The term garum and other fish sauces modified by these and other adjectives, such as *primum* (first quality), even more commonly appear in veterinary treatises.[37] These modifiers are similar to or reproduce exactly the phraseology appearing frequently in painted inscriptions, called *tituli picti*, on fish sauce amphorae. These labels were used for two purposes: to identify the product in the vessel and to advertise the sauce to a potential buyer.[38] The literary references are few in number and for the most part appear in treatises of late or of uncertain date, but the similarity in wording to product labels seems more than mere coincidence. Although reference simply to garum or allec is found, frequently the quality of sauce assumes an importance of its own. Not merely liquamen is recommended, but *liquamen optimum*; garum will not do, *garum primum* is required. It is significant that the references appear only in medical or, more often, in veterinary sources and in the Edict of Diocletian of A.D. 301, each one a source of practical and utilitarian character as were the amphorae.[39] What, if any, influence on medical and veterinary writers can be traced to commercial fish sauce *tituli picti* is difficult to say. The evidence, however, is suggestive and recalls to us the fundamental point that salted fish products were not only materia medica but also commodities of trade.

---

[37] See, for example, Vegetius *Mulomed.* 1.10.1, 17.10, 17.16; 2.22.8, 91.2, 108.2, 132.4; 3.28.10; Pelagonius *Ars vet.* 1.11,13; 6.98; 30.428; 32.467; the 9th century compilation *Corpus Hippiatricorum Graecorum* 11.11 (= *Corpus Hippiatricorum Graecorum*. Eugenius Oder and Carolus Hoppe, eds. 2 vols. [Leipzig 1924]). They are not completely absent from human medicine, but again the sources are late. Cf. Marcellus Empiricus *De med.* 9.14, 36, 112; 16.89 (*gari flos*, for tuberculosis); 30.47; and Paul of Aegina 3.59.10 (γάρον πρωτεῖον, for hemorrhoids). Galen's recommendation of "Spanish garum" (τὸ Σπανὸν γάρος) to treat ear problems may refer to the famous and expensive garum sociorum. Galen *De compositione medicamentorum secundum locos* 3 (= 12.622K). Cf. 12.637K for a possible reference to the same sauce (γάρος μέλαν). See also Zahn, s.v. "garum" *RE*, cols. 842–43.

[38] See below pp. 159–70.

[39] *Edict. Diocl.* III.6–7. For this study I have used the text of Siegfried Lauffer, *Diokletians Preisedikt* (Berlin 1971).

CHAPTER FOUR

PRODUCTION AND COMMERCE

Sources and Problems

Difficulty in interpreting the significance of literary and archaeological evidence hinders any investigation of commerce in salted fish products. The literary sources will be treated in the discussion of the individual provinces, but a preliminary statement should be made here concerning the nature of the archaeological evidence. The material remains take several forms, such as salting factories excavated in several provinces of the Mediterranean basin, but by far the most abundant is the large quantity of amphorae found in various cities, such as Rome and Pompeii, on or near the site of fish salteries, and particularly in shipwrecks. The growth of interest in underwater archaeology and the increased attention given to amphora studies have yielded results which have contributed significantly to our knowledge of Roman commerce in salted fish products.[1]

The study of amphorae is not new. It began in earnest in the late nineteenth century, particularly with Heinrich Dressel's publication of amphorae discovered in Rome near the Praetorian camp, and has especially accelerated during the past fifty years.[2] The major thrust of amphora studies was initially in the direction of establishing a typology of shapes based on a comparison of lip form, size, type of spike, and other characteristic details of the individual container. The purpose of this typology was to establish a chronology of forms which could be used to date the archaeological material in which they were found. Today, amphorae possess histor-

---

[1] See, for example, Keith Muckleroy, *Maritime Archaeology* (Cambridge 1978), esp. the bibliography, pp. 255–67. For a good general survey of the growth of underwater archaeology in the Western Mediterranean see Pierre Jarnac, *Épaves et cités sous la mer* (Paris 1977). See also *Marine Archaeology*. D. J. Blackman, ed. (London 1973), and Joan du Plat Taylor, *Marine Archaeology* (New York 1965). As of 1984, 821 shipwrecks dating to the ancient and medieval periods had been discovered in the Mediterranean and Black Seas. Most of the wrecks date to the late Roman Republic and the early imperial period. In the Mediterranean the most common type of cargo was amphorae. Anthony J. Parker, "Shipwrecks and Trade in the Mediterranean," *Archaeological Review from Cambridge* 3 (1984): 99–113. These transport vessels have increasingly received separate treatment in archaeological site reports and are frequently being made the subject of separate monographs. See, for example, Paul R. Sealey, *Amphoras from the 1970 Excavations at Colchester Sheepen*. BAR British Series, 142 (Oxford 1985), and, most recently, *Amphores Romaines et Historie Économique. Dix Ans de Recherche*. Collection de l'École Française de Rome, 114 (Rome 1989).

[2] Heinrich Dressel, "Di un grande deposito di anfore rinvenuto nel nuovo quartiere del Castro Pretorio," *BCAR* 7(1879): 36–112, 143–95. For a brief overview of the development of amphora studies see Josine M. Schuring, "Studies on Roman Amphorae I–II," *BABesch* 59,2 (1984): 137–47, and D. P. S. Peacock and D. F. Williams, *Amphorae and the Roman Economy. An Introductory Guide* (London 1986), esp. pp. 2–19.

ical importance in and of themselves, since they provide valuable information on Roman commerce. It is generally held, for instance, that shape provides information useful in identifying the contents and point of origin of a vessel. Study of these vessels and their contents additionally may shed light on trade routes for perishable commodities, reveal industrial and commercial policies and the fortunes of specific geographic areas, and elucidate organization and mechanisms of commerce. The fact that many shipwrecks have mixed cargoes, for instance oil, wine, and garum, implies not only the presence of merchants in those products and shipping agents but also transshipping and harborside activities.[3]

Amphora study is, however, still evolving. Recent typological studies have concentrated on classifications which take into consideration vessel shape, chemical and fabric analysis, and epigraphical evidence. One need not read the literature too long to realize that much about the topic, particularly typology, remains unknown, or at best controversial. Beginning with Dressel, who apparently did so unintentionally, separate typologies of amphorae have been established and designated by the name of the person defining the criteria, such as Pelichet and Beltrán, or the site where the vessels were located, such as at Camulodunum in Britain or at Ostia in Italy. The difficulty of assigning an amphora to one form or another based

---

[3] A. K. B. Evans, "Pottery and History," in *Roman Pottery Research in Britain and North-West Europe. Papers Presented to Graham Webster*, Part ii. A. C. Anderson and A. S. Anderson, eds. BAR International Series, 123 (Oxford 1981), pp. 528–29; Parker, "Shipwrecks and Ancient Trade," pp. 102–03; and Peacock and Williams, *Amphorae and the Roman Economy*, pp. 9–19. For a wreck carrying oil, wine, and garum see Dali Colls et al., *L'épave Port-Vendres II et le commerce de la Bétique à l'époque de Claude. Archaeonautica*, 1 (Paris 1977); and Anthony J. Parker and Jennifer Price, "Spanish Exports of the Claudian Period: the Significance of the Port Vendres II Wreck Reconsidered," *IJNA* 10,3 (1981): 222–24. It is frequently difficult to establish with certainty whether salt-fish vessels, if only a few are found with a wreck, formed part of the cargo or of the ship's provisions. See, for example, La Chrétienne H wreck of the first century A.D., found at Saint-Raphaël (Var), which carried several hundred wine amphorae of Dressel Form 2–4 but only four salt-fish vessels of Dressel Forms 7 and 9–10. The Dressel Form 7 amphora still contained fish vertebrae and scales. Since this ship originated in Tarraconensis, the salt-fish containers, at least the Dr. Form 7 amphora, may have been imported from Baetica where most of these types of vessels were produced. See Claude Santamaria, "L'épave 'H' de la Chrétienne à Saint-Raphaël (Var)," *Archaeonautica* 4 (1984): 9–52, esp. pp. 39–40. Fos 1, a first century B.C. wreck of a ship out of Cosa in Italy, carried a cargo of wine amphora (Dr. Form 1 B) and some common ceramic. Among its provisions for captain and crew, besides some Campanian and other common ceramic, was a single fish sauce vessel (Dr. Form 12), found at the center of the ship among its inner-planking. Since, as will be shown below, literary sources speak frequently of Spanish exports to Italy and elsewhere, nothing denies the possibility that the crew of Fos 1 may have purchased the Spanish salt-fish amphora in Italy. On this wreck, see Marie-France Giacobbi-Lequément, "La céramique de l'épave Fos 1," *Archaeonautica* 7 (1987): 167–91. A possible example of transshipping may be seen in the late first century B.C. wreck Cap Béar 3, found in 1982 off Port Vendres. Containing wine vessels of Italy (Dressel 1B) and of Northern Spain or Southern Gaul (Pascual 1) along with salt-fish amphorae (Dressel 12) of Southern Spain, the ship appears to have been bound for Narbo. The excavators surmise that the less numerous fish sauce vessels may have been taken aboard at Barcino or Baetulo in Northern Spain where they had earlier been imported from Baetica in the south. See Bernard Liou and P. Pomey, "Informations archéologiques. Pyrénées-orientales: Port-Vendres," *Gallia* 43 (1985): 547–49.

on the shape of the whole vessel or of part of the vessel (for example, rim profile) is evident from the need felt by many scholars to abandon, to alter, or to add to previous typological schemes.[4] Although many questions of detail remain unanswered, enough information has been collected with a reasonable degree of certainty that one can trace at least the outlines of commerce. A word on the state of our understanding of these vessels will be helpful in establishing on what foundation these outlines have been drawn.

A relationship between amphora shape, contents, and point of origin does seem to exist, but scholars have yet to agree completely on its nature. The association of Dressel Form 1 with wine from Italy and of Dressel Form 20 with oil from Baetica in Spain is generally accepted.[5] Fausto Zevi argues convincingly that Dressel Forms 7–13 contained fish sauce and other salted fish products from Baetica in Spain.[6] He bases his conclusion on the study of painted inscriptions (*tituli picti*) found on amphorae. These labels, according to Zevi, show characteristics similar to those found on amphorae of Dressel Form 20, known to have originated in Southern Spain. That these amphorae commonly held fish sauce can be seen from a study of the containers from the Praetorian camp in Rome. Of 62 fish sauce amphorae (identified as such by *tituli picti*) 48, or 78 percent, were of Dressel Forms 7–13.[7]

Amphorae probably designed for one product but reused for another, however, complicate matters. Some Catalan Dressel 7–11 vessels found at La Longarina in Italy, for example, may have held wine, as did also a Bae-

---

[4] Schuring ("Studies on Roman Amphorae I–II," p. 147) asserts that shape alone as a criterion for grouping amphorae according to provenance or chronological sequence is inadequate. He calls for the abandonment of typologies based soley on shape and draws attention to the technology of pottery production as more fruitful. The present study is concerned only with forms identified as having held a salted fish product and as deriving from a specific point of origin, rather than with the reasons for assigning a certain amphora to a particular form. It seeks, therefore, to synthesize the information obtained from the researches of scholars expert in amphora studies and using this material to draw certain conclusions about commerce in salted fish products.

[5] André Tchernia, "Les amphores romaines et l'histoire économique," *JS* 65 (1967): 226–34.

[6] Zevi, "Appunti," pp. 231–33. I regret that I was unable to consult Ricardo Pascual Guasch, "Ánforas de garum en Culip," *Rivista de la Mar* 6 (1959): 10–11, cited by Javier Nieto, "El pecio *Culip IV*: observaciones sobre la organización de los talleres de *terra sigillata* de la Graufesenque," *Archaeonautica* 6 (1986): 81.

[7] *CIL* XV.4686–99, 4701, 4703–31, 4737–39. Zevi's conclusions have not, however, gained universal support. Anthony J. Parker, for instance, in his review of Beltrán Lloris's book on amphorae in Spain, expresses reservations and cites in particular the discovery in Mainz of an amphora identified usually with Baetican fish sauce which contained instead olive oil. Miguel Beltrán Lloris, *Las ánforas romanas en España*. Monografías arqueológicas (Anejos de "Caesaraugusta"), No. 8. (Zaragosa 1970). Anthony J. Parker, "Roman Amphoras: A Review Article," *IJNA* 1 (1972): 226. M. H. Callender, writing prior to the publication of Zevi's article, denies that a rigid relationship exists among all amphora forms and specific products but seems to accept such a connection between fish sauce and, at least, Dressel Forms 7–9. See Callender, *Roman Amphorae*, pp. 17–18.

tican Dressel 7–11 amphora from Rome. Some Beltrán II amphorae held *defrutum*, others contained olives. The reverse also holds true. A Baetican Dressel 2–4 amphora, normally containing wine and found in London, held *mur*(ia), and a variant of the same type vessel held *liquam*(en).[8] It seems, therefore, that the association of fish sauce with Dressel Forms 7–13 is strong but not without exception, indicating that a direct and rigid relationship between all amphora shapes and a specific product cannot be proven. The sixty-two inscribed fish sauce amphorae found at the Praetorian camp account for twelve different forms.[9]

Although much work remains to be done to connect the point of origin with a particular amphora shape, the association of Dressel Forms 7–14 with Spain seems secure.[10] The Spanish origin of these amphorae is confirmed by the discovery of potter's kilns in Baetica at Algeciras, where fragments of several of these forms were found.[11] In addition, the use of petrology, the study of mineral content of clay, promises to contribute significantly to linking amphora form to point of origin. D. P. S. Peacock, for example, has studied the petrology of Spanish amphorae from Baetica

---

[8] Sealey, *Colchester Sheepen*, pp. 63–64, 83–84; Peacock and Williams, *Amphorae and the Roman Economy*, p. 106; Raymond Boyer, "Conserve d'olives dans deux amphores trouvées dans les fouilles de La Bourse, à Marseilles," *Gallia* 44 (1986): 229–33. It is frequently difficult to assign an amphora to a specific form within the group Dressel 7–11, thought to derive from Baetica but copied in other parts of Spain. On Catalan Dressel 7–11 amphorae, see Jordi Miró, *La Producción de ánforas romanas en Catalunya. Un estudio sobre el comercio del vino de la Tarraconense (siglos I a.C.-I d.C.)*. BAR International Series, 473 (Oxford 1988), esp. pp. 99–104, 177–80.

[9] Fish sauce amphorae at the Praetorian camp included the following Dressel Forms: 7, 8, 9, 10, 11, 12, 13, 14, 16, 18, 28, 39. Six were of unknown form due to the mutilated state of preservation. Callender, *Roman Amphorae*, pp. 7–22, has shown that many other amphora forms held an assortment of different products. Anthony J. Parker ("The Evidence Provided by Underwater Archaeology for Roman Trade in the Western Mediterranean," in *Marine Archaeology*. D. J. Blackman, ed. [London 1973], p. 366), notes that different amphora shapes were made in the same potter's workshop and concludes from this that different forms were destined to hold different products. He would not, however, conclude that these products have been identified for all amphora shapes, and certainly not for Dressel Forms 7–13. André Tchernia ("Les amphores romaines," p. 226), although admitting that the relationship between form and contents has never been rigorously proven, does in general lean toward acceptance of a relationship, however ill-defined at present.

[10] Ricardo Pascual Guasch ("El Pecio Gandolfo [Almería]," *Pyrenae* 4 [1968], p. 146) argues that Dressel Form 14 should be included among fish sauce amphorae from Spain. He reports that a Roman kiln found in the vicinity of Calahonda in Andalusia contained a complete example of an amphora of Dressel Form 14. See *idem*. "Underwater Archaeology in Andalusia (Almeria and Granda)," *IJNA* 2 (1973): 112–13, and esp. fig. 9E, p. 115. See also Guilherme Cardoso, "Ânforas romanas no Museu do Mar (Cascais)," *Conimbriga* 17 (1978): 63–78. Pascual Guasch prefers to connect Dressel Form 12 with Italy, while Peacock supports Zevi's association of this form with Baetica in Spain. See Ricardo Pascual Guasch, "Algunos aspectos del comercio antiguo según las ánforas," in *Comunicaciónes a la I reunion de historia de la economía antigua de la península ibérica*. Papeles del laboratorio de arqueología de Valencia, no. 5 (Valencia 1968), pp. 72–74; and D. P. S. Peacock, "Amphorae and the Baetican Fish Industry," *ANTJ* 54 (1974): 232–43.

[11] M. Sotomayor, "Hornos romanos de ánforas en Algeciras," in *X° Congreso nacional de arqueología. Mahon, 1967* (Saragossa 1969), pp. 389–99. See also Peacock and Williams, *Amphorae and the Roman Economy*, pp. 73–76.

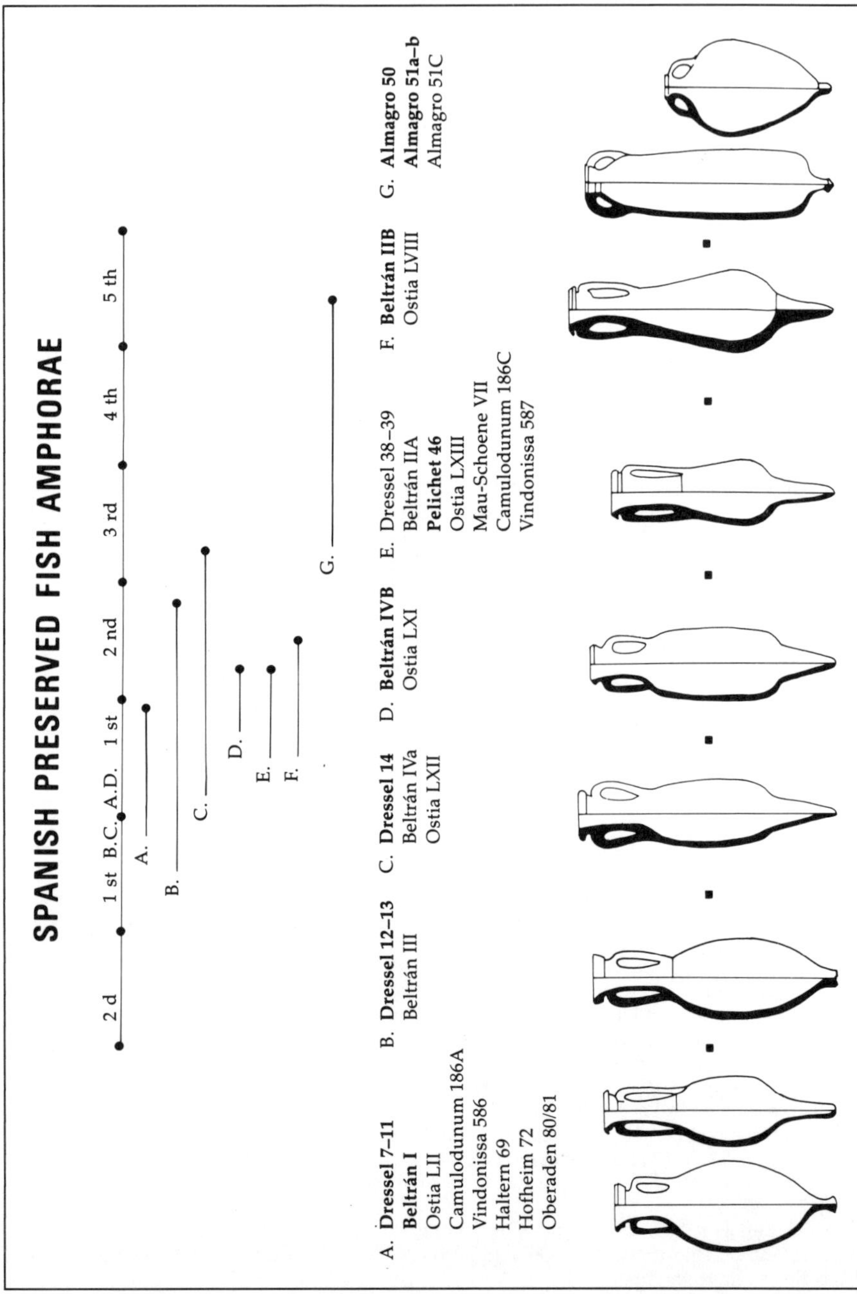

Figure 1: Chronology of Spanish Salt-fish Amphora Forms (vessels not drawn to scale)

and has distinguished vessels made at two different sites.[12] Anthony J. Parker has recognized several Lusitanian amphorae and would place the origin of Beltrán Form IVb, roughly similar to Dressel Form 14 and distinct from the Baetican Beltrán IVa, at potters' kilns near Setúbal on the Atlantic coast of Portugal.[13] Much work, however, remains to be done. Although the identification of potters' stamps on amphora handles has aided scholars in identifying the point of origin of some amphora forms, this is of little use for Dressel Forms 7–14, since they rarely bear stamps. In addition, no fish sauce amphora form has yet been conclusively identified as Gallic in origin, and no more than two may be considered as African.[14]

In summary, it cannot be considered as proven that each individual amphora shape always contained a specific product, or even a specific type of product, and many forms cannot yet be associated with a particular place of manufacture. One can safely say, however, that the majority of amphorae of Dressel Forms 7–14 contained fish sauce and other salted fish products. These vessels were manufactured in Baetica, with variants, such as that of Form 14 (Beltrán IVb), from other areas of Spain. Other provinces, such as Africa and Gaul, exported salted fish products, but at present little is known of their amphora forms. Since throughout this study reference will frequently be made to Spanish salt-fish amphorae included in various typologies, it will be helpful to describe these vessels in general terms, to list the designations assigned to them, and to indicate as far as is presently possible their chronological range.

Amphorae containing garum and salsamenta do not form a homogeneous group but do possess the following general characteristics: a large, articulate, and generally rounded lip, a broad and high neck, banded handles with a vertical profile having a straight elbow characterized by fur-

---

[12] Peacock, "Baetican Fish Industry," p. 241; Miguel Beltrán Lloris, "Problemas de la morfología y del concepto histórico-geográfico que recubre la noción tipo. Aportaciones a la tipología de las ánforas beticas," in *Méthodes classiques et méthodes formelles dans l'étude des amphores* (Actes du Colloque de Rome, 27–29 Mai 1974). Collection de l'École Française de Rome, no. 32 (Rome 1977), pp. 97–131; and Peacock and Williams, *Amphorae and the Roman Economy*, pp. 73–76.

[13] See Anthony J. Parker, "Lusitanian Amphoras," in *Méthodes classiques et méthodes formelles dans l'étude des amphores* (Actes du Colloque de Rome, 27–29 Mai 1974). Collection de l'École Française de Rome, no. 32 (Rome 1977), pp. 35–46. See also A. M. Dias Diogo, "Fornos de ânforas do Monte da Enchurrasqueira e do Vale da Cepa. Notícia preliminar," *Conimbriga* 22 (1983): 209–15, and J. C. Edmondson, *Two Industries in Roman Lusitania. Mining and Garum Production*. BAR International Series, 362 (Oxford 1987), pp. 157–64.

[14] Fausto Zevi, [Review of *Roman Amphorae* by M. H. Callender] *JRS* 57 (1967): 237; Fausto Zevi and André Tchernia, "Amphores de Byzacène au Bas-empire," *AntAfr* 3 (1969): 173–214. For a possible Gallic fish sauce amphora see R. P. Wright and M. W. C. Hassall, "Roman Britain in 1973: II. Inscriptions," *Britannia* 5 (1974): 467, no. 44 and note 41. For a variant of a Dressel Form 2–4 vessel found in London with a *titulus* identifying its contents as liquamen from Antipolis see M. W. C. Hassall and R. S. O. Tomlin, "Roman Britain in 1983: II. Inscriptions," *Britannia* 15 (1984): No. 37, p. 344; illustrated in Peacock and Williams, *Amphorae and the Roman Economy*, frontispiece. Dressel Form 2–4 amphorae were made in several provinces, Italy, Spain and Gaul. See *ibid.*, pp. 105–06. Dressel 6B and 6C amphorae may have been produced in Histria in Cisalpine Gaul. See Peacock and Williams, *Amphorae and the Roman Economy*, pp. 99–100.

rowing or a longitudinal channeling, and an ovoid or pyriform body coming to a point, frequently hollow, at the foot. Often these vessels, coated on the inside with pitch and bunged with a pottery disc, vary in size but are generally large, measuring up to 1.15 meters in height, and have a capacity of between 12 to 18 liters.[15] Figure 1 presents a general picture of the major typological schemes and their chronological ranges.[16]

Not all amphorae bear *tituli picti* identifying their contents. This is particularly true for salsamentum. The physical remains of fish bones, scales and meat are often the only sure means of recognizing these products. Mackerel (*scomber*) bones have been found in two Camulodunum 186a vessels from the Port Vendres II wreck, while tunny bones were recovered from Beltrán III vessels from the first century B.C. Titan wreck. Many other examples could be cited. Whether vessels contained processed fish or fish sauce is frequently difficult to establish.[17]

Although most extant amphorae lack any identifiable marks, many bear painted inscriptions identifying the contents as one of the four Roman fish sauces.[18] These inscriptions, which served as a safeguard in case the label, called the *pittacium* (Petronius *Sat.* 34), became lost, provide invaluable information relating to commerce. The inscriptions usually furnish some, but not all, of the following information: name and quality of the product contained in the vessel, merchant or proprietor, the consignee, and the consig-

[15] Jean-Pierre Joncheray, *Essai de classification des amphores* (Fréjus 1970), pp. 24–25; and A. Carandini and Clementina Panella, *Le Terme del Nuotatore: Ostia III* (Parte seconda). Studi Miscellanei 21 (Rome 1972), p. 507. On the capacity of five Beltrán Form I and II vessels found in Britain and on pottery discs see Sealey, *Colchester Sheepen*, p. 81. For fish sauce amphorae coated on the interior with a layer of degraded rosin or pitch, see especially Robert Lequément, "Etiquettes de plomb sur des amphores d'Afrique," *MEFRA* 85 (1975): esp. p. 678 and note 3. See also *BT. Kelim* 10.5 (Epstein, p. 54). For a chemical analysis of the lining material, see C. Heron and A. M. Pollard, "The Analysis of Natural Resinous Materials from Roman Amphoras," in *Science and Archaeology, Glasgow 1987*. BAR, British Series, 196 (ii). Elizabeth A. Slater and James O. Tate, eds. (Oxford 1988), pp. 429–47.

[16] No one typology is all inclusive and there exists among scholars no complete agreement on synchronizing the various forms of the many typological schemes. For this chart I have followed with a few changes and additions the synchronization of forms and chronological ranges presented in Peacock and Williams, *Amphorae and the Roman Economy*, passim. I wish to thank the authors for their permission to use the drawings found in Fig. 1.

[17] Mackerel: Colls et al., *L'épave Port-Vendres II*, pp. 40–42; tunny: Sealey, *Colchester Sheepen*, p. 83; and Fernand Benoit, "Nouvelles épaves de Provence," *Gallia* 16 (1958): 5–8. Heinrich Dressel, in his commentary on the *titulus pictus* of *CIL* XV.4782 found in the Praetorian camp on an amphora similar to Form 9, reads the inscription ABDOMC as ABDO(mina) (sc. thynni) M(embratim) C(aesa). To support this reading, he cites Pliny *HN* 9.48, who in referring to tunny says, *hi membratim caesi cervice et abdomine commendatur atque clido, recenti dumtaxat, et tum quoque gravi ructu*. Cf. *ILS* 9446 (note). See also Lucilius 50: *abdomina thynni*. Amphorae found at Magdalensberg in Noricum may have contained salted fish: SAL(samenta). See Rudolf Egger and Walter Görlich, "Der Lebensmittelimport aus Italien auf den Magdalensberg," *Carinthia* 1 (1969), p. 413. Cf. Félix Pareja, "Marques sur une amphore de l'île de Fraile (Aguilas)," *Cahiers d'Archéologie Subaquatique* 1 (1972): 107–08. Dressel notes in his commentary to *CIL* XV.4757 that an amphora of Form 7 or 9 found in Rome contained fish scales. Cf. *CIL* IV.9804: ὄψ(ον).

[18] See, for example, *CIL* IV.5663–67, 2589–94, 5721–25, 9407–11; XV.4686–94, 4713–22, 4730. See also Robert I. Curtis, "Product Identification and Advertisement on Roman Commercial Amphorae," *AncSoc* 15–17 (1984–86): 209–28.

nor. Although abbreviations were frequently used, the identification of the product presents only a minor difficulty. The letters G F, for example, identified G(ari) F(los), while LIQ F denoted LIQ(uaminis) F(los). The correct interpretation of names and numbers on the vessels, however, is not so easily resolved and complete unanimity on their interpretation has yet to be achieved.[19] A related difficulty is the proper identification of the origin of the person named. The resolution of part of the problem no doubt lies in the determination of the origin of the amphora. But to what destination is the product bound? Must the merchant always be a native of Spain if his name appears on a Baetican amphora? Can he possibly be a merchant from Pompeii, for example, trading in Southern Spain? This part of the overall problem of amphora studies is far from resolution.

With a background in Roman salted fish products established and bearing in mind certain caveats in interpreting the archaeological evidence, we can now turn our attention to a survey of the Roman provinces which produced these products and whose merchants engaged in their trade. Production and commerce in these products made some individuals wealthy and provided a livelihood for many inhabitants throughout the Roman Empire. A significant amount of what follows will of necessity concentrate on fish sauce, since most literary and much archaeological evidence concerns garum, not salsamenta. The reason for this is difficult to explain, but may relate to the fact that some kinds of garum were considered luxury products and all sauces in general had a rather strong odor and bizarre preparation process which attracted more attention than the other more common and cheaper salted fish products. Additionally, the more varied uses of garum as a condiment and medicine combined with the ease of transport and storage made it a product more highly visible than salsamentum. Little will be lost, however, in focusing on fish sauce since Roman salteries manufactured several products from a single fish and a merchant in one product would most likely deal as well in the others. This survey is intended to do no more than to place the available archaeological material within the context of literary evidence relating to the Roman salting industry and to commercial activity. Since ancient authors frequently discuss more than one geographical area in commenting upon the fish salting industry, some repetition in my discussion becomes unavoidable. Conclusions will of necessity be tentative ones because of the nature of the evidence and frequently can do no more than to point out possible areas where further study can be profitable.

---

[19] For a full discussion of names appearing in product labels and their significance, adopted here, see Appendix 3, previously published in Robert I. Curtis, "A. Umbricius Scaurus of Pompeii," in *Pompeiana et Classica in Honor of Wilhelmina F. Jashemski*. 2 vols. (New Rochelle, N.Y. 1988–89), 1: Appendix, pp. 37–39. I wish to thank the publisher, Aristide D. Caratzas, for permission to reprint, with slight alteration, this Appendix here. For *pittacia* in the form of lead tesserae attached to amphorae, see below notes 118 and 200.

The Western Provinces of the Roman Empire

Spain[20]

The earliest literary evidence for fish salting establishments in the West comes from references in Attic comedy writers of the fifth and fourth centuries B.C., such as Eupolis, Nicostratus, and Antiphanes, who mention salted fish from Gades in Spain.[21] The salting industry must have begun long before this if, by the late fifth century B.C., Spanish salteries were sufficiently established to export processed fish to Greece. In fact, as Nicostratus implies, the Gaditanian product was considered nearly on a par with that from the area of Byzantium. Although no direct evidence exists for Spanish garum specifically, there is no reason to doubt that at this time it was one of several products imported from Spanish salteries.

The *communis opinio* has for a long time held that commercial exploitation of salteries in the Western Mediterranean was a Phoenico-Punic institution.[22] The primary basis for this conclusion is the numerous Phoenico-

[20] The best work on Spanish production centers remains that of Ponsich and Tarradell, *Garum*, esp. pp. 81–90. Although it includes little on commerce in Spanish fish products and focusses discussion primarily on Baetica and Mauretania Tingitana across the Strait in Africa, the conclusions reached therein remain the bases upon which finds in other provinces are discussed. My debt to their efforts will become obvious as this book proceeds. The recent Spanish edition by Michel Ponsich (*Aceite de Oliva y Salazones de Pescado. Factores geo-economicos de Betica y Tingitana.* Madrid 1988) expands the discussion of ancient fishing methods and their modern counterparts, updates the earlier work, incorporates many additional sites discovered since 1965, and describes more fully those only mentioned in the first edition. Ponsich devotes more discussion to Spain than was done earlier and revises upward the period of destruction for many factories in Africa and Spain. I will cite the recent edition only where it differs from or expands upon the earlier work. See also Maria Luisa Sanchez Leon, *Economía de la Hispania meridional durante la dinastia de los Antoninos* (Salamanca 1978), pp. 225–38; and the excellent monograph by Gabriela Martin and Maria Dolores Serres, *La factoría pesquera de Punta de l'Arenal y otros restos romanos de Jávea (Alicante).* Valencia 1970. For the salteries of Portugal see especially Jorge de Alarcão, *Roman Portugal.* 2 vols. Warminster, England 1988; and Maria Luísa Estácio da Veiga Affonso Dos Santos, *Arqueologica romana do Algarve.* Vol. I. Lisbon 1971. An old, but still valuable survey is that of Antonio Mesquita de Figueiredo, "Ruines d'antiques établissements à salaisons sur le littoral sud du Portugal," *Bulletin hispanique* 8 (1906): 109–21 Add to these Francesco Pellati, "I monumenti del Portogallo romano," *Historia* 5 (1931): 214–16; Alberto Iria, "As ruínas de tanques de salga de peixe encontradas recentemente em Olhão," *Industria portuguesa* 273 (1950): 727–32; O. Da Veiga Ferreira, "Algumas considerações sobre as fábricas de conservas de peixe da antiguidade encontradas em Portugal," *Archivo de Beja* 23–24 (1966–67): 123–34, and Edmondson, *Two Industries*, pp. 100–51.

[21] The adjective "Gaditanian" may apply not only to products from the city of Gades itself but also to those from all of Southern Spain and the coast of North Africa opposite. See Ponsich and Tarradel, *Garum*, p. 99 and below, pp. 61–62. See Hesychius s.v. Γαδειρικὸν τάριχος; Eupolis fr. 186 Edmonds: πότερ ἦν τὸ τάριχος Φρύγιον ἢ Γαδειρικόν; Nicostratus frs. 4, 5 Edmonds: Βυζάντιόν ⟨ τε ⟩ τέμαχος ἐπιβακχευσάτω Γαδειρικόν θ' ὑπογάστριον παρεισίτω; and Antiphanes fr. 77 Edmonds: τάριχος ἀντακαῖον εἴ τις βούλετ' ἢ/ Γαδειρικόν, Βυζαντίας δὲ θυννίδος/ ⟨ἐν ⟩ εὐφροσύναις ὀσμαῖσι χαίρει. Cf. Euthydemus (*ap.* Athen. 3.116c): 'Ιόνιον δ' ἀνὰ κῦμα φέρων Γαδειρόθεν ἄξει βρέττιος ἢ Καμπανὸς ἢ ἐκ ζαθέοιο Τάραντος ὀρκύνοιο τρίγωνα, τά τ' ἐν στάμνοισι τεθέντα ἀμφαλλὰξ δείπνοισιν ἐνὶ πρώτοισιν ὀπηδεῖ. Ps-Aristotle *De mirabilibus auscultationibus* 136 notes that Gades sent salted tunny to Carthage.

[22] For the Phoenico-Punic origins of Spanish salteries see Miguel Tarradell, "Economía de la colonizzación fenica," in *Estudios de economía antigua de la península ibérica* (Barcelona 1968), p.

Punic colonies established in North Africa and Southern Spain dating from the eighth to the sixth century B.C. It may be more than coincidence that Phoenico-Carthaginian colonial population centers frequently precede the siting of Roman fish salteries.[23] On the other hand, a Greek origin has been proposed as well.[24] According to this theory, in the sixth century B.C. Phocaeans of Asia Minor, bringing the knowledge of the salting process from the East where fish preservation in the Black Sea area had been practiced since the early seventh century B.C., imparted it to the Tyrian colonists of Southern Spain. But as the Spanish peninsula became more Punicized, these inhabitants forgot the Hellenic origins of the salting industry.

More recently, a western origin, at least for the area around Gades, has been put forward. Near the city of Cadiz, archaeologists have found for the first time remains of Punic fish salting installations.[25] The four salting factories are identified as such by finds of tunny bones, fish hooks, and amphorae containing fish bones. The vessels are primarily of Punic type Mañá-Pascual A-4, similar to ones found in Corinth (Pl. 8) which also held remains of tunny, and type Mañá D, plus some local ceramic containers. In one instance a small square basin in a poor state of preservation had its interior coated with a mortar of lime and sand. The best of the sites so far discovered was at Las Redes, near Puerto de Santa Maria, Cadiz. Here a building, roughly square and measuring 10.7 x 10.6 meters, has five sections: a main entrance, a possible storeroom, a separate room possibly for making fish sauce, a room for cutting up and preparing fish for processing, and a fermentation room containing two vats, one rectangular and the

96; Ponsich and Tarradell, *Garum*, p. 113; E. Cuadrado, "Corrientes comerciales do los pueblos ibéricos," in *Estudios de economía antigua de la península ibérica* (Barcelona 1968), p. 127; and Antonio García y Bellido, "La industria pesquera y conserva española en la Antiquëdad," *Investigación y progreso* 13 (1942): 5. The name Malaca may derive from the Punic word for "salting place" or "to salt." See Smidth, "Historical Observations," p. 16. More recent work, however, sees it as a word derived from Mulucha, a Mauretanian river. See Jacques Alexandropoulos and Jean Gran Aymerich, "Recherches sur Malaga Phénicienne et Punique," *MCV* 24 (1988): 438.

[23] Tarradell, "La colonizatión fenica," p. 96, and Edmondson, *Two Industries*, pp. 105–07. For a discussion of Punic and Greek colonization in Spain see Antonio García y Bellido, *Las colonizaciones púnica y griega en la península ibérica* (Madrid 1954). Cf. Yu. B. Tsirkin, "Economy of the Phoenician Settlements in Spain," in *State and Temple Economy in the Ancient Near East. II.* Edward Lipinski, ed. Orientalia Lovaniensia Analecta, 6 (Leuven 1979), pp. 547–64. Many Phoenician cities in Spain, such as Gades, Sexi, and Abdera, minted coins showing on their reverse side the image of the tunny. Gades maintained this representation on its coins even during the Roman period. See Ponsich and Tarradell, *Garum*, pp. 110–11; and Barclay V. Head, *Historia Numorum*. 2d ed. (Oxford 1911), p. 3.

[24] Robert Étienne, "A propos du 'garum sociorum'," *Latomus* 29 (1970): 298–99.

[25] G. de Frutos, G. Chic, and N. Berriatua, "Las anforas de la factoria prerromana de salazones de 'Las Redes' (Puerto de Santa Maria, Cadiz)," in *Actas 1er Congreso Peninsular de Historia Antigua* (Santiago de Compostela 1988), 1: 295–306, and Ángel Muñoz Vicente, Gregorio de Frutos Reyes, and Nerea Berriatua Hernández, "Contribución a los orígenes y difusión comercial de la industria pesquera y conservera Gaditana a Través de las recientes aportaciones de las factorías de salazones de la Bahía de Cadiz," in *Actas de Congreso Internacional el Estrecho de Gibraltar Ceuta – Noviembre 1987* (Distancia 1989 [?]), pp. 487–508.

other square.[26] The floor of the preparation room sloped slightly seaward and was composed of small stones mixed with lime and crushed ceramic. The room for making fish sauce was identified as such from the dark color of the earth on its floor, possibly a result of the decomposition of organic matter, and the presence of a small hearth. These installations await fuller publication, but preliminary investigations indicate that the factories began operation in the late fifth century B.C., realizing their greatest period of activity during the years 430–325 B.C. They declined rapidly afterward and ceased operation in ca. 200 B.C. Corinthian amphorae found in the remains of the factories and Punic type Mañá-Pascual A-4, commonly found in the area around Gades and discovered in Corinth in a fifth century B.C. context, imply commercial links with the Greek East. Other local ceramic, which are not found at great distances from Gades, were also used for storage of salt-fish products.[27] Remains of these salting installations and ceramic evidence suggest, therefore, that fish salting in the West, if not introduced by Punic settlers from Carthage, may have been indigenous to the area of Gades. Although these recent discoveries are promising, more work remains to be done before this theory can be accepted.

Based upon the state of the evidence known at this time, therefore, the question of the origin of commercial fish processing must remain unanswered. It seems probable that the knowledge of fish processing entered the West through the medium of Phoenicians (and by extension, Carthaginians) and subsequently of Greeks. Both, experienced in fish preservation, would have introduced it, where appropriate, into their areas of colonization. In any case, the question of who introduced the knowledge first, though an interesting one, is relatively of minor importance. What is significant is that the salting industry seems to have been transported into the West from the East. The Romans apparently derived their knowledge of it from the Greeks, since the Latin word garum came from the Greek γάϱον. The scant remains of Phoenico-Punic salteries (and none for Greek installations) in the West are perplexing, and no convincing theory has yet to account for it adequately.[28]

Excavations in Spain and Portugal have unearthed many large and small Roman fish salting establishments (Figs. 7, 9). Salteries extended along the coast from Lisbon and ancient Caetobriga on the Atlantic coast to Rhode on the Mediterranean Sea, including the island of Scombraria and the Balearic Islands. Many of those in Portugal (ancient Lusitania) were located

---

[26] The rectangular vat measured 1.0 x 2.0 meters; the square one, 1.0 x 1.0 meter.

[27] The Greek vessels were of types Koehler A and B. For the Corinthian evidence see below p. 115. For the Punic vessels see Muñoz Vicente et al., "Contribución," esp. pp. 497–502 and the bibliography cited therein.

[28] Ponish and Tarradell (*Garum*, p. 114), writing prior to the discovery of the Punic material at Gades, suggest that the process of Roman industrialization was so complete that it obliterated any pre-Roman installations. Cf. O. Da Veiga Ferreira, "Algumas notas acerca da pesca na Antiguidade," *O Arqueologo português*. 3rd ser. 2 (1968): 130. Punic transport vessels which date from the fourth to the third century B.C. and which probably held salt-fish (Mañá D) have

just north and south of the Sado River, for example, at Lisbon, Setúbal, Rasca, Troia, Creiro, and Portinho da Arrábida, and on the littoral of the Algarve, for instance, at Boca do Rio, Senhora da Luz, Vau-Alvor, Portimão, Armação de Pera, Quarteira, Torre de Ares (ancient Balsa), Olhão, and Cacela. The saltery at Caetobriga in Northwestern Lusitania at the mouth of the Sado estuary in Troia was exceeded in size only by Baelo in Baetica.[29] Spanish sites concentrated in the area of Baetica in Southern Spain and in portions of Tarraconensis and included, from west to east, Cerro del Trigo, Sanlúcar de Barrameda, Cadiz (ancient Gades), Barbate (ancient Baesippo), Bolonia (ancient Baelo), Villavieja (ancient Mellaria), Carteia, San Pedro de Alcantara (ancient Silniana), Torremolinos, Malaga (ancient Malaca), Torrox, Almuñécar (ancient Sexi), Mazarrón, Abdera, Villaricos (ancient Baria), and Cartagena (ancient Carthago Nova).[30] Literary

---

been found at several sites in Sicily, indicating perhaps Punic salting activity. The sparse remains of vats at these sites, however, are probably Roman and so throw no light on the earlier installations. See below p. 100. Punic sites in Spain may have suffered heavily during the Second Punic War.

[29] Other Portuguese sites in the Algarve include Quinta de Commenda, Foz da Ajuda, Forte di Montguellas, Forte di Prasca, Salema, Burgau, Paul de Lagos, Ferragudo, Cerro da Vila, Loulé Velho, Faro, and Muro; with possible sites at Areia, Cabo Espichel, Ponta da Paleeria, and Praia do Murtinal. This list does not claim to be all inclusive. For sites on the Portuguese coast see Alarcão, *Roman Portugal*, passim; Ponsich, *Aceite de Oliva y Salazones de Pescado*, pp. 221–28; Da Veiga Ferreira, "Algumas considerações," pp. 123–34; Carlos Tavares da Silva and Mateus Gonçalves Cabrita, "O problema da destruição da povoação romana de Tróia de Setúbal," *Revista de Guimarães* 76 (1966): 147–55; and Cardoso, "Museu do Mar (Cascais)," pp. 63–78. According to some scholars ancient Caetobriga lies in the Troia peninsula on the left bank of the Sado River, for others it corresponds to Setúbal, southeast of modern Lisbon, on the right bank. See J. Alarcão, "Troia," *The Princeton Encyclopedia of Classical Sites* (Princeton 1976), pp. 935–36, and Edmondson, *Two Industries*, pp. 124–28.

[30] Other Spanish sites, continuing west to east, include Mar Menor, Santa Pola, the island of Tabarca, Tossal de Manises (ancient Lucentum), the island of Campello, Calpe, Punta del Castell, Punta de l'Arenal, possibly Denia (ancient Dianium), Rhode, and Ibiza in the Balearic Islands. Again, not every site has been listed. See Ponsich, *Aceite de Oliva y Salazones de Pescado*, pp. 169–218; Martin and Serres, *Punta de l'Arenal*, passim; García y Bellido, "La industria pesquera," p. 2; Raymond Thouvenot, *Essai sur la province romaine de Bétique* (Paris 1940), pp. 540–42; Gabriela Martin, "Las pesquerías romanas de la costa de Alicante," *Trabajos de arqueología dedicados a D. Pío Beltrán*. Papeles del laboratorio de arqueología de Valencia No. 10 (Valencia 1970), pp. 139–53; and M. Sotomayor, "Neuva factoría de salazons de pescado en Almuñécar (Granada)," *Noticiario arqueológico hispánico* 15 (1971): 147–48 (I regret that I was unable to consult either J. M. Fontana, *Una nota de Hispania económica. Los salazones y salsas de Almuñécar*, cited by Alberto Prieto in "Estructura social del 'Conventus Gaditanus'," *HAnt* 1 [1971]: 151, n. 14, or F. Molina Fajardo and S. Jimenez Contreras, "La factoría de salazones El Majeulo," in *Almuñécar. Arqueología e Historia* [Granada 1983]: 279–90, cited in Aurelio Padilla Monge, *La provincia romana de la Betica (253–422)* [Écija 1989], p. 154); Sanchez Leon, *Economía*, pp. 225–38; Fernando Amores, "Una nueva factoría romana de salazones en Trafalgar (Cádiz)," *Habis* 9 (1978): 441–53; Daniel Woods, *Carteia*. Excavaciones arqueológicas en España, No. 58 (Madrid 1967), esp. pp. 23–28; Jean-Gérard Gorges, *Les villas hispano-romaines. Inventaire et problématiques archéologiques* (Paris 1979), passim; Gustav Gamer, "Antike Anlagen zur Fischverarbeitung in Hispanien und Mauretanien," *AW* 18,2 (1987): 19–28; J. M. Nolla and F. J. Nieto, "Una factoria de salaó de peix a Roses," *Fonaments* 3 (1981): 187–200, and J. M. Nolla-Brufau, "Excavaciones recientes en la ciudadela de Roses. El edificio Bajo-imperial," in *Papers in Iberian Archaeology*. T. F. C. Blagg, R. F. J. Jones, and S. J. Keay, eds. BAR International Series, 193 (ii) (Oxford 1984), pp. 430–59.

sources attest to salting establishments at Baelo, Carteia, Gades, Sexi, Malaca, Mellaria, New Carthage, and the island of Scombraria, and perhaps Barcino.[31] Some factories, such as at Baelo and Caetobriga, were large, while others possessed only a few salting facilities.[32]

Without exception, sites for Spanish fish processing centers possessed three basic characteristics. First, there had to be an abundance of fish. Since tunny enter the Mediterranean from the Atlantic by passing through the Strait of Gibraltar, it was no accident that many of the Spanish salteries lay along the coast of Turdetania and Baetica.[33] Tunny and other fish, such as the mackerel, mullet, and eels (murena and anguilla) were plentiful, as were also certain shellfish, such as the murex, oyster, and squid.[34] Second, salteries required a steady supply of fresh water for cleaning the fish, preparing the brine for salting, and cleaning the installation. Spanish salteries, therefore, invariably lay at the mouth of a river, stream or lagoon. Cerro del Trigo, for example, lay at the mouth of the Guadalquivir (ancient Baetis) River, Baelo on the Rio del Valle, Santa Pola on the Rio Vinalopo, and Jávea on the Rio Gorgos. Salteries located near rivers lay close to the water's edge, while those near the sea were frequently sited high enough to avoid

---

[31] Baelo and Mellaria (Strabo 3.1.8): Εἶτα Μενλαρία, ταριχείας ἔχουσα, καὶ μετὰ ταῦτα Βελὼν πόλις καὶ ποταμός. ἐντεῦθεν οἱ διάπλοι μάλιστά εἰσιν εἰς Τίγγιν τῆς Μαυρουσίας καὶ ἐμπόρια καὶ ταριχεῖαι; New Carthage and the Island of Scombraria (Strabo 3.4.6): κἀνταῦθα (in New Carthage) δὲ καὶ ποῖς κλησίον τόποις πολλὴ ἡ ταριχεία. . . .εἶθ' ἡ τοῦ Ἡρακλέους νῆσος ἤδη πρὸς Καρχηδόνι, ἣν καλοῦσι Σκομβραρίαν ἀπὸ τῶν ἁλισκομένων σκόμβρων, ἐξ τὸ ἄριστον σκευάζεται γάρον.See also Pliny *HN* 31.94. Gades (above note 21); Carteia (Pliny *HN* 9.92; 31.94). Sexi and Malaca (Strabo 3.4.2): πόλις δ' ἐστὶν ἐν τῇ παραλίᾳ ταύτῃ πρώτη Μάλακα, ἴσον διέχουσα τῆς Κάλπης, ὅσον καὶ τὰ Γάδειρα˙ ἐμπόριον δ' ἐστὶ νῦν τοῖς ἐν τῇ περαίᾳ Νομάσι, καὶ ταριχείας δὲ ἔχει μαγάλας. . . . ἐφεξῆς δ' ἐστὶν ἡ τῶν Ἐξιτανῶν πόλις, ἐξ ἧς καὶ τὰ ταρίχη ἐπωνύμως λέγεται.Barcino (Ausonius *Ep*. 25): *Barcinonensis muriae condimento*. Mention of Turdetanian salteries in general, which would include those of the Algarve, appear in Strabo 3.2.6: Ἐξάγεται δ' ἐκ τῆς Τουρδητανίας σιτός τε καὶ οἶνος πολὺς καὶ ἔλαιον οὐ πολὺ μόνον, ἀλλὰ καὶ κάλλιστον˙ καὶ κηρὸς δὲ καὶ μέλι καὶ πίττα ἐξάγεται καὶ κόκκος πολλὴ καὶ μίλτος οὐ χείρων τῆς Σινωπικῆς γῆς τά τε ναυπήγια συνιστᾶσιν αὐτόθι ἐξ ἐπιχωρίας ὕλης, ἅλες τε ὀρυκτοὶ παρ' αὐτοῖς εἰσι καὶ ποταμῶν ἁλμυρῶν ῥεύματα οὐκ ὀλίγα, οὐκ ὀλίγη δὲ ουδὲ ἐκ τῶν ὄψων ταριχεία ούκ ἔνθεν μόνον, ἀλλὰ καὶ ἐκ τῆς ἄλλης τῆς ἐκτὸς Στηλῶν παραλίας, οὐ χείρων τῆς Ποντικῆς.

[32] For small installations having few salting vats the use of the term "factory" perhaps implies rather more than was the reality. For those the size of Baelo, Lixus (in Mauretania Tingitana), and others, where man-made structures of a permanent nature were built, where the potential output would obviously exceed the requirements of fishermen alone, and where at least part of the finished product was probably intended for sale elsewhere, it is, I believe, a quite appropriate term, even in the modern sense of the word. At what point a mere installation deserves the appellation factory is impossible to say. For convenience, I will use the terms factory, installation, and center interchangeably, fully aware that some, wishing for more precision than can be applied, will object.

[33] The distance between Gades in Spain and Tingis on the Moroccan coast is only about thirty miles (Strabo 17.3.2). For the route followed by the tunny entering the Mediterranean Sea see Jean Bourge, "Étude sur les migrations du 'scomber thynnus' (thon commun) dans le bassin occidental de la Méditerranée," *Revue tunisienne* 22 (1915): 85–97. See especially the discussion in Ponsich, *Aceite de Oliva y Salazones de Pescado*, pp. 30–43.

[34] Adolf Schulten, *Geografía y etnografía antiguas de la península ibérica*. 2 Vols. (Madrid 1959, 1963), 2: 529–41. Caetobriga, in Portugal, may have gotten its name from the Greek word for tunny, ὁ κῆτος (*ibid*., p. 535).

the tides.[35] Third, the processing centers required a ready supply of salt. Consequently, most were established near salt mines or salt marshes. The installations of the Algarve, for instance, obtained salt from the Turdetanian salt mines or from salt-water streams. The saltery at Punta de l'Arenal in Jávea had a salt marsh nearby, as did that at Santa Pola.[36] The availability of salt would be critical, requiring for those at a distance from a ready supply prior planning to insure the accumulation of sufficient stock-piles, particularly for the time-frame of the regular tunny migrations in late spring and late summer when large amounts of fish would need to be processed quickly.

A thorough discussion of every Spanish site is unnecessary to form a general idea of how a Roman saltery functioned, since Spanish salting installations show a remarkable degree of homogeneity. The size and complexity of a saltery naturally depended upon the size of the population, the abundance and type of available fish, and the accessibility of salt. Baelo is the best preserved Roman salting installation and offers an excellent example with which to compare others, less well-known, found elsewhere.

The city of Baelo had at least two areas devoted to fish preservation: one, located to the south of the city on the beach, probably outside the walls; the other, in a commercial sector within the city, to the west of the macellum and facing the decumanus.[37] The former area is composed of six separate groups of salting vats. Two groups, containing respectively six and nine salting vats, were linked by a central room in which fish were scaled, cleaned, and cut up before being placed into vats (Fig. 2 and Pl. 2).[38] The floor of this room sloped slightly in the direction of the sea, and along one wall lay an oblong sump. The sloping floor aided in the cleaning of the room after the fish had been prepared, while the sump may have served as a refuse container. A peristyle house lay between groups two and four but did not connect directly with either. Opposite this house and across a large

[35] Ponsich and Tarradell, *Garum*, p. 102. In some cases aqueducts could directly supply the large amounts of fresh water needed by the salting installations. See, for example, Alfonso Jiménez, "Los acueductos de Bellone Claudia (Bolonia, Cadiz)," *Habis* 4 (1973): 285.

[36] Turdetania (Strabo 3.2.6); Punta de l'Arenal (Martin and Serres, *Punta de l'Arenal*, p. 8); and Santa Pola (Ponsich and Tarradell, *Garum*, p. 82). For salt resources in Spain and Portugal, see also R. J. Forbes, *Studies in Ancient Technology*. Vol. 3 (Leiden 1955), p. 173; and Ponsich, *Aceite de Oliva y Salazones de Pescado*, pp. 44–48. I regret that I was unable to consult Luís F. Baltazar, "Indústrias romanas de salga em Portugal," *Al-madan* 1 (1983): 12–14, cited in Alarcão, *Roman Portugal*, p. 127.

[37] On the shore: Pierre Paris et al., *Fouilles de Belo (Bolonia, province de Cádiz) (1917–1921)*: I. *La ville et ses dépendances* (Bordeaux 1923), pp. 119ff.; Thouvenot, *Essai*, pp. 541–42; Ponsich, *Aceite de Oliva y Salazones de Pescado*, pp. 192–99; Michel Ponsich, "A propos d'une usine antique de salaisons à Belo (Bolonia-Cadix)," *MCV* 12 (1976): 69–79; and Manuel Martin-Bueno et al., "Baelo Claudia: Sector sur 1981–1983 (Avance)," *MCV* 20 (1984): 487–96. Inside the city: Sylvie Dardaine and Jean-Noël Bonneville, "La campagne de fouilles d'Octobre 1979 à Belo," *MCV* 16 (1980): 386–403; and Jean-Noel Bonneville et al., "La dix-huitième campagne de fouilles de la Casa de Velázquez à Belo en 1983 (Bolonia, province de Cadix)," *MCV* 20 (1984): 470–76.

[38] Generally accepted criteria to determine how to distinguish separate factories among the groupings of vats have not been established. The incompleteness of excavation of most of the

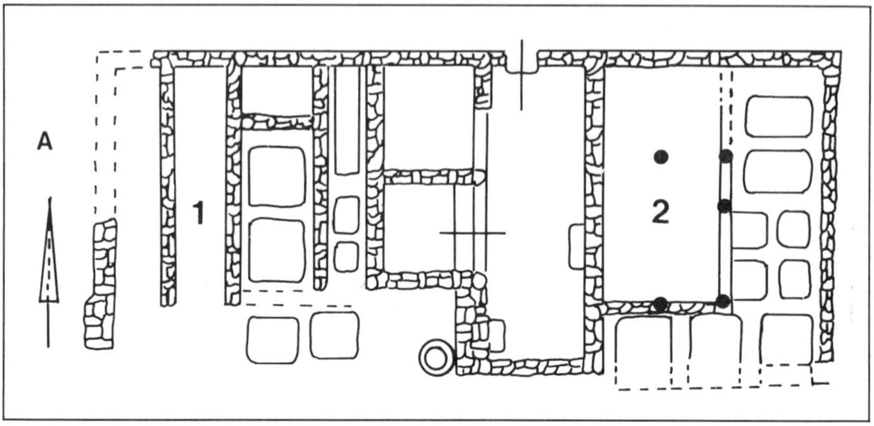

Figure 2: Baelo: Factories No. 1 and No. 2
(after Ponsich and Tarradell, *Garum*, Fig. 53)

colonnaded street stood a villa. To the north of the villa lay the sixth group. At Baelo the vats were built in rooms with a roof to protect the products from the sun and rain, but with windows to provide ventilation, and were arranged in two or three ranks, grouped either parallel or in a square formation. There was no access between the vats, but one could approach any of the basins by walking around on top of the partitions which separated them. The vats in all but one group were square or rectangular in shape and varied in size, but can be categorized generally as large and small ones. Group Number 5 had three large cylindrical vats, measuring 3.10 m. in diameter and 2.50 m. deep, and one smaller one. Ponsich and Tarradell suggest that the large basins served to salt fish, while the small ones were probably reserved for making garum.[39]

Baelo is almost unique, so far as is known up to now, in that it possessed a salting factory within the city itself.[40] This shop facing directly onto the portico of the decumanus had rooms for cleaning and salting fish. A long north-south room contained vats of various sizes lined with a reddish-orange mortar and constructed in a manner similar to those on the shore. The room was roofed and had a window at the rear to provide aeration.

---

sites is the major problem. For example, both Antonio García y Bellido ("La industria pesquera," p. 6) and Paul MacKendrick (*The Iberian Stones Speak* [New York 1969], p. 208) treat these as one factory of fifteen vats, while Ponsich (*Aceite de Oliva y Salazones de Pescado*, p. 194, Fig. 101) separates them into Groups One and Two.

[39] Ponsich, *Aceite de Oliva y Salazones de Pescado*, pp. 78, 197–98, and Fig. 101, p. 94. For the cylindrical vats, see esp. *ibid.*, p. 40, Fig. 14. See also Martin-Bueno et al., "Baelo Claudia," p. 491, note 8. Although the huge size of the large circular vats suggested to Ponsich that whales could have been processed here, they may have also served to prepare fish sauce. The round shape would have facilitated stirring, an important step in insuring a well-autolysized mixture.

[40] But cf. Tyritake in the Black Sea area, below pp. 122–24, and the Byzantine zoning regulation, below p. 189 and note 18.

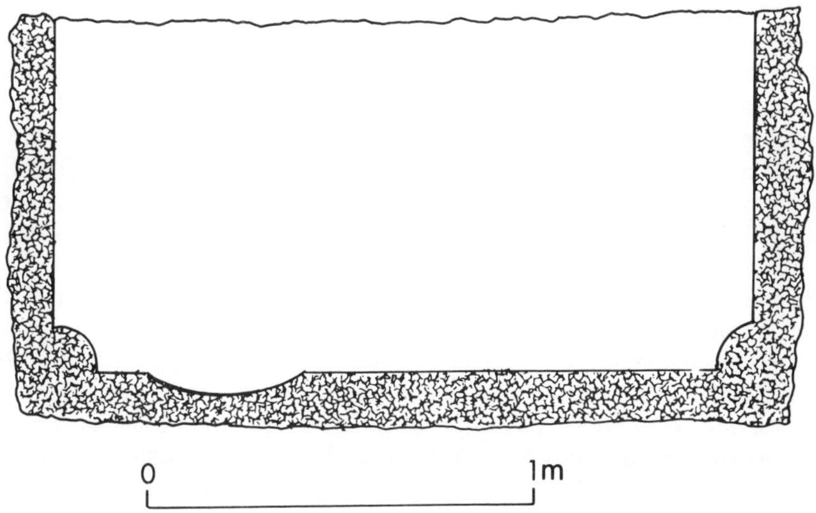

Figure 3: Punta de l'Arenal: Salting Vat
(after Martin and Serres, *Punta de l'Arenal*, Fig. 20)

This factory functioned from the reign of Claudius up to the latter part of the third century A.D.[41]

The salteries lying along the coast of Alicante between Santa Pola and Jávea in Hispania Tarraconensis, exhibit some characteristics different from those in Baetica. Invariably located in rocky areas, the Alicantan factories frequently include a pond (*piscina*) cut into the rock and provided with access to the sea by means of channels. These so-called "Baños de la Reina" are a typical feature of these salteries and apparently served to keep fish alive until processed.[42] The fish tanks were faced with a fine mortar of lime and broken tile, typically used to create water-tight containers, such as cisterns.

The distinctive element of any saltery was the salting vat (Fig. 3), called a *cetaria*.[43] Construction of the vats followed a general plan; the size and

---

[41] Dardaine et al., "La campagne de fouilles," p. 398.

[42] Martin, "Las pesquerías romanas," pp. 144–51, esp. Fig. 3. Cf. below p. 87, the piscina at Cosa in Italy. Several perplexing constructions have come to light in the waters along the coast of Baetica, for example, near Barbate. They appear in various shapes, rectangular, semicircular, or, like the one at Barbate, circular. These structures may have functioned in the following manner. The incoming tide would bring fish within the "corrals," but the outgoing tide would trap them within the confining walls where they could then be easily caught by fishermen. Consequently, these constitute ponds, or holding areas, for live fish until processed in a nearby saltery. A. Moreno Páramo and L. Abad Casal, "Aportaciones al estudio de la pesca en la antiquëdad," *Habis* 2 (1971): 209–21.

[43] Pliny *HN* 9.92: *Carteiae in cetariis adsuetus exire e mari in lacus eorum apertos atque ibi salsamenta populari– mire omnibus marinis expetentibus odorem quoque eorum, qua de causa et nassis inlinuntur–,*

shape varied. Some vats at Vao, for example, measured 1.50 x 1.03 x 1.85 meters, while others at Caetobriga measured 4.00 x 3.70 x 2.00 meters. Most vats were square or rectangular, but some, such as at Baelo, were cylindrical. Some round, shallow basins found at Jávea and Calpe contained fragments of dolia. This latter find suggests a parallel with the preparation of garum described by Manilius in *Astronomica* 5.676–81. The round vats of Jávea, which probably held fish sauce, varied in size from 0.95 x 1.15 meters to 0.87 x 1.07 meters.[44] While the vats of Baetica and Lusitania were usually grouped by twos in a series or in a square, those at Punta de l'Arenal are scattered about.[45]

There were three basic types of vats depending upon the location of the saltery; that is, whether the vats lay on or near the beach and often roofed in some basic fashion, on a rocky promontory, or were constructed within a building of some sort. Those of Baetica and Lusitania were generally of the first and third types, while those along the Alicantan coast present examples primarily of the second. Vats in sandy areas were usually sunk into the ground and constructed of mortar and rubble composed of broken tiles, bricks, or small rocks (Pl. 2). The interior was faced with a mortar of lime and finely-broken tiles (*opus signinum*), but the exterior remained rough. Rocky areas required vats to be cut into the rock or to sit like a tub on the rocky ground. The interiors likewise had a facing of fine mortar.[46] All three types of vats possessed rounded angles at the top; at the interior angles an ovolo served to reinforce the sides and to aid in periodically cleaning the vats. Since there usually existed no way to drain the basins, many, but by no means all, contained a small depression in the bottom to

---

convertit in se custodum indignationem adsiduitate furti inmodicam. The *lacus apertus* was obviously a vat containing salsamenta, not live or fresh fish. Pliny's use of the plural *cetariis* implies a collection of *cetariae*. Since fish were salted in vats, not fish ponds (*piscinae*), *cetaria* must refer to the vat. Hence, the saltery was viewed as a collection of salting vats. Cf. Pliny *HN* 31.94; and *ibid*. 9.49: *Hispaniae cetarias hi replent, thynnis non commeantibus*. Horace (*Sat*. 2.5.44) uses a neuter plural form: *plures adnabunt thynni et cetaria crescent*. This is usually taken to refer (erroneously, I think) to *piscinae*. The scholiast to this passage certainly sees it otherwise: *cetaria dicuntur proprie loca, in quibus salsamenta fiunt*. And again: *officina, in qua liquamen conficitur*. See Schol. Horace *Sat*. 2.5.44 (*PseudoAcron* [Keller, ed.], vol. 2, p. 172). In the sixth century A.D., Cassiodorus (*Variae* 12.22.4) refers to the salteries of Histria as *garismatia*, a word which brings to mind the association of salteries with the production of garum. Cf. *CGL* III. 477, 30: *liquaminarium* γάρερουν.

[44] Vao: Pellati, "I monumenti," p. 216; Jávea: Martin and Serres, *Punta de l'Arenal*, pp. 40–43, 85. Martin and Serres convincingly demonstrate that the saltery at Punta de l'Arenal displays characteristics remarkably similar to salting installations in Baetica and North Africa. Yet after presenting evidence which suggests the presence of garum production, such as finds of large and small vats and certain types of amphorae which frequently were used to transport fish sauce (Dressel Form 7), they conclude that their factory produced not garum, but a similar tunny product (*ibid*., pp. 84–86). Even if the saltery at Punta de l'Arenal was much smaller than many of those in Baetica and North Africa, garum production would still have had an important place in the salting activity. Manilius' description of fishermen preparing their catch of tunny on the shore shows that regardless of the size of the salting operation all parts of the fish were utilized, some for fish sauce, others for salsamenta. The use of dolia for producing fish sauce was apparently not unheard of elsewhere. See below pp. 92–94, 122–23.

[45] Martin and Serres, *Punta de l'Arenal*, p. 85.

[46] Some vats at Jávea, rested like a tub on the surface of the ground. *Ibid*., pp. 39–41.

collect the remains and to help in the cleaning process (Fig. 3 and Pl. 3). At Rhode (Rosas) in Hispania Tarraconensis, one room of the salting factory contained five roughly square vats coated on the interior with *opus signinum* and arranged in a semi-circle about a central space. The floors of the vats were higher than that of the room itself and sloped slightly in the direction of the center of the room. At the bottom of at least three of them (and possibly a fourth) a conduit extended through the front wall which faced the interior of the room. This conduit was capable of being plugged and, when opened, emptied into a small round catch-basin cut into the floor of the central space.[47] These vats lacked both the quarter-round in the angles and the depression in the floor. At least one large vat (3.65 x 1.45 x 0.90m.), typical of the types of vat found in Baetica and North Africa, was found in another room located to the southwest.

Buildings contiguous to salteries form another general characteristic of Spanish fish processing centers. Dried fish was probably typical among products processed in salting installations. Identification of drying facilities, such as drying racks, no doubt made of wood and so perishable with time, is difficult. A small salting factory, lying at a point on the east coast of the Cabo de Trafalgar (Cadiz), comprises two distinct parts.[48] The first area has a group of two small salting basins of the usual type, except for what appear to be benches or shelves of unknown purpose constructed in the interior. The second area, some 600 meters away, has a small structure with four entrances, thus providing an airy enclosure. Cavities in the ground may have held braces for the drying racks. The excavators date this installation from the late first century B.C. to the early second century A.D.

Large houses or villas formed contiguous parts of many salteries, such as at Portimão, Torre de Ares, Calpe, San Pedro de Alcantara, and Jávea.[49] Permanent lodgings of a nature befitting the social status and in a quantity sufficient to accommodate the large number of workers required to operate

---

[47] Nolla-Brufau, "Excavaciones recientes," pp. 430–59, esp. Figs. 15–2 and 15–3; and Nolla and Nieto, "Roses," pp. 193–96. The vats measured between 1.60 x 1.65 meters and 1.85 x 1.80 meters; the small circular catch-basins had diameters varying between 0.8–0.85 meters, with a depth ranging between 0.25–0.30 meters. The collective capacity of all of the vats was about 9.50 cubic meters. One of the square vats had at some time been subdivided into two smaller ones of rectangular shape. A small semi-circular basin was excavated into the floor against the south wall of the room and apparently had no direct relationship to the salting vats. An arrangement similar to the one at Rosas appears at Alcazarsegher in North Africa, although there the catch-basin is semi-circular. Ponsich and Tarradel, *Garum*, pp. 72–73 and Fig. 48. Modern vats used to produce Filipine *patis* and Vietnamese *nuoc-mam* are also fitted with a valve near the bottom to drain out the finished product. See Steinkraus et al. *Handbook*, pp. 506 (*patis*), 517 (*nuoc-mam*).

[48] Amores, "Una nueva factoría," pp. 441–53.

[49] For villas and their frequent proximity to salting installations see especially Gorges, *Les villas hispano-romaines*, pp. 184 (Punta de l'Arenal), 260 (Tossa de Mar), 305 (Marbella), 306 (San Pedro de Alcántara, at Las Torres), 307 (Torrox, at El Faro), 317 (Los Nietos, at Las Mateas, and Puerto Mazarrón), 456 (Lavra, at O Fontão), 457 (Póvoa de Varzim, at Alto de Martim Vaz), 481–82 (Mexilhoeira Grande, at Abicada), 482 (Olhão, at Quinta do Marim, and Portimão), and 482–83 (Quarteira, at Cerro da Vila). For fish salteries and landed estates in the Algarve, see Edmondson, *Two Industries*, pp. 129–30.

a saltery, however, have not been found at any site so far excavated. Temples and modest graves do provide some evidence for the presence of workers at these installations. Apparently, in most places, workmen were seasonal employees who lived in temporary lodgings while engaged in salting activities during the period from July through August when the migratory route of the tunny took the commercial fish along the Spanish coast. Having finished in one place the workers may have moved on to another saltery farther down the coast or else undertook other work, such as agriculture, until the next tunny migration. An off-season occupation would for most workers be a necessity as well, since the abundance of fish resources probably varied from year to year.[50]

The salting factories at Senhora da Luz and San Pedro de Alcantara possessed structures nearby, perhaps baths, with heating facilities.[51] The saltery at Sanlúcar de Barrameda had a small furnace near one of its salting rooms.[52] Attached to this room, though on the outside of the building itself, was a small square vat with the basic characteristics of a salting basin. The furnace may have served also as a kiln, since numerous fragments of ceramic, amphorae, and terra sigillata were found in the same room. A saltery would naturally need a supply of containers to bottle its product for processing and for sale or for export. Many producers probably found it more convenient to manufacture their own amphorae rather than purchase them elsewhere. Five amphora kilns lay near the saltery at Gades, and Carteia possessed two.[53] Many amphorae discovered at these two sites were of the shape normally associated with fish products. Baetica was a major supplier of oil and wine to Rome, as the remains of amphorae at Monte Testaccio attest, and the Valley of the Guadalquivir in Baetica is littered with numerous remains of amphorae produced in kilns scattered along the river.[54] If wine producers manufactured their own amphorae, it seems logical to conclude that fish processors did likewise. The evidence of kilns at Algeciras in Spain, Caetobriga and Beja in Portugal, and elsewhere shows this to have been the case.[55]

---

[50] Ponsich, "Une usine antique de salaisons à Belo," pp. 70–71. See also *idem*, "Pérennité des relations dans le circuit du Détroit de Gibraltar," *ANRW*, Vol. II, pt. 3, pp. 676–77, and Edmondson, *Two Industries*, pp. 127–34. For the inconsistency of Mediterranean fish resources see below p. 149.

[51] Ponsich and Tarradell (*Garum*, p. 103) see a connection between these so-called baths and the salting process, if they contained a method of heating but lacked a room for water. There may also have been one at Punta de l'Arenal. See Martin and Serres, *Punta de l'Arenal*, p. 85.

[52] M. Esteve Guerrero, "Sanlúcar de Barrameda (Cádiz): fábrica de salazón romana en La Algaida," *Noticiario arqueológico hispánico* 1–3 (1952): 127.

[53] Peacock, "Baetican Fish Industry," pp. 232–42.

[54] J. J. Van Nostrand, *Roman Spain*, Vol. 3 (1937) of *ESAR*, pp. 184–85. See also Robert Étienne, "Les amphores du Testaccio au IIIe siècle," *MEFRA* 61 (1949): 151–81, and George Edward Bonsor, *The Archaeological Expedition Along the Guadalquivir*. Clara L. Penney, transl. (New York 1931), passim.

[55] See esp. Peacock, "Baetican Fish Industry," pp. 232–42; Cardoso, "Museu do Mar (Cascais)," pp. 63–78; Parker, "Lusitanian Amphoras," pp. 35–46; Peacock and Williams, *Amphorae and the Roman Economy*, pp. 72–76; and Dias Diogo, "Fornos de ânforas," pp. 209–15.

Roman fish salteries were complexes of salting vats, villas, temples, baths, and temporary structures. Among these facilities excavators have found amphorae, dolia, terra sigillata, and other ceramics. Many sites, such as Lucentum, Baria, Vao, Silniana, Carteia, Baelo, and Caetobriga, have yielded the dried remains of fish bones and scales, either still in the vats or scattered throughout the factory. At Cerro del Mar at the mouth of the Rio de Vélez excavators uncovered what may have been the site of a first century A.D. warehouse for garum amphorae (Dressel Forms 7–11) awaiting shipment to markets elsewhere. The considerable remains of fish bones, both contained in amphorae and scattered about in a 10 cm. thick deposit, included especially those of the sardine (*Engraulis encrasicholus*), mackerel (*scomber scombrus*), and various types of sea bream. Remains of a saltery have not been discovered.[56] Murex shells found at Baria and Caetobriga indicate that salteries there may also have produced purple dye. The Balearic Islands had an active purple dye industry, even into the late empire when an official textile establishment operated there.[57] As one would expect in a fishing region, excavators frequently found fishhooks, weights, nets, and tools designed to repair nets.[58]

The extent of excavations accomplished to date is insufficient to establish a firm chronological framework for the functioning of Roman salteries in Spain and Portugal. Punic salting establishments dating between the fifth and third centuries B.C. have come to light at Cadiz, thereby substantiating contemporary Greek sources for Spanish salting activity in the pre-Roman period. Strabo attests Roman salting operations in the late first century B.C. and archaeological evidence from Baelo, at least, seems to confirm it. A sounding beneath the southern extremity of the portico of the macellum revealed a salting vat containing rubbish dated to the late first century B.C.[59] The latest Spanish saltery (Rhode) dates to the sixth century A.D. The most active period, however, falls mainly in the first and second centuries A.D. Many salteries seem to have ceased functioning or, at best, to have reduced industrial activity in the third century. Some witnessed a rebirth or, like the one at Rhode, only began operation in the fourth century A.D.[60]

---

[56] Oswaldo Arteaga, "Vorbericht über die Grabungskampagne 1976 auf dem Cerro del Mar," *MDAI(M)* 18 (1977): 103–05, and Angela von den Driesch, "Osteoarchäologische Auswertung von Garum-resten des Cerro del Mar," *MDAI(M)* 21 (1980): 151–54.

[57] Baria: García y Bellido, "La industria pesquera," p. 8; Caetobriga: Pellati, "I monumenti," p. 216; and Edmondson, *Two Industries*, pp. 118–21; Balearic Islands: Blümner, *Die gewerbliche Thätigkeit*, pp. 136–37. See also *Not. dign. occ.* 11.71 (Seeck, ed. p. 151).

[58] See Ponsich and Tarradell, *Garum*, passim; and Antonio Mesquita de Figueiredo, "Contribuições para a historia da pesca, em Portugal, na epocha luso-romana," *O archeologo português* 4 (1898): 53–58.

[59] Strabo 3.1.8 (Mellaria and Baelo), 3.2.6 (Turdetania), 3.4.2 (Malaca), 3.4.6 (New Carthage and Scombraria). One of Strabo's major sources was Poseidonius (*ca.* 135–50 B.C.) who may have provided him with information on Spanish salteries dating back to the second century B.C. See Bonneville et al., "La dix-huitème campagne," pp. 473–75. Otherwise there is no evidence for this period.

[60] Ponsich, *Aceite de Oliva, y Salazones de Pescado*, pp. 233–34; Nolla-Brufau, "Excavaciones recientes," pp. 444–48.

Apparently, events of the third century seriously affected most Roman fish salteries in Spain, although according to evidence of the *Expositio Totius Mundi et Gentium* and of Ausonius, Spanish salteries were still producing fish sauce in the fourth century.[61] The installation at Baelo flourished into the fifth century or later, while that at Rhode operated into the late sixth century.[62]

As early as the fifth century B.C., Spain was exporting its salted fish products to Greece where, by the following century at least, they compared favorably with the products of Byzantium.[63] Nothing further is known of Spanish fish sauce commerce, however, until the first century B.C. The cargo of the mid-first century B.C. wreck Titan A found off the coast of the île du Levant included several Dressel 12 amphorae, completely intact, even to the presence of the stopper in the mouth. Inside were found heads, tails, and small bones of tunny preserved in muria.[64] Although earlier Greek and Latin authors mention salted fish and fish sauce, Horace is the earliest author to mention Spanish garum specifically.[65] Strabo provides the best evidence for the presence of an active Ro-

---

[61] Ponsich and Tarradell, *Garum*, pp. 116–17. See also Josè Maria Blázquez, "La crisis del siglo III en Hispania y Mauretania Tingitana," *Hispania* 28 (1968): 5–37 (=*Economía de la Hispania romana* [Bilboa 1978], pp. 461–83). See also *Expositio totius mundi et gentium* 59 (Rougé, ed.): *Deinde a Gallia Spania terra lata et maxima et dives, viris doctis ⟨ et omnibus bonis ornata et ⟩ in omnibus negotiis ⟨ pollens ⟩, quorum ex parte dicemus: oleum enim et liquamen et vestem variam et lardum et iumenta mittens, omni mundo sufficiens*; and Ausonius *Ep.* 25: *Quanto me adfecit beneficio non delata equidem, sed suscepta mea querimonia, Pauline fili! veritus displicuisse oleum, quod miseras, munus iterasti, addito etiam Barcinonensis muriae condimento cumulatius praestitisti. scis autem me id nomen muriae, quod in usu vulgi est, nec solere nec posse dicere, cum scientissimi veterum et Graeca vocabula fastidientes Latinum in gari appellatione non habeant. sed ego, quocumque nomine liquor iste sociorum vocatur,*

Iam patinas implebo meas, ut parcior ille
Maiorum mensis applaria sucus inundet.

Robert Étienne suggests that Ausonius' reference should be interpreted to mean that the production of garum sociorum had shifted from New Carthage to Barcelona (Barcino) in response to the crisis of the third century A.D. See Étienne, "Garum sociorum," p. 309. That the "crisis" was more a general economic decline, beginning perhaps in the late second century and brought on by growing insecurity, than a result of invasions is still unclear. Cf. Richard Reece, "The Third Century: Crisis or Change?" in *The Roman West in the Third Century*. Anthony King and Martin Henig, eds. BAR International Series, 109 (Oxford 1981), pp. 27–38; Simon J. Keay, "The *Conventus Tarraconensis* in the Third Century A.D.: Crisis or Change," *ibid.*, pp. 451–86; and Padilla Monge, *La provincia romana de la Betica (253–422)*, p. 37.

[62] Ponsich, *Aceite de Oliva y Salazones de Pescado*, p. 198. Ceramic evidence shows that many places were at least inhabited, if not actively processing fish, in the sixth century A.D. See also Edmondson, *Two Industries*, pp. 108–09. The factory at Rhode initiated operations in the second half of the fourth century A.D. and apparently functioned until abandoned suddenly in the late sixth or early seventh century. There is no evidence to suggest the abandonment resulted from violence of any kind. Nolla-Brufau, "Excavaciones recientes," pp. 444–48.

[63] For possible exportation of salted fish from Spain to Corinth in the fifth century B.C., see below p. 115. For the comparison with processed fish from Byzantium see Nicostratus frs. 4,5 Edmonds; Antiphanes fr. 77 Edmonds.

[64] Benoit, "Nouvelles épaves de Provence," pp. 5–8; and Phillippe Tailliez, "Travaux de l'été 1958 sur l'épave du 'Titan' à l'île du Lévant (Toulon)," in *Atti del II Congresso Internazionale di Archaeologia Sottomarina Albenga 1958* (Bordighera 1961), p. 197.

[65] Horace *Sat.* 2.8.46: *garo de sucis piscis Hiberi.*

man fish salting industry along the coasts of Turdetania and Baetica. Although he never visited Spain and apparently learned of the production centers from his sources, Strabo no doubt spoke from first-hand knowledge of Spanish products available to him in Italy. He remarks that Turdetanian merchants were active in great numbers in both Puteoli and Ostia.[66]

More is known about Spanish commerce in fish products in the first two centuries A.D. than for any other province in the Roman Empire. Literary sources are few in number, but the archaeological and epigraphical evidence is significant. Pliny states that the best garum was produced from the mackerel by the *socii* of New Carthage, and Martial devotes an entire epigram to garum made by the same organization.[67] Obviously, garum sociorum, "garum of the allies" (or, more accurately, "of the partners"), was a delicacy highly regarded in Rome. Pliny reports a price of 1,000 sesterces for two congii, or approximately 4,000 sesterces for one amphora.[68] Some Spanish fish sauce may have been expensive, but most of it certainly was not. Were it so, Spanish exports would not have practically controlled the processed fish market in Italy.

Recent excavations in the "Baths of the Swimmer" in Ostia have uncovered a large quantity of salt-fish amphora fragments. This material forms the basis for a typology of shapes which can be generally assigned a date based upon the strata in which they were found.[69] A comparison of the relative quantities of these types yields a fairly clear picture of the fortunes of Spanish exports to Ostia.[70] Dressel Forms 7–13, Beltrán Form IIB, and Dressel Forms 38–39 (Pelichet 46) appear in great quantity during the Flavian era, the period during which the bath was constructed. The Trajanic and Hadrianic strata show a diminution in the numbers of Dressel Forms 7–13, but an increase in other types. By the late Antonine period Dressel Forms 7–13 disappear, Beltrán Form IIB containers decrease, while all others remain abundant. The Severan strata, however, contain few of the usual Spanish salt-fish amphorae, but there does appear a new form, Almagro 50, which may have been a Lusitanian fish sauce vessel. In the late third century Almagro 50 amphorae appear in modest numbers, but there is an increase in the presence of North African amphorae, some of which may have held salt-fish. This picture also holds true for the fourth century.

[66] Strabo 3.2.6. For Strabo's travels in the Western Mediterranean see G. C. Richards, "Strabo," *G & R* 10 (Feb. 1941): 79–90.

[67] Pliny *HN* 31.94. In an epigram (13.102), entitled *Garum Sociorum*, Martial writes: *Expirantis adhuc scombri de sanguine primo/ accipe fastosum, munera cara, garum*.

[68] The amphora as a unit of measure equalled approximately eight congii, or six gallons and seven pints. For the expense of fish sauce in general see below, pp. 170–75.

[69] Fede Berti et al., *Le Terme del Nuotatore: Ostia II*. Studi Miscellanei 16 (Rome 1968–69), esp. pp. 120–26; Carandini and Panella, *Ostia III*, esp. pp. 506–15, 664–96; L. Anselmino et al., *Ostia IV*. Studi Miscellanei 23 (Rome 1977), esp. pp. 120–280, 359–83; and Clementina Panella, "Annotazione in margine alle stratigrafie delle Terme ostiensi nel Nuotatore," in *Recherches sur les amphores romaines*. Collection de l'École Française de Rome, No. 10 (Rome 1972), pp. 69–106.

[70] Carandini and Panella, *Ostia III*, pp. 506–15; Panella, "Annotazione," pp. 69–106.

The wreck Sud-Lavezzi 1, found off the southern coast of Corsica, had a small cargo of 450 amphorae. Of these, 194 were of type Almagro 51. To judge from the amphora of this type which was found in a wreck off the coast of Marseilles and which contained the bones of the scomber colias, Sud-Lavezzi 1 confirms continued commerce in Spanish fish products in the 4th or early 5th century A.D.[71]

In summary, it seems that Spain exported huge quantities of salted fish products to Ostia during the first two centuries A.D.[72] Coming primarily from Baetica, Spanish salt-fish met with little competition from other areas producing fish sauce, including the Italian salteries.[73] Certain amphora forms were phased out over the years, but they were replaced with others which also held salt-fish products. Why these forms varied so much remains a mystery. Whether a result of general economic decline brought on by insecurity resulting from the wars following the death of Commodus in A.D. 192 is uncertain, the instability of the third century apparently seriously interrupted, but did not end, trade between Spain and Italy. Spanish exports in fish sauce never fully recovered and, although some reached Ostia in a new type of container, the North African salteries apparently assumed much of the Spanish trade in these products. This scenario coincides well with the chronology established for Spanish and, as will be seen later, North African salteries. The Spanish salteries, for the most part, either reduced production activity or ceased it altogether in the third century A.D. Perhaps only Northeastern Spain, in the area of Barcino and Rhode in particular, continued to be commercially active; others may have contented themselves with satisfying local needs alone.

Spanish merchant ships carried fish products to all parts of the Western Mediterranean. Many never reached their destination and came to rest on the bottom of the sea. The Pecio Gandolfo wreck, off Punta de las Entinas

[71] Panella, "Annotazione," pp. 101–04; and Andrea Carandini and Clementina Panella, "The Trading Connections of Rome and Central Italy in the Late Second and Third Centuries: the Evidence of the Terme del Nuotatore Excavations, Ostia," in *The Roman West in the Third Century*, pp. 487–503. For the Sud-Lavezzi I wreck, see Bernard Liou, "Informations archéologiques. Corse du Sud," *Gallia* 40 (1982): 439–44. For the wreck off the coast of Marseilles, see *idem*, "Recherches sous-marines," *Gallia* 31 (1973): 585–86. See also Edmonson, *Two Industries*, pp. 165–72. For an Almagro 50 amphora found at Arles, see Liou, "Inscriptions peintes sur amphores: Fos (suite)," 120–22.

[72] Whether it was, according to Berti et al. (*Ostia II*, pp. 125–26), the major import of the first century A.D., surpassing even oil, may be doubted, but cf. R. Pascual Guasch, "La evolución de las exportaciones béticas durante el Imperio," in *Produccion y comercio del aceite en la antigüedad. Primer Congreso Internacional*. José María Blázquez Martínez, ed. (Madrid 1980), pp. 233–42. Pascual's study of 78 shipwrecks dating between the first and third centuries A.D. included 57 completely or partially laden with Baetican products. He concludes that salt-fish exports exceeded that for oil and metals in the first and second centuries A.D. For the Augustan period see A. Hesnard, "Un dépôt augustéen d'amphores à La Longarina, Ostie," in *The Seabourne Commerce of Ancient Rome: Studies in Archaeology and History*. J. H. D'Arms and E. C. Kopff, eds. MAAR, vol. 36 (Rome 1980), pp. 141–56.

[73] Spanish exports of salted fish products to Pompeii were also significant. See Daniele Manacorda, "Anfore spagnole a Pompei," in *L'instrumentum domesticum di Ercolano e Pompei nella prima età imperiale*. Quaderni di cultura materiale, 1 (Rome 1977), pp. 121–33.

near Almeria, for example, contained Dressel Form 14 vessels, as did the wreck from the Bay of San Antonio off the island of Ibiza in the Balearic Islands. Both finds yielded Dressel Form 14 amphorae which still contained fish bones.[74] Near the southern coast of Majorca, the Rápita wreck contained amphorae of Pelichet 46.[75] Among those found off the coast of Gaul are La Chrétienne B at Antheor near the île Sainte Marguerite, the Titan wreck near the île du Levant, and Planier 5 near Marseilles. Perhaps the most important recent find is that of Port Vendres II, discovered in 1972. The wreck, which dates between A.D. 41 and 50, contained various Baetican products, including ingots of tin and amphorae of wine, oil and salted fish products.[76] Several wrecks have been discovered near Corsica in the strait of Bonifacio. The Lavezzi 2 wreck, near the island of the same name, and the Tour Sainte-Marie wreck, off Cape Corsica, held Dressel Form 7–11 amphorae.[77] Apparently, these ships were bound for Ostia but never made it past the treacherous strait between Corsica and Sardinia.

Spanish salt-fish amphorae have been found in many provinces of the Western Roman Empire, bearing witness to the wide-flung commercial activity of Spanish merchants. Those found at Mogador and in many areas of Mauretania Tingitana across the strait from Baetica may represent the exportation of Spanish fish products to North Africa. The most impressive series of finds occurred in the northern provinces of Gaul, both Germanies, Raetia, and Britain, while Spanish salt-fish amphorae are beginning to appear in excavations in the Greek East.[78]

Spanish salt-fish merchants were active throughout the Western Roman

[74] Pascual Guasch, "El Pecio Gandolfo (Almería)," pp. 143–46, and *idem*, "Dos ánforas del Pecio Gandolfo (Almería)," *Zephyrus* 11 (1960): 208. Shipwrecks containing Baetican fish products have been discovered along the coast of Andalusia near Roquetas del Mar, Guardias Viejas in the Bay of San Miguel, off the coast of ancient Abdera, with possible sites near Las Plameras, Los Percheles, and the Bay of La Higuera. See *idem*, "Underwater Archaeology," pp. 107–19. Another site at Riells-La Clota near Ampurias has also yielded fish sauce amphorae. See Federico Foerster, "Spain: Riells-La Clota," *IJNA* 7,2 (1978): 163. The wreck near the island of Ibiza, another one off the coast of the island of Cabrera, and others may indicate that a major sea route from Spain to Italy lay to the south of the Balearic Islands. See most recently, Dali Colls, Claude Domergue, and Victor Guerrero Ayuso, "Les lingots de plomb de l'épave romaine *Cabrera 5* (île de Cabrera, Baléares)," *Archaeonautica* 6 (1986): 31–35. Perhaps the inhabitants of Ibiza participated in this trade. Cf. Gamer, "Antike Anlagen zur Fischverarbeitung," pp. 19–28.

[75] Maria Pilar G. Serrano, "Ánforas romanas en las costas de Mallorca," *AEA* 36 (1963): 207–10. Fish sauce amphorae were also included among the cargo of a shipwreck found at Ses Salines in Majorca. See Anthony J. Parker, "Lead Ingots from a Roman Ship at Ses Salines, Majorca," *IJNA* 3 (1974): 148.

[76] La Chrétienne B and the Titan: Fernand Benoit, "Épaves de la côte de Provence. Typologie des amphores," *Gallia* 14 (1956): 29–32; Planier 5: *idem*, "Nouvelles épaves de Provence (III)," *Gallia* 20 (1962): 156; Port-Vendres II: Colls et al., *L'épave Port-Vendres II*, pp. 40–43, 78–83.

[77] André Tchernia, "Direction des recherches archéologiques sous-marines," *Gallia* 27 (1969): 494–99. For a summary of shipwrecks found near Corsica see W. Bebko, *Les épaves antiques du sud de la Corse* (Bastia 1971), passim.

[78] André Jodin, *Les établissements du roi Juba II aux îles Purpuraires (Mogador)* (Tanger 1967), pp. 178–80. See also Michel Ponsich, *Recherches archéologiques à Tanger et dans sa région* (Paris 1970), pp. 252–54. Ponsich (*Tanger*, pp. 253–54) suggests that Spanish kilns may have furnished

Empire, but it seems unlikely that this commerce was organized on a provincial level or that there existed a consortium which monopolized the salted fish products of both Baetica and Mauretania Tingitana combined. Michel Ponsich, in noting the nearness of the two areas with each other, the marked physical similarities, and the close historical ties, treats the Atlantic coasts of Southern Spain and Morocco almost as a single economic unit, with the former exercising superiority over the latter. He believes that the salteries and other industries near the Strait of Gibraltar formed a consortium or cooperative and shipped their products to Gades where they were distributed to other parts of the Roman world under the label "Gaditanian."[79] A monopoly exercised by a societas of Gades, he continues, would explain the silence of the ancient sources on Tingitanian salteries and the high reputation of Gaditanian products.[80] Ponsich's suggestion remains for the present unproven. He readily admits that purple dye was retained in Africa and, as an export product, achieved renown throughout the Roman world, but he does not explain why this should be so, particularly if the monopoly was as all-pervading as he implies. It remains possible that many individual merchants, for instance those from Lixus or Cotta in Mauretania Tingitana or from Lusitania on the Atlantic coast, may have preferred to sell their products to the large companies in Gades, Malaca, Baelo, or even in New Carthage rather than to export them to other provinces.[81] The large companies could have then added these products to their own and exported them to Gaul, Italy, and elsewhere under a common label. This is not the same as a monopoly, since it does not exclude the existence of small societates or individuals operating independently of the large companies. Until they can be definitely associated with a large organization, names appearing in *tituli picti* on Spanish salt-fish amphorae should be considered as identifying independent merchants or shippers. Small societates may be represented in *tituli picti* by names appearing in the plural, such as A. A. Atinii, C. C. Atinii, and Licinii.[82]

---

most, if not all, of the amphorae used in African salteries in the area up to the mid-third century A.D., when the crisis in Spain interrupted commercial activity.

[79] Ponsich, *Tanger*, p. 336: "Certaines industries, communes des deux côtés du détroit, firent partie d'un consortium pour faciliter leur groupage et leur transport, et leur productions, poisson salé, garum, huile par exemple, étaient envoyées à Gadès, d'où elles étaient distribuées sous l'étiquette de 'gaditaines.' D'autres, en revaunche, la pourpre en particulier, restaient des marchandises maurétaniennes, comme le blé et les plantes potagères, et avaient une certaine renommée dans tout le monde romain." See also *idem*, "Détroit de Gibraltar," pp. 670–79.

[80] Ponsich ("Détroit de Gibraltar," p. 680) concludes, "Le label de gaditain donné au garum semble annexer toute la production du circuit du détroit en enlever aux productions africaines l'opportunité d'être appréciées."

[81] Strabo (3.4.2) implies that a certain degree of trade relations existed between the two areas. See also Martin P. Charlesworth, *Trade Routes and Commerce of the Roman Empire*. 2nd ed. (Cambridge 1926), pp. 141–42. For Lusitania see Edmondson, *Two Industries*, pp. 186–87.

[82] *CIL* XV.4689–90 (Licinii); 4695–4700 (A. A. Atinii); 4701–02 (C. C. Atinii).

Large companies dealing in salted fish products did exist. Perhaps the most noted is the *societas* of New Carthage, mentioned by Pliny, Martial, and Ausonius and recorded in *tituli picti* on fish sauce amphorae found at Pompeii and Rome.[83] The connection of Spanish salt-fish commerce with the *Corpus Negotiantium Malacitanorum*, which maintained a headquarters in Ostia, is assured by the fact that the *quinquennalis* of this organization, P. Clodius Athenio, was a *negotians salsarius*.[84] The Malacan merchants probably serviced their own city and nearby salteries and competed freely with the *socii* of New Carthage and with merchants from other salt-fish producing areas for the export market.[85] Imperial salteries were apparently operating in Spain in the late first century or early second century A.D. The *titulus pictus* of a Dressel Form 7–11 amphora found at Fos-sur-Mer identifies the vessel's contents as [garum] SCOMBRI/ FLOS and proclaims that it came [e]x OF(ficina) AUGG(ustorum).[86] This unique inscription implies that imperial salteries operated independently of large corporations. Insufficient information exists, however, to determine the degree of market control exercised by either.

---

[83] Pliny *HN* 9.66, 31.93; Martial 13.102; Ausonius *Ep.* 25; *CIL* IV.5651(?), 5659; XV.4730; and possibly Galen *De compositione medicamentorum secundum locos* 3 (12.637K). There is no need to question the association of New Carthage with garum sociorum as does A. Balil; Pliny's meaning is sufficiently clear. See A. Balil Illana, "Economía de la Hispania romana," in *Estudios de economía antigua de la península ibérica* (Barcelona 1968), p. 353, note 196. See also Étienne, "Garum sociorum," pp. 297–313, and Javier R. Garcia del Toro, "*Garum Sociorum.* La industria de salazones de pescado en la Edad Antigua en Cartagena," *Anales de la Universidad de Murcia* 36 (1979): 27–57.

[84] *CIL* VI.9677: D(is) M(anibus)/ P(ublius) CLODIUS ATHENIO/ NEGOTIANS SALSARIUS/ Q(uin)Q(uennalis) CORPORIS NEGOTIANTIUM/ MALACITANORUM ET/ SCANTIA SUCCESSA CONIUNXS EIUS/ VIVI FECERUNT SIBI ET LIBERIS SUIS ET/ LIBERTIS LIBERTABUSQUE SUIS POSTERISQUE EORUM/ IN FRONTE P(edes) XIII IN AGRO P(edes) XII.

[85] Van Nostrand (*Roman Spain*, pp. 184–98) concludes that most of the Spanish export trade was in the hands of private individuals and that free competition prevailed, at least until the early third century A.D. The *titulus pictus* of an amphora of Dressel Form 9 (CIL XV.4570), found near the Praetorian camp, seems to identify garum from Gades. It lacks a product identification, but the amphora shape may imply a fish product from Spain. The inscription, however, contains a consular date, a feature common to wine amphorae. If it is a garum container, then apparently Gaditanian merchants shipped fish sauce independently of those from New Carthage or Malaca. Heinrich Dressel believes that the contents of an amphora of Dressel Form 7 (*CIL* XV.4737) was (muria) MAL(acitana), a sauce coming specifically from Malaca. There is no evidence, however, to support the contention of J. J. Van Nostrand (*Roman Spain*, pp. 199–200) that the company of merchants from Malaca served as distributors of fish sauce from New Carthage.

[86] Bernard Liou and Robert Marichal, "Les inscriptions peintes sur amphores de l'anse Saint-Gervais à Fos-sur-mer," *Archaeonautica* 2 (1978): 131–35. The last element can be clearly read as AUGG. For the expression *ex officina* cf. below, p. 95. Since Dressel Form 7–11 vessels date to the first century B.C. and first century A.D., the most likely imperial owners would be the Flavians, specifically Vespasian and Titus, known to have had extensive connections with Spain. See C. H. V. Sutherland, *The Romans in Spain, 217 B.C.–A.D. 117* (London 1939), pp. 182–200. The vessel, however, may have had a long life, with the label dating to the reign of Marcus Aurelius and Lucius Verus, the earliest attested period for the abbreviation AUGG in inscriptions. See B. E. Thomasson, "Zum Gebrauch von Augustorum, AUGG. und AUG. als Bezeichnung der Samtherrschaft zweier Herrscher," *ZPE* (1983): 125–35.

A fragmented and undated Greek inscription found in Malaca seems to refer to a group of *negotiatores* from Asia and Syria.[87] Their purpose in Spain is uncertain, but a connection with Malacan salt-fish products is feasible, since Spanish products did penetrate the Eastern Mediterranean. Greece, Cyrenaica, and Egypt, for instance, imported Spanish salt-fish.[88]

In summary, Spanish producers and merchants dominated commerce in salted fish products in the Western Mediterranean between the first and third centuries A.D. and may even have competed in the eastern markets. Spanish merchants transported fish products to Italy, Gaul, Africa, and many places along the *limes* of the northern provinces, including Britain. These merchants operated as individuals, as members of small *societates*, and as part of large companies having representatives in various cities in the western provinces. The most famous of these large companies was the *societas* of New Carthage, producers of garum sociorum. There seems to have been free competition among Spanish salt-fish merchants, but several large companies, perhaps in some way connected with the state, and imperial factories may have captured much of the market.

Africa

Literary sources are almost silent on fish salteries in Africa.[89] The *Periplus* of Ps-Scylax, dating to the middle of the fourth century B.C., mentions

[87] *CIL* II, p. 251 (= *IGRR* I/II.26). The inscription probably dates to the imperial period. See Antonio García y Bellido, "Los 'mercatores', 'negotiatores', y 'publicani' como vehiculos de romanizacion en la España romana preimperial," *Hispania* 26 (1966): 506.

[88] Daniel Sperber ("Some Observations of Fish and Fisheries in Roman Palestine," *ZDMG* 118 [1968]: 267) does not believe that Palestine imported Spanish salt-fish products because of the distance involved. But cf. F. M. Heichelheim, *Roman Syria,* Vol. 4 (1938) of *ESAR*, p. 201, and Libanius *Decl*. 32.28, writing from Palestine in the fourth century A.D.: καὶ κρεῶν μὲν ἢ ᾠῶν ἢ τούτων τινὸς τῶν πολυτελῶν οὐδ᾽ οὕτως ἂν ἐπριάμην, οὐδ᾽ οὕτως, εἰ μυρίοι με ἐκέντουν Ἔρωτες, εἰωθὼς δὲ ἐνίοτε τοῦ Βυζαντίου ταρίχους ἐσθίειν, ἴστε δὲ ὡς καὶ χρηστὸν ὄψον οἱ σκόμβροι καὶ εὔωνον, τοῦ Γαδειρικοῦ ποτ᾽ ἂν ἐπεθύμησα καὶ στένων μέν, ἐπριάμην δ᾽ ἂν ὅμως, εἶτ᾽ ἐλθὼν οἴκαδε οὐκ ὀπτήσας συνέφαγον ἄρτῳ ξηρῷ, ὅ μοι δεῖπνον ἀεὶ τὸ ἥδιστον ἦν, ἀλλ᾽ ἐπέσταξα ἂν ἐλαίου καὶ ὄξους ἐπέχεον καὶ ῥαφανίδας συνέφαγον, ὧν καὶ ἓν ἤρκει πρότερον δεῖπνον ποιῆσαι πολυτελές. Elizabeth Lyding Will, who is preparing for publication in the Athenian Agora Series a book on amphorae found in Greece (Athens, Corinth and Delos) and Alexandria, informs me that she has about twenty-five examples of Spanish salt-fish amphorae, designated as Will Type 16, from these areas of the Eastern Mediterranean. Type 16 corresponds to Dressel Forms 7–14, Pelichet 46, and other Spanish amphorae typologies. I am grateful to Prof. Will for apprising me of this material and allowing me to cite it before her book has appeared. Spanish salt-fish exports to Cyrenaica, begun only in the first century A.D., was never significant and declined in the second century A.D. See J. A. Riley, "The Coarse Pottery from Berenice," in Vol. 2 of *Excavations at Sidi Khrebish Benghazi (Berenice)*. Suppl. 5 to *Libya Antiqua* (Tripoli 1979), pp. 114, 157–59. For Spanish salt-fish in second century A.D. Athens see Lucian *Navigium* 22. Spanish exportation of salted fish products to the East will be discussed in more detail in Chapter 5.

[89] For this discussion Africa will be defined as that area which includes both Africa Proconsularis and Mauretania. The former stretched from Cyrenaica to the Ampsaga River and included Tripolitania, Byzacena, and Numidia; the latter covered the area from the Ampsaga River to the Atlantic Ocean and included Caesariensis and Tingitana. This expanse, covering North Africa from the Atlantic Ocean to the province of Cyrenaica, encompasses the modern countries of Morocco, Algeria, Tunisia, and a large portion of Libya.

salteries in the vicinity of the island of Meninx.[90] On the western coast of the Greater Syrtis lay a city called, in Phoenician, *Magom Malahat*, "city of salteries."[91] Pliny speaks of salteries and garum production at Leptis, but whether he means Leptis Minor in Byzacena or Leptis Magna in Tripolitania is unknown. The former seems more likely, since Strabo states that the islands of Taricheiae lay between Hadramentum and Thapsus.[92] Leptis Minor also lay between these two cities, and the name of the islands implies the presence of a fish saltery. Strabo is also our source for the only other African saltery known from literary records. He states that Zuchis, probably Praesidium Zuchis lying near the Lesser Syrtis, possessed a dye factory and "all kinds of fish salteries."[93]

Archaeology has confirmed the existence of other African salteries in Northern Morocco at Thamusida, Lixus, Kouass, Tahadart, Cotta, Sahara, Alcazarsegher, and Sania e Torres and in the Purple Islands off Mogador in Tingitana (Figs. 7, 9).[94] The appearance of murex shells at Kouass and elsewhere strengthens the notion that dye works formed a regular part of salteries where shellfish were available.[95] The discovery of a saltery at Mogador lends further confirmation, since Pliny adds the additional information that Juba II (d. ca. A.D. 23) established a dyeing industry on some small islands off the coast of Tingitana.[96] The process of extracting dye from the

---

[90] Ps-Scylax *Periplus* 110 (Müller, I, pp. 86–87): ἀπὸ δὲ ᾿Αβροτόνου Ταριχεῖαι, πόλις καὶ λιμήν. Παράπλους ἀπὸ ᾿Αβροτόνου ἡμέρας μιᾶς. κατὰ δὲ ταῦτά ἐστι νῆσος, ᾗ ὄνομα βραχείων, μετὰ Λωτοφάγους κατὰ Ταριχείας.

[91] Stéphane Gsell, *Histoire ancienne de l'Afrique du Nord*. 2nd ed. Vol 4: *La civilisation carthaginoise* (Paris 1924), p. 51.

[92] See Pliny *HN* 31.94. Strabo 17.3.16: εἶτα ᾿Αδρύμης πόλις, ἐν ᾗ καὶ νεώρια ἦν. εἶθ' αἱ Ταριχεῖαι λεγόμεναι, νησία πολλὰ καὶ πυκνά. εἶτα Θάψος πόλις, καὶ μετὰ ταύτην νῆσος πελαγία Λοπαδοῦσσα.

[93] Strabo 17.3.18: μετὰ δὲ τὴν Σύρτιν Ζοῦχις ἐστι λίμνη σταδίων τετρακοσίων στενὸν ἔχουσα εἴσπλουν καὶ παρ' αὐτὴν πόλις ὁμώνυμος πορφυροβαφεῖα ἔχουσα καὶ ταριχείας παντοδαπάς. In an address, probably before a bishop's council, Synesius (ca. 370–413 A.D.), Bishop of Ptolemaïs, denigrates Andronicus, the governor, as a man of mean background who "has arrived at the praefectureship from a tunny watch." If this accusation is true, there may have been, at least in the late fourth century A.D., a fish processing installation near Berenice (Benghazi), the city of Andronicus' birth, in Cyrenaica. See Synesius *Ep.* 57 (Hercher, ed., pp. 667–68): ἄναμνήσθητε γάρ ὑμεῖς τίς ἦν πρὸς ἐμὲ τόν εἰ μηδὲν ἄλλο, ἐξ ἐκείνων γενόμενον, ὧν ἀπ' Εὐρυσθένους τοῦ καταγαγόντος Δωριέας εἰς Σπάρτην μέχρι τοὐμοῦ πατρὸς αἱ διαδοχαὶ ταῖς δημοσίαις ἐνεκολάφθησαν κύρβεσιν, ἄνθρωπος οὐκ ἔχων εἰπεῖν ὄνομα πάππου, ἀλλ' οὐδὲ πατρός, φασί, πλὴν ὅσον εἰκάσαι, ἀπὸ θυννοσκοπείου δὲ ἐπὶ τὴν ἡγεμονικὴν ἀπήνην ἁλάμενος. See *Epistolographi Graeci*. Rudolf Hercher, ed. (Paris 1873; rpt. Amsterdam 1965).

[94] Ponsich and Tarradell, *Garum*, pp. 9–77; and Jodin, *Les établissements du roi Juba II*, pp. 68–71, 173–80, 256–61. See also René Rebuffat, *Thamusida III*. Supplement 2 of *Mélanges d'archéologie et d'histoire* (Rome 1977), pp. 284–85. For the suggestion that the *titulus pictus* COD TING VE, and similar ones found at Vindonissa and Pompeii, may refer to co(r)d(ula) ting(itana) ve(tus) and that COD LIX VE, and the like found at Pompeii, may pertain to co(r)d(ula) Lix(itana) ve(tus), see Liou, "Inscriptions peintes sur amphores: Fos (suite)," pp. 66–69.

[95] Ponsich and Tarradell, *Garum*, pp. 39, 102.

[96] Pliny *HN* 6.201. The location of Juba's factory received the name "Purple Islands" for this reason (*ibid.* 6.203). For murex and purple on the Gaetulian coast see also *ibid.* 5.12; 9.127. An unknown number of imperial textile factories (*bafia*) operated in Africa during the late empire. See *Not. dign. occ.* 11.69–70 (Seeck ed., p. 151). For a possible garum or purple factory in Tin-

murex closely approximates the production methods for garum, and so would naturally use similar facilities. The dye-carrying veins of the murex, which were allowed to macerate in salt for three days, formed a liquid which was transferred to lead pots and heated for six more days. At the end of this period, the liquid was strained into another container for use.[97] Other African salteries include those at Cartenna and Tipasa in Mauretania Caesariensis (Plate 5), Neapolis and Sullecthum in Byzacena, and perhaps Rusicade in Numidia.[98]

African salteries show characteristics similar to those in Spain and Portugal. The availability of fish, especially the tunny, was the determining factor.[99] Salt marshes were closely associated with the processing centers at Kouass and Tahardart, and many salteries lay at or near the mouth of rivers. Lixus lay on the mouth of the Loukos River, Kouass on the Garifa, Tahadart on the Tahadart, Cotta on the Khil, Sahara and Alcazarsegher near the El Kazar, Thamusida on the Sebou, and Sania e Torres near the Smir. Several salteries apparently employed cisterns to collect rain water for use in the production process.[100]

The most complete and best preserved African saltery is that at Cotta. It measured fifty-six by forty meters and possessed four basic areas: a preparation room in the form of a long corridor, the salting area, an area for the storage of amphorae, and a tower used for a tunny watch. The long corridor, open to the street, probably held tables upon which fish were cut up. The salting area (Pl. 4a) comprised twelve large and four small vats ar-

---

gitana see Alexis Denis, "L'auge aux trois bassins du toufri de Tingui (Maroc)," *AntAfr* 3 (1969): 215–24. Pliny likewise seems to verify the presence of a saltery on the island of Meninx when, in *HN* 9.127, he names it as one of two places in Africa from which the Romans obtained purple. See also Strabo 17.3.18 for Zuchis.

[97] Pliny *HN* 9.133: *capi eas* (purpuras) *post canis ortum aut ante vernum tempus utilissimum, quoniam, cum cerificavere, fluxos habent sucos. sed id tinguentium officinae ignorant, cum summa vertatur in eo. eximitur postea vena quam diximus, cui addi salem necessarium, sextarios ferme centenas in libras; macerari triduo iustum, quippe tanto maior vis, quanto recentior, fervere in plumbo, singulasque amphoras* [centenas] *aquae, quingentenas medicaminis libras aequali ac modico vapore torreri et ideo longinqueae fornacis cuniculo. ita despumatis subinde carnibus, quas adhaesisse venis necesse est, decimo ferme die liquata cortina vellus elutriatum mergitur in experimentum et, donec spei satis fiat, uritur liquor.*

[98] Cartenna: Marcel Leglay, "Cartennae," *Fasti Archaeologici* 9 (1956): 377. Tipasa: Wilhelm Schleiermacher, "Tipasa," *Germania* 43 (1965): 165–68; Jean Baradez, "Quatorze années de recherches archéologiques à Tipasa (1948–1961)," *Revue Africaine* 105 (1961): 235, 241–42; and *idem*, *Tipasa. Ville antique de Maurétanie* (Alger 1952), esp. pp. 39–40. Neapolis: Jean-Pierre Darmon, "Néapolis," *Africa* 2 (1968): 271–83. Darmon (p. 275, note 4) also mentions a possible site (unpublished) at Beni Khiar, a few kilometers from Nabeul. Sullecthum: Louis Foucher, "Note sur l'industrie et le commerce des salsamenta et du garum," *Actes du 93e Congrès National des Sociétés Savantes, Tours 1968. Section d'archéologie* (Paris 1970), pp. 17–21. Rusicade: Jean Lassus, "Chronique l'archéologie algerienne en 1956," *Libyca* 5 (1957): 147.

[99] Ponsich, *Aceite de Oliva y Salazones de Pescado*, pp. 30–43. Strabo 17.3.16 mentions a tunny watch near the promontory of Ammon Balithon, in Byzacena below Thapsus. Cf. Synesius *Ep.* 57 (Hercher, pp. 667–68).

[100] On salt see Ponsich and Tarradell, *Garum*, pp. 100–01; on cisterns, Leglay, "Cartennae," p. 377; Jodin, "Les établissements du roi Juba II," pp. 66–75; Foucher, "Note," p. 18; and Ponsich and Tarradell, *Garum*, p. 57.

ranged in a U-shaped formation about an open area which contained an impluvium and cistern.[101] The salting room was roofed, but the compluvium let in rain water used for cleaning and fresh air for aeration.[102]

Vats in African salteries generally conformed in size, shape, and construction to those found in Spain. Rectangular in shape, they were usually placed at ground level, made of cement and tile, covered with *opus signinum* to prevent drainage, and reinforced with an ovolo in the interior angles. Many had the small depression in the floor to aid in cleaning. At Cotta, of the sixteen basins found about the central work area, four, grouped together, were smaller than the rest. Ponsich and Tarradell identify these as basins for the preparation of garum or some other fish product.[103] It is significant that many factories, such as at Tahadart, Lixus (Fig. 4 and Pl. 4b), and Cartenna, had an arrangement of basins similar to that used at Cotta, that is, an open court surrounded on three sides by salting vats.

Furnaces, as in several of the Spanish salteries, formed an important part of African installations. Next to the salting area at Cotta was a furnace which had a foyer, warm room, and cool room. Garum could be heated in pots in the warm room until reduced to the proper level and then cooled before being transferred to commercial containers which were kept in a storeroom occupying two sides of the salting area. In the factories of Cotta and Tahadart which contained furnaces, the presence of many heating pots also attests to the use of artificial heat to prepare garum.[104] The saltery at Mogador had a villa with a furnace room which could easily have served a similar purpose.[105] Sullecthum possessed a bath nearby which may likewise have been used, and the saltery at Tipasa expanded to include a bath which had been destroyed in the third century A.D.[106]

As in Spain, the finds of small materials reveal much about the activity at

---

[101] A similar arrangment appeared in Factory No. 1 at Tahadart (Ponsich and Tarradell, *Garum*, pp. 43–44).

[102] The importance given to aeration can be seen in many factories where the salting area, though roofed to protect the open vats, have windows to let in air. Cf. for example, Factory No. 1 at Cotta (*ibid.*, pp. 43–44) and, in Spain, at Baelo (Ponsich, "A propos d'une usine antique," pp. 73–75, and Dardaine and Bonneville, "La campagne," p. 392).

[103] Ponsich and Tarradell, *Garum*, p. 57. This division between small and large vats, frequently encountered in Spanish salteries, appears also at Lixus and Tahadart. Lixus also had an intermediate size basin which Ponsich and Tarradell suggest was used in periods of slackened saltery activity for processing murex, sponges and other marine animals (*ibid.*, p. 37).

[104] Although no furnace was found at Kouass, the discovery of several cooking pots indicates that one may have existed there (*ibid.*, p. 39). A pre-Roman potter's kiln was found about 500 meters from the saltery. See J. H. Van Der Werff, "Amphores de tradition punique à Uzita," *BABesch* 52–53 (1977–78): 182, note 70. See also Michel Ponsich, "Note préliminaire sur l'industrie de la céramique préromaine en Tingitane (Kouass, Région d'Arcila)," *Karthago* 15 (1969–70): 77–97. Cf. below, p. 115, note 18.

[105] Jodin, "Les établissements du roi Juba II," p. 257. Villas, though lacking a bath or other heating apparatus, were found at Tipasa and Cotta.

[106] Sullecthum: Foucher, "Note," p. 18; Tipasa: Baradez, "Quatorze années," p. 235. A nearby fish pond had its walls elevated and channels constructed to connect it with the expanded garum factory. See Lassus, "Chronique l'archólogie algerienne," pp. 138–39.

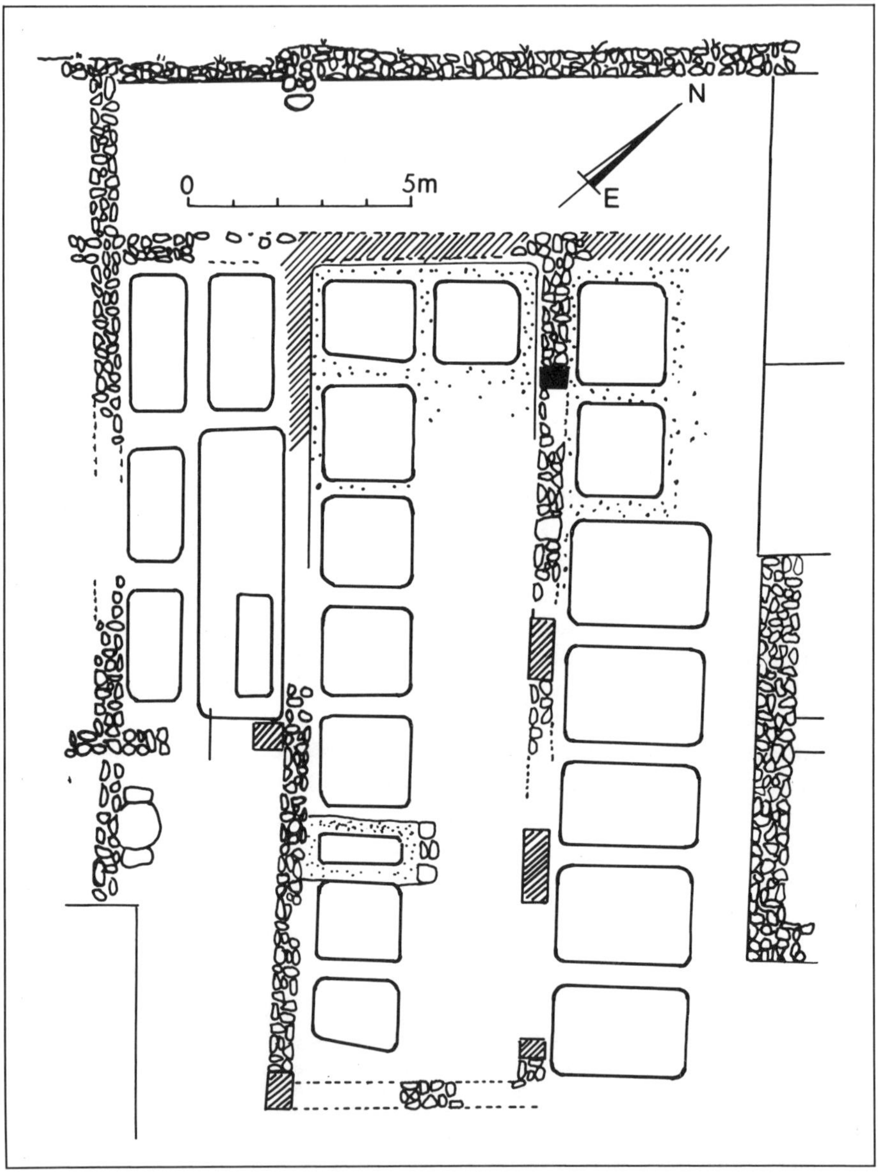

Figure 4: Lixus: Factory No. 9 (after Ponsich and Tarradell, *Garum*, Fig. 19)

the salteries. Remains of fish bones and scales, murex shells, fishhooks, and lead weights were found at Mogador, Tipasa, Cartenna, Alcazarsegher, and Tahadart. In Cotta and Tahadart, where furnaces formed part of the salting factory, cooking pots of various sizes and shapes were abundant. Some were mere bottles or pitchers, while others were large vessels with wide mouths.[107] Glass phials, similar to ampullae, found at some factories recall Ps-Rufius Festus' recipe for garum, in which the freshly made sauce was stored in a glass ampulla until used.[108]

Archaeologists have found no African saltery which antedates the late first century B.C., while the latest dates to the fifth or early sixth century A.D. The period of greatest attested activity was the first century A.D. Those begun during the late Republic include Lixus, Kouass, Cotta, and Mogador. At Lixus, of the eight datable factories, at least six began operation during the reign of Juba II (d. A.D. 23).[109] Other first century A.D. salteries include Tahadart, Sahara, Sania e Torres, Alcazarsegher, and probably Neapolis. Some of the salteries either ceased to function entirely or else drastically reduced their activity in the third century A.D. This was true for Cotta, Sahara, Mogador, and probably Neapolis.[110] Lixus, and possibly Kouass, Tahadart, and Alcazarsegher, functioned into the fifth century A.D. or later.[111] The decline in salting activity in Tingitana may have mirrored the "crisis" being experienced at the same time across the strait in Spain.

Evidence relating to the commerce of African salted fish products is not plentiful. Archaeological excavations indicate that many African salteries were operating in the first century B.C., and Pliny (*HN* 31.94) implies that by the middle of the first century A.D. Leptis was noted for its garum. Epigraphic evidence of the same period shows that at least one African merchant transported his product to Rome.[112] Whatever may have been the situation in Mauretania Tingitana, the merchants of Africa Proconsularis

[107] Ponsich and Tarradell (*Garum*, p. 108) postulate that the former may have held liquid garum, while the latter probably contained garum in thicker form. For garum containers see esp. Ponsich, *Aceite de Oliva y Salazones de Pescado*, pp. 55–77, esp. Figs. 21 and 27.

[108] Ponsich and Tarradell, *Garum*, p. 109. See also Ps-Rufius Festus *Brev.* (Appendix I-4). Vietnamese *nuoc-mam* and Philippine *patis* are often placed in glass bottles to age. See Mackie et al., *Fermented Fish Products*, p. 4; and Steinkraus et al., *Handbook*, p. 506.

[109] Ponsich, *Aceite de Olivia y Salazones de Pescado*, pp. 103–36.

[110] The installation at Cotta reduced its production of salted fish products in the third century and converted to oil production, utilizing the same vats and installing oil presses. See Ponsich, *Tanger*, p. 284.

[111] Lixus apparently sustained heavy damage in the third century, but was rebuilt in the fourth. See Ponsich and Tarradell, *Garum*, p. 37. In the mid-fourth century the northern part of the House of the Frescoes in Tipasa was renovated into a fish sauce factory, utilizing large dolia. Fire destroyed the house in the fifth century. Schleiermacher, "Tipasa," pp. 165–68; Jean Baradez, "Nouvelle fouilles à Tipasa," *Libyca* 9 (1961): 92–96.

[112] *CIL* VI.9676: D(is) M(anibus)/ TI(berius) CLAUDIUS DOCIMUS/ FECIT SIBI ET SUIS LIBERTIS/ LIBERTABUSQUE/ POSTERISQUE EORUM/ NEGOTIANS SALSAMENTARIUS/ ET VINARIARIUS MAURARIUS.

apparently competed independently with the Spaniards in the western markets. How well they competed remains unknown. Perhaps only Leptis was able to penetrate the near-monopoly of Spanish merchants with any success during the first century A.D. African amphorae are not well enough known to allow any conjecture on African salt-fish commerce until the third century A.D., when Spain began to lose its grip on the market.

No African amphora can be definitely associated with salted fish products, but two types found at Ostia, designated Africana I (type "Africano Piccolo") and Africana II (type "Africano Grande"), may have held fish sauce.[113] This conclusion was based on the stamp ASYL incised into the handle and connected with Sullecthum in Byzacena, where excavations have uncovered salting installations and amphorae with similar stamps.[114] The dating of these amphorae is uncertain but seems to fall into the middle or late third century A.D.[115] Containers from Africa Proconsularis and, to a lesser degree, Mauretania appear in significant quantities in Ostia in the second half of the third century A.D.[116] The mosaics of the Piazzale delle Corporazioni in Ostia indicate clearly that African products formed an important part of Ostian imports at this time. Most of the extant mosaics which indicate the origin of the shipper (*navicularius*) who rented the stall in the square date to the early third century, and the majority identify African shippers.[117] Among those represented are Carthage, Hippo Diarrytus, Gummi, and Sullecthum. Mosaic advertisements for Spanish shippers are conspicuously absent but may have been represented among those mosaics no longer extant. The preponderance of African shippers, nevertheless, is significant. The majority of shippers from Africa traded in grain. Sullecthum, however, probably sent oil, and possibly fish sauce. One mosaic bears the inscription M C, which may designate Mauretania Caesariensis. Oil may have also been the chief product from here, but again fish sauce cannot be excluded as a possibility, since both Tipasa and Cartenna operated salteries. Africana I and II amphorae have been found in fourth and fifth century A.D. contexts in Rome and other parts of Italy, while a shipwreck, found in the Bay of Pampelonne in Gaul near the île de Saint Tropez and dated to the late empire, contained many amphorae similar to

[113] Zevi and Tchernia, "Amphores de Byzacène," pp. 182–85. Byzacene amphorae found in an early fifth century A.D. deposit at the Schola Praeconum in Rome contained olive oil. David Whitehouse et al., "The Schola Praeconum II," *PBSR* 53 (1985): 200–03. But see also below, n. 118.

[114] Foucher, "Note," pp. 17–21. The factory remains unpublished.

[115] Zevi and Tchernia, "Amphores de Byzacène," p. 185.

[116] Panella, "Annotazioni," p. 101; Carandini and Panella, "Trading Connections," pp. 487–503.

[117] For the Piazzale delle Corporazioni see Russell Meiggs, *Roman Ostia*. 2nd ed. (Oxford 1973), pp. 283–88; Joël Le Gall, *Le Tibre dans l'antiquité* (Paris 1953): 238–42; and R. M. Haywood, *Roman Africa*, Vol. 4 (1938) of *ESAR*, pp. 62–64.

ones from Sullecthum. Apparently African salteries at this time were sending their products to Italian and Gallic markets.[118]

Although amphorae of Dressel Forms 7–13 found at Carthage show that Africa Proconsularis imported Spanish salted fish products, there is no reason to think that all of it came from Spain.[119] Many salteries operated in close proximity, such as at Neapolis, Leptis Minor, and probably Rusicade. Intra-provincial trade in fish sauce must have been a thriving business to support so many salteries. The tariff found at Zarai, a city on the border of Numidia and Mauretania Caesariensis, contains a reference to garum. Dating to A.D. 202 in its extant form and probably representing a modification of a tariff promulgated earlier, it seems to list locally produced products.[120] The fish sauce may have come from any number of salteries in Africa Proconsularis or Mauretania Caesariensis.

In summary, little can be said concerning African commerce in salted fish products. Leptis Minor had acquired a reputation for its garum in the first century A.D., but there is insufficient evidence to trace its commercial activity. Nothing can be said concerning the organization for commerce of any African province, except perhaps Mauretania Tingitana. Even here the evidence provides little more than a base for speculation. By the third century there were many shippers operating in Ostia, but there is no certainty that any carried salted fish products. The possibility is strong, however, since by this time Spanish trade in those items was declining and African commerce over-all was on the rise, at least with Italy. The salteries of Africa Proconsularis, perhaps especially Sullecthum in Byzacena, may account for the bulk of African salt-fish products sent to Italy and elsewhere at this period.

---

[118] For African amphorae in Italy, see Andrea Carignani and Francesco Pacetti, "Anfore tardo-antiche dagli scavi del Palatino," in *Amphores Romaines et Histoire Économique. Dix Ans de Recherche.* Coll. de l'École Française de Rome, 114 (Rome 1989), pp. 610–15; Dorica Manconi, "Anfore Romane in Umbria alla sinistra del Tevere," in *ibid*, pp. 590–93; and Marinella Pasquinucci, Linda Cherubini, Antonella Del Rio, Simonetta Menchelli, Simonetta Storti, and Maria Adelaide Vaggioli, "Ricerche archeologico-topographiche nella fascia costiera Tirrenica (*Ager Pisanus* e *Volaterranus* occidentale): risultati preliminari," in *ibid.*, pp. 620–25. For the shipwreck in the Bay of Pampelonne, see Robert Lequément, "Une épave du Bas-Empire dans la Baie de Pampelonne (presqu'île de Saint-Tropez)," *RAN* 9 (1976): 177–88. The fact that most of the amphorae, as well as similar ones found at La Luque at Marseille, contained shells of crustaceans indicates that the "Africano Grande" type amphora, which Zevi and Tchernia believe held oil, may have also held fish products. See also *idem*, "Étiquettes de Plomb," pp. 667–80, where Lequément had earlier arrived at the same conclusion based on inscribed lead tesserae attached to amphorae of this type. Parker tentatively suggests that, based on African amphoras found in an early third century A.D. wreck near Syracuse, African amphorae lined with pitch carried fish products; unlined, they contained olive oil. See D. J. L. Gibbins and A. J. Parker, "The Roman Wreck of c. AD 200 at Plemmirio, Near Siracusa (Sicily): Interim Report," *IJNA* 15,4 (1986): 287–90. A few African amphorae may have made their way to Britain, but the trade, if it existed at all, was insignificant.

[119] Zevi, "Appunti," p. 241.

[120] *CIL* VIII.4508. See also J. P. Darmon, "Note sur le Tarif de Zaraï," *Les cahiers de Tunisie* 48 (1964): 6–23.

Gaul

No literary evidence for fish salteries or for garum production in Gaul antedates the first century A.D., although the salting industry operated well before then. Fish salting in the area of the Étang de Berre on the Mediterranean coast north of Marseilles dates at least to the Bronze Age, and along the Narbonnese coast fish were being salted during the La Tène period.[121] Apparently, Gauls in all eras were partial to fish, and fish preservation was continuously practiced by the inhabitants residing along the Atlantic and Mediterranean coasts.

Fishing formed an important part of life in Roman Gaul. Fish caught in the waters off the southern coast of Gaul find mention in Aelian, Strabo and Pliny; Ausonius devotes a lengthy passage in the *Mosella* to enumerating the many kinds of fish caught in the Moselle River.[122] Tunny were caught off Massilia (Marseilles) and near the mouth of the Rhone River, while mullet were plentiful near Ruscino (Perpignan) and Massilia. A corporation of Gallic fishermen (*conductores piscatus*), probably from the Atlantic coast of Armorica, dedicated an inscription to a local goddess at Leeuwarden in the Netherlands.[123] Shellfish, such as oysters, came from Médoc, near Burdigala (Bordeaux), as well as Massilia and the Atlantic coast of Armorica. In fact, an industrial complex of the first century A.D. in Narbo may have even prepared garum from oysters.[124] Gallic fishermen extracted dye from shellfish, and in the late empire Narbo and Telo (Toulon) each possessed official textile factories (*baphia*).[125]

Excavation has confirmed literary references to fish processing activity at Forum Iulii and Antipolis.[126] A Gallo-Roman villa, not far from Forum Iulii at Villepey-le-Reydissard, may have included provisions for the production of garum. The remains at Antipolis are more significant, though by no means large. Between 1953 and 1964 excavators uncovered several small salting installations at various points around the bay of Antipolis. The salting vats show the usual characteristics, and small finds of fishhooks, small

[121] Fernand Benoit, *Recherches sur L'Hellénisation du Midi de la Gaule* (Aix-en-Provence 1965), p. 210.

[122] Aelian *NA* 13.16; Strabo 4.1.8; Pliny *HN* 9.59; Ausonius *Ep.* 5; *Mosella* 75–149.

[123] *CIL* XIII.8830: DEAE HLUDANAE/ CONDUCTORES/ PISCATUS MANCIPE/ Q VALERIO SECU/NDO V(otum) S(olvit) L(ibens) M(erito). The inscription cannot be dated.

[124] Tunny: Aelian *NA* 13.16; Oppian *Halieutica* 3.625–28. Mullet: Cassius Dio 40.54.3; Strabo 4.1.6. Oysters: Ausonius *Ep.* 5; and Michel Labrousse, "Recherches sur l'alimentation des populations gallo-romaines: escargot, huîtres et fruits de mer à Montmaurin," *Pallas* 8 (1959): 57–84. For a discussion of seafood available from Gaul see Louis C. West, *Roman Gaul, The Objects of Trade* (Oxford 1935), pp. 63–67; Camille Jullian, *Histoire de la Gaule*. Vol. 5 of *La civilisation gallo-romaine* (Paris 1908–26), pp. 197–200; Olwen Brogan, *Roman Gaul* (London 1953), pp. 136–37; and Patrick Galliou, *L'Armorique romaine* (Braspars 1984), pp. 115–20. Narbo: Y. Solier, "Dépôt d'huîtres au Boulevard de 1848," *Bulletin de la Commission archéologique de Narbonne* 38 (1964–65): 73–76.

[125] Vitruvius *De arch.* 7.13.2; *Not. dign. occ.* 11.72–73 (Seeck, ed., p. 152).

[126] Forum Iulii: Pliny *HN* 31.94–95; Antipolis: *ibid.*; Martial 4.88.5; 13.103.

heating vessels, and dolia, some half-buried, bespeak the fishing industry as well as indicate garum production in the area. A large basin of about ten meters on the sides, complete with small channels directed toward the sea, was probably used as a holding tank for fish.[127] Within the Gulf of Lyon salteries operated in the vicinity of the Étang de Vendres just north of Narbo, at Sète, at Argentiere near Scamandre, Châteauneuf-lez-Martigues, in the Camargue, especially at Notre-Dame-d'Amour on the Étang de Vaccares, at Carrelet, and in the vicinity of the Étang de Berre between Massilia and the mouth of the Rhone River.[128] Salting basins in the vicinity of the lakes of Berre and of Camargue exhibit characteristics analogous to those seen in Baetica and in the Algarve; that is, cement walls with an ovolo at the angles and a small depression or hole in the bottom.[129]

Archaeological excavations have discovered the remains of salting basins on the Atlantic coast in the Department of Charente-Maritime. At Le Gua at a place called le Fief de Chalons excavators uncovered two basins separated by a wall fifty centimeters thick.[130] The basins, constructed of a rubble of small stones, were covered with a reddish mortar. One of the two had in its corners and at the bottom the typical convex molding. Near Nieul-sur-Mer two other basins, better preserved than those at le Fief de Chalons, were found between two branches of a marsh.[131] The vats, also composed of a rubble of small stones, are likewise covered with a reddish mortar. An ovolo reinforces the angles in the same manner as at le Fief de Chalons. At the bottom, the vats have a small hole scooped out in the manner similar to

---

[127] A. Donnadieu, "Les fouilles des ruines gallo-romaines de Villepey (Villa Podii) près Fréjus (Forum Julii)," *Mémoires de l'institute des fouilles de Provence et des Préalpes* 1 (1926–29): 129–49; Raymond Lantier, "Ausgrabungen und neue Funde in Frankreich aus der Zeit von 1915 bis 1930 (Paläolithikum bis Römerzeit)," *Deutsches archäologisches Institut. Römish-germanische Kommission zwanzigster Bericht 1930* (Frankfurt am Main 1931), p. 125; and Albert Grenier, "Le garum de Fréjus," *REA* 34 (1932): 291–92. In the mid-1970s, on a hill to the west of the port of Fréjus excavators uncovered two small basins made of cement and tile and constructed on a pebble floor. In a nearby furnace were found some fish bones and pottery fragments, evidence leading the excavators to postulate the presence of a small garum factory. See Paul-Albert Février, "Les récents travaux archéologiques effectués à Fréjus (Var)," *BSAF* (1976): 26–27. For Antipolis see J. H. Clergues, "Les fouilles de la plaine d'Antibes: Vaugrenier. Note préliminaire," *RSL* 35 (1969): 178, and *idem*, "Fichier d'archéologie sous-marine du secteur d'Antibes," *Cahiers d'archéologie subaquatique* 1 (1972): 53–62.

[128] Benoit, *L'Hellénisation*, pp. 210–11. See also *idem*, "L'économie du littoral de la Narbonnaise à l'époque antique: le commerce du sel et les pêcheries," *RSL* 15 (1959): 104; *idem*, "L'archéologie sous-marine en Provence," *RSL* 18 (1952): 290–97; *idem*, "Les abbayes du sel. L'Héritage antique du delta au moyen-âge," *Delta* (*Revue économique et littéraire du delta du Rhône*) 3 (1961): 17–32, and *idem*, "Châteauneuf-lez-Martigues," *Gallia* 22 (1964): 578. For Sète, see G. Barruol, "Sète," *Gallia* 27 (1969): 400, and *idem*, *Gallia* 37 (1979): 533–34.

[129] Benoit, "Les abbayes du sel," p. 31. On the île Sainte-Marguerite in the Lérin Islands, opposite Cannes, there may have existed a fishery or saltery. See Jules Formigé, "La station antique de Lero à l'île Sainte-Marguerite (Alpes-Maritimes)," *Gallia* 5 (1947): 146–55.

[130] Gerard Nicolini, "Charente-Maritime: Le Gua," *Gallia* 35 (1977): 376; and *idem*, "Charente-Maritime: Le Gua," *Gallia* 37 (1979): 391–92.

[131] Nicolini, "Charente-Maritime: Le Gua," *Gallia* 35 (1977): 376–77. See also *idem*, "Charente-Maritime: Nieul-sur-mer," *Gallia* 37 (1979): 392.

many salting vats in Spain. A furnace was found nearby. Other sites of basins in the area include Saint-Nazaire-sur-Charente, Chateau d'Oleron, Germignac, and Brives-sur-Charente.[132]

The best information on Gallic fish processing comes from extensive archaeological work accomplished in Armorica (Brittany), in the departments of Côtes-du-Nord, Morbihan, and especially around the Bay of Douarnenez in the Department of Finistère. Since the publication in 1973 of about fifteen separate fish salteries in the area, archaeological work has further expanded our knowledge of these establishments, plus uncovered additional ones.[133] Included among the sites of fish salteries in Armorica are Audierne, Combrit at Kerobestin, Kerlaz at Lanevry, Plonevez-Porzay at Tréfeuntec, Poullan at Kerandraon, and Telgruc at Caon. Roads which seem to connect the salteries with each other converge on the area of Douarnenez, where most of the remains exist. Between Douarnenez and the beach of Sainte-Anne-la-Palue vestiges of fish salting activity appear approximately every five hundred meters.[134]

Remains of salteries at Douarnenez exist near the town itself and on the beach at Ris, but the most important site is at Plomarc'h, where saltery owners may have controlled the whole of the salting complex situated in the vicinity.[135] This factory is composed of three separate areas. The best excavated section, designated No. 2, contains sixteen vats arranged in two groups of seven basins with the groups separated by two central vats.[136] These vats were constructed within an enclosed 30 x 18 meter rectangular area which was once roofed. The basins, sunk into the ground and surrounded by an open area of fine gravel used as work space permitting easy access to the vats, measured approximately 3.6 meters on each side and were coated with *opus signinum* and reinforced at the angles. The vats of No. 1, though not as completely excavated as those of No. 2, show similar characteristics, except that whereas the angles of the former were reinforced with an ovolo the reinforcement of the latter was rather flat. To the north of the five vats of No. 1 are traces of a furnace. Although Armorican salteries show characteristics common to those found in Spain and North

---

[132] Nicolini, "Charente-Maritime: Le Gua," *Gallia* 35 (1977): 376, note 11.

[133] René Sanquer and Patrick Galliou, "Garum, sel et salaisons en Armorique gallo-romaine," *Gallia* 30 (1972): 199–223. See also Patrick Galliou, "Les industries de salaisons en Armorique romaine," *Caesarodunum* 10 (1975): 141–47; René Sanquer, "Bretagne: Douarnenez," *Gallia* 33 (1975): 349–50; *idem*, "Bretagne: Douarnenez," *Gallia* 35 (1977): 355–60; *idem*, "Bretagne: Plonevez-Porzay," *Gallia* 37 (1979): 365; and *idem*, "Bretagne: Plomodiern," *Gallia* 37 (1979): 365. Galliou, *L'Armorique romaine*, pp. 126–31, gives a summary of possible and confirmed sites of Armorican salteries.

[134] René Sanquer, "Une nouvelle lecture de l'inscription à Neptune trouvée à Douarnenez (Finistère) et l'industrie du garum armoricain," *Annales de Bretagne* 80 (1973): 216.

[135] Pierre Merlat, "Ploaré-Douarnenez," *Gallia* 15 (1957): 186–90; Sanquer and Galliou, "Garum," pp. 209–11; and Sanquer, "Douarnenez," *Gallia* 35 (1977): 355–60.

[136] Unit No. 2 at Plomarc'h comprised 750 $m.^3$ of salting space, while all the Armorican salteries combined totaled several thousand cubic meters. See Galliou, *L'Armorique romaine*, p. 133.

Africa, with the exception of small vats found at Kerandraon-en-Poullan, they generally do not vary between large and small ones. The vats at Kerobestin averaged 2.60 x 2.94 x 3.34 meters, while those on the beach at Ris near Douarnenez averaged 3.70 x 2.80 x 1.60 meters. Many of the Armorican vats, when excavated, yielded broken tiles which probably served to press down the material during fermentation.[137]

Remains of processed animals were found in several vats in Armorica. Most of the remains were of fish, such as eels and sardines found at Combrit and sardines, sprats, and perhaps a sea-pike at Plomarc'h.[138] At the latter site one vat in Section No. 1 yielded a carmelized layer of brownish material one or two millimeters in thickness and strongly impregnated with the odor of fish. This may be the desiccative remains of garum.[139] At Pointe du Guet, of eight vats grouped in a U-shape, three contained vertebrae, scales, and bones of sardines and bream along with remains of beef and sheep. These latter discoveries are not totally unexpected. Since Strabo remarks that Gaul exported salted pork and sheep to Rome and other parts of Italy and Columella notes that the method of salting pork was similar to that for preserving fish, the salting of meat other than marine animals in fish salteries is not surprising. This also helps to explain Dioscorides' remark that garum could be made from meat other than fish.[140] Meat may have been salted in these installations when fish were unavailable.

Gallic salteries, like those in Spain and Africa, were located on sites which allowed access to fresh water and salt. Salteries near Étang de Berre could obtain water from tributaries of the Rhone River, and those near Villepey could acquire it from the Reydissard, a small stream nearby. The Armorican salteries all lay near small streams or deep estuaries. Salt was for Gaul among the least of its worries. Its many salt marshes, especially in the Gulf of Lyon, provided the province with a lucrative export product.[141] Armorican salteries appear to have produced salt by evaporation of salt water through a system of shallow ditches lined with tiles and heated by a nearby furnace.[142] The salteries of Gallia Narbonensis and of coastal Armorica, with one exception, lay near beaches or large saltwater lakes, but on a level

[137] *Ibid.*, pp. 207, 212, 219; and cf. *ibid.*, p. 131. For the tiles see Sanquer and Galliou, "Garum," p. 219.

[138] Kerobestin: Sanquer and Galliou, "Garum," p. 207. Plomarc'h: Sanquer, "Douarnenez," *Gallia* 35 (1977): 359.

[139] Sanquer, "Douarnenez," *Gallia* 35 (1977): 359. Cf. above, p. 21.

[140] Strabo 4.4.3: οὕτως δ' ἐστὶ δαψιλῆ καὶ τὰ ποίμνια καὶ τὰ ὑοφόρβια, ὥστε τῶν σάγων καὶ τῆς ταριχείας ἀφθονίαν μὴ τῇ Ῥώμῃ χορηγεῖσθαι μόνον, ἀλλὰ καὶ τοῖς πλείστοις μέρεσι τῆς Ἰταλίας. Columella *Rust.* 12.55.4; Dioscorides *De mat. med.* 2.32. For Pointe de Guet see René Sanquer, "Informations archéologiques. Bretagne (Finistère). Douarnenez," *Gallia* 41 (1983): 291–92. Vats at Kerobestin have also yielded bones of cattle cut into quarters, and a basin at Telgruc contained sheep bones.

[141] For Gallic salt resources see Benoit, "Le commerce du sel," pp. 87–110.

[142] Sanquer and Galliou, "Garum," pp. 221–23; Galliou, "Les industries de salaisons," pp. 145–46; and *idem*, *L'Armorique romaine*, pp. 120–25.

high enough to avoid the tides.[143] In Armorica a small factory of four large vats, covered by a roof and preceded by a court on two sides of which was a warehouse complex, operated at Lanester (Morbihan) on the banks of the estuary of Blavet.[144] Two watertight vats could have served to prepare salt-fish, while two uncoated vats may have been used to dry fish or store them before salting. This factory seems designed to prepare river fish, such as mullet, eel and trout.

Gallic salteries are almost always found with subsidiary structures. Villas appear contiguous to salteries at Villepey-le-Reydissard, on the Étang de Berre, and in Armorica at Trequer and Douarnenez which had three villas nearby. Furnaces accompanied Armorican salting facilities at Plomarc'h, Ris, Lanevry, Camezen and Trefeuntec, as well as the one at Nieul-sur-Mer in Charente-Maritime. These furnaces may have served to produce salt needed in the salting process or, perhaps, to accelerate the garum production process. Small containers commonly used in Spain and Africa to concentrate garum, however, are, with the exception of Plomarc'h and Antibes, generally lacking from Gallic salteries. At Ris in Douarnenez the saltery was preceded by a cement ramp sloping toward the sea, which may have served for drying fishermen's nets. At Curnic in Guissény (Finistère) a 6.0 x 5.32 meters fish pond lay on the beach.[145] Though not demonstrably connected with a saltery, it does recall the installations found at Antibes.

Archaeological investigation has yielded only scanty evidence for establishing a firm chronology for the Gallic salteries. The earliest saltery so far excavated is that at Villepey-le-Reydissard and dates to the late first century B.C. Those of Armorica which can be dated belong to the period between the first and fourth centuries A.D., but flourished primarily in the second and third centuries A.D.[146] Sanquer and Galliou believe that the Romans took over and improved upon a salting process practiced by the Gauls in the proto-historic period and added to it the production of garum, a product unknown to the Gauls. Benoit earlier had come to a similar conclusion with respect to Gallic salting activity in the Gulf of Lyon.[147] It remains true,

---

[143] Sanquer and Galliou, "Garum," p. 220. The vats at Kerandraon lay farther up on a cliff near a small stream. Only four small vats, measuring 1 x 1 meter, give evidence for fish processing activity. *Ibid.*, p. 217.

[144] Patrick André, "Les pêcheries romaines du Blavet," *Archéologie en Bretagne* 32 (1981): 43–45; René Sanquer, "Informations archéologiques, Bretagne. Morbihan: Lanester," *Gallia* 39 (1981): 316–18; and *idem*, "Informations archéologiques. Bretagne. Lanester," *Gallia* 41 (1983): 289–90.

[145] Galliou, "Les industries de salaisons," p. 145; Clergues, "Fichier," p. 55. For Ris and Curnic see Galliou, *L'Armorique romaine*, p. 117.

[146] Donnadieu, "Villepey," pp. 146–47; Sanquer and Galliou, "Garum," passim; Sanquer, "Douarnenez," *Gallia* 33 (1975): 349; and *idem*, "Douarnenez," *Gallia* 35 (1977): 359. See also Patrick Galliou and René Sanquer, "L'industrie du garum et des salaisons en Armorique romaine," *Caesarodunum* 10 (1975): 158; Patrick Galliou, "Western Gaul in the Third Century," in *The Roman West in the Third Century*. Anthony King and Martin Henig, eds. BAR International Series, 109 (Oxford 1981), p. 267; and Galliou, *L'Armorique romaine*, pp. 134–35.

[147] Sanquer and Galliou, "Garum," p. 223; Benoit, *L'Hellénisation*, p. 209.

however, that regardless of the actual antiquity of the salting process in Gaul the oldest salting facilities so far excavated date to the Roman period, and these no earlier than the Augustan era.

The latest date for Gallic salting activity perhaps comes also from Villepey-le-Reydissard where the villa near the salting installation was destroyed in the late fourth or early fifth century A.D. It is uncertain, however, if the vats were in use at that time. The Armorican salteries show a marked decline in activity by the late third century, with a few functioning into the mid-fourth.[148] The determination of a *terminus post quem non* for fish sauce production in Gaul is complicated by references to garum found in official documents dating to the sixth century A.D. and later.[149] Near the Étang de Berre several basins for salting fish were found in close proximity to a villa dating to the Carolingian period.[150] Although these vats may have only been utilized by the owners of the Roman villa which preceded the Carolingian one, the possibility of Carolingian salting activity seems a strong one. It is certain, however, that the Gallic salteries were at best operating at a much reduced level of activity possibly as early as the late-third century and definitely by the mid-fourth century A.D.[151] The cause for this decline should probably be sought, as in Spain, in the increasing insecurity and general economic decline of the third and fourth centuries.

Commerce in Gallic fish products has left few remains. Although the remarks of Pliny and Martial concerning fish sauce in Antipolis and Forum Iulii imply that Gaul did export salted fish products, the extent of this activity will remain a mystery until more is known about Gallic amphorae. A variant of a Dressel Form 2–4 amphora, dating to the Flavian period and found in Southwark, London, bore a *titulus pictus* identifying its contents as liquamen from Antipolis. Another one of the same form and with a similar *titulus* has come to light at Ostia.[152]

---

[148] As at Plomarc'h and Lanevry. See Sanquer and Galliou, "Garum," pp. 211 and 213, respectively; Galliou, "Western Gaul," p. 275; *idem*, *L'Armorique romaine*, pp. 249–52; and *idem*, "Celtic Permanence or Roman Change? Roman Brittany Revisited," *Oxford Journal of Archaeology* 5,1 (Mar. 1986): 73.

[149] See below, pp. 184–86.

[150] Benoit, "Le commerce du sel," pp. 104–05.

[151] The salting establishment at Kerobestin on the Bay of Douarnenez was destroyed in A.D. 270, although the town continued to be inhabited into the fourth century A.D. See Sanquer and Galliou, "Garum," p. 208.

[152] Hassall and Tomlin, "Roman Britain in 1983," p. 344; Peacock and Williams, *Amphorae and the Roman Economy*, p. 106, with a photograph of the *titulus* as frontispiece. For the vessel at Ostia, still unpublished, see Fanette Laubenheimer, "Les amphores Gauloises sous l'Empire: recherches nouvelles sur leur production et leur chronologie," in *Amphores Romaines et Histoire Économique. Dix Ans de Recherche*. Coll. de l'École Française de Rome, 114 (Rome 1989), pp. 106–07. D. P. S. Peacock states that an amphora of G(ari) F(los) S(combri) found near Hadrian's Wall at Vindolanda shows similarities in fabric and form to vessels in the northwest area of the Gulf of Lyon. See Wright and Hassall, "Roman Britain in 1973," p. 467, no. 44. Wright and Hassall, in contrast to Peacock, would rather place the origin of the amphora in Lusitania in Spain. Alarcão, *Roman Portugal*, 1: 146, note 108, suggests that the vessel came from Esuris, probably Castro Marim, along the River Tagus. Cf. Stéfanie Martin-Kilcher, "Fischsaucen und Fischkonserven aus dem römischen Gallien," *Archäologie der Schweiz* 13 (1990): 37–44.

The salteries of Gaul's Atlantic coast appear to be an anomaly. Besides a few examples in Charente-Maritime (Le Gua and Nieul-sur-Mer, for instance), they concentrate in the Bay of Douarnenez (Finistère), probably because of the abundance of fish in the area. One, however, has been found in the department of Morbihan at Lanester and a few possible sites have come to light in Côtes-du-Nord. Perhaps there is a connection between the conventus of Roman citizens residing in the area of Douarnenez and possibly engaging in the commerce, if not also the production, of salted fish products, and the salting installations in Spain or in Provence.[153] The need to supply food to the army camps in Gaul and especially in Britain provides reason enough to establish at this particular point an industry analogous to those in Spain, Africa and the Mediterranean coast of Gaul. The Armorican salteries probably also supplied local markets, and possibly engaged in more wide-ranging interprovincial trade.[154] Perhaps future excavation will show the Armorican salteries not to have been so anomalous. Recent finds of salting basins in the department of Charente-Maritime hold out promise of finding more sites on the Atlantic coast of Gaul.

The large number of shipwrecks which contained Spanish fish sauce amphorae discovered along the Mediterranean coast and the many similar amphorae found in the interior of Gaul and along the *limes* indicate that Gallic merchants, at least in the first two centuries A.D., imported significant amounts of Spanish fish products. They probably served in the capacity of middlemen by transferring the products from sea-going vessels to smaller ones which could traverse the Rhone, Saone and Rhine Rivers. Marcus Primus Secundianus, who lived in Lugdunum, was not only a member of a corporation of Rhodanian sailors (*nautae*) but was also a fish sauce merchant (*negotians muriarius*).[155] The major port for this exchange of Spanish for Gallic transportation was Fos, located near the mouth of the Rhone River. Excavations in the vicinity of this city have uncovered frag-

---

[153] Sanquer, "Inscription à Neptune," pp. 215–36; and *idem*, "Les industriels des salaisons en Armorique romaine," *Caesarodunum* 10 (1975): 148–56. In the latter article Sanquer notes the discovery of a similar inscription to Neptune found near a salting installation on the beach in the province of Pontevedra. These two inscriptions seem to indicate a close, but not surprising, relationship between Neptune, the god of the sea, and Roman fish salting installations. Cf. *CIL* V.7850, where fishermen make a dedication to Neptune.

[154] Many amphorae found in Armorica indicate that the area did have trading contacts outside Western Gaul. How active was this trade is unknown. See Nora K. Chadwick, *Early Brittany* (Cardiff 1969), pp. 101–12. For an Atlantic commercial route from Spain and the Mediterranean to Northwest Gaul and Britain see Galliou, *L'Armorique romaine*, pp. 170–75. Although wine and oil amphorae are abundantly represented, Dressel Form 7–13 vessels are not numerous, a fact which may imply that local salt-fish production sufficed in Brittany (*ibid.*, p. 178). The capacity of the salting installations at Plomarc'h alone, over 1,000 cubic meters, probably allowed for exportation. See Galliou, "Western Gaul in the Third Century," p. 267.

[155] *CIL* XIII.1966(= *ILS* 7028): D(is) M(anibus)/ ET MEMORIAE AETERNAE/ M(arci) PRIMI SECUNDIANI IIIIII VIR(i) AUG(ustalis)/ C(oloniae) C(opiae) C(laudiae) AUG(ustae) LUG(duno) CURATOR(is) EIUSD(em) COR/POR(is) NAUTAE RHODANI(ci) ARARE NA/VIGANT(is) CORPORAT(i) INTER FABROS/ TIGN(arios) LUG(duni) CONSIST(entis) NEGOT(iantis) MURIAR(ii)/ M(arcus) PRIMUS AUGUSTUS FIL(ius) ET HERES PATRI/ KARISSIM(O) PONEND(um) CUR(avit) ET SUB ASC(ia) DED(icavit). Spanish garum and liquamen vessels have been found at Lugdunum and garum amphorae at Saint-

ments of over 24,000 amphorae, many of which contained fish products from Spain and Italy.[156] Two fish sauce vessels, urcei of Pompeian Form VI, found at Fos bear *tituli picti* identifying the contents as fish sauce made by Aulus Umbricius Scaurus, Pompeii's leading fish sauce producer (Pl. 7b).[157] Commerce in salted fish products passing through Gaul en route to the northern provinces was apparently a thriving and well organized business.

Britain and the Northern Provinces

Up to this point allusion has been made to extensive commercial traffic in Mediterranean salt-fish products in the northern provinces and Britain.[158] Before elaborating on this a word should be said concerning the production of preserved fish products in these areas. No evidence exists for extensive fish salteries of the types found in Spain, Africa, and Gaul. Perhaps small installations of the size found at Lanester (Morbihan) in Armorica also existed along the Thames River in England or on the continent along the Rhine and Danube Rivers and their tributaries, but, if so, they have left few remains.

Fish and salt were abundantly available in northern waters and were certainly utilized in the medieval period in France and England.[159] The herring inhabits almost exclusively the Northeastern Atlantic, while a closely related species, the anchovy, inhabits the Mediterranean and migrates in the spring along the French, Belgian, and Dutch coasts to the East Frisian littoral. In the fall they migrate to the northern part of the English Channel along the English coast. Other related species, such as sprat and sardine, were available in northern waters and the shad could be found in inland rivers. In Britain, near Richborough, along the North Kent and Essex coasts, and in the Thames estuary oysters were plentiful, so much so that they were exported to Rome as early as the first century B.C.[160] Salt-making sites existed at several places along the Belgian coast in the Iron Age and

Romain-en-Gal, at Vienne also on the Rhone River. See Armand Desbat, Robert Lequément and Bernard Liou, "Inscriptions peintes sur amphores: Lyon et Saint-Romain-en-Gal," *Archaeonautica* 7 (1987): 154–59 (Lyon), 164–66 (Saint-Romain-en-Gal); and Christine Becker, Claudine Constantin, and Françoise Villedieu, "Types d'amphores en usage à Lugdunum du Ier au VIe siècle," in *Amphores Romaines et Histoire Économique. Dix Ans de recherche*. Coll. de l'École Française de Rome, 114 (Rome 1989), pp. 656–59.

[156] Robert Diot, "La route des amphores," *Aventure sous-marine* 21 (1959): 25; Benoit, "Provence (III)," pp. 147–50; L. Monguilan, "Geographie commerciale de la Gaule. Un port romain dans le Golfe de Fos," *Caesarodunum* 12 (1977): 359–70; Liou and Marichal, "Les inscriptiones," pp. 109–81; and Robert I. Curtis, "Spanish Trade in Salted Fish Products in the 1st and 2nd Centuries A.D.," *IJNA* 17,3 (1988): 205–10.

[157] For Spanish and Pompeian fish sauce vessels found at Fos see Liou and Marichal, "Les inscriptions," pp. 131–45, 165–67. For possible evidence of Gallic import of African fish products in the late empire see Lequément, "La Baie de Pampelonne," pp. 177–88.

[158] The term "northern provinces" refers to those lying along the Rhine and Danube Rivers: Pannonia, Noricum, Raetia, Germania Superior, Germania Inferior, and Gallia Belgica.

[159] See below, p. 186.

[160] Bernard Grzimek, *Grzimek's Animal Life Encyclopedia*. English Edition (New York 1973), 4: 199; and Curtis, "*Negotiatores Allecarii*," pp. 154–55. Sprats and sardines went into the salting

Roman periods and there is increasing evidence for pre-Roman and Roman salt-works on the east and south coasts of England, as well as inland.[161] The areas offering the best hope for discovering northern salting installations are the coastal areas of Britain, Gallia Belgica, and Germania Inferior.[162] As yet, however, only London has yielded firm evidence for Roman fish preservation.

Excavations along the waterfront of Roman Londinium have revealed a structure, called the Peninsular House, which dates from the first century A.D. and which apparently housed commercial activities through the early fourth century.[163] Located near the waterfront quay it had easy access to ships docking there. On the third century floor lay a three-inch layer of fish bones, primarily of herring and sprat. Also nearby was a broken South Spanish salt-fish vessel (Camulodunum 186), dating to the late first century A.D. and probably reused for the local product. Since herring are not indigenous to the Mediterranean, the fish bones must have been of North Atlantic origin. It has been suggested that what existed here was a local fish processing center of the third century A.D. which utilized a timber tank and drain arrangement for the fermentation process. If fish processors in Britain and Northern Europe used wood, a highly perishable item, for their salting vats, it would help to explain the lack of evidence for salting installations in those provinces. On the other hand, it seems more likely that the structure served as a central warehouse where fish sauce prepared elsewhere in more permanent facilities of the kind found in Armorica, perhaps farther up (or down) the Thames River, was collected for shipping elsewhere.[164]

Spanish salt-fish amphorae appear as far north as Vindolanda, just south of Hadrian's Wall in Britain.[165] Spanish merchants had three potential routes to Britain from which to choose. The fastest and probably least ex-

---

vats in Armorica at Plomarc'h and Combrit. See Sanquer and Galliou, "Garum," p. 207, and Sanquer, "Informations archéologiques: Douarnenez," *Gallia* 35 (1977): 355–60. For oysters see J. Winder in Gustav Milne, *The Port of Roman London* (London 1985), pp. 91–95.

[161] *Salt. The Study of an Ancient Industry.* K. W. De Brisay and K. A. Evans, eds. (Colchester 1975), passim.

[162] Discovered at Aardenburg in Gallia Belgica was a dolium with a pre-firing incised inscription: ALIIC XI S(emis), or "Allec, 11.5 amphorae." Whether the sauce was locally produced or imported cannot be determined. See J. E. Bogaers, "Nehalennia en de epigrafische Gegevens," in *Deae Nehalenniae* (Leiden 1971), p. 40. Roman fishing activity in the Netherlands in the first century A.D. is attested at Leeuwarden in the Dutch province of Friesland, where a Roman citizen, Q. Valerius Secundus, a *manceps* of a *societas* of *conductores piscatus*, dedicated an altar to Hludana, a local goddess. See *CIL* XIII.8830; and Diedrich Bohlen, *Die Bedeutung der Fischerei für die antike Wirtschaft* (Hamburg 1937), p. 46.

[163] Nic Bateman and Alison Locker, "The Sauce of the Thames," *The London Archaeologist* 4 (1982): 204–07; Milne, *Port of Roman London*, pp. 87–91.

[164] Cf. the finds at Cerro del Mar in Spain, above p. 57, and a possibly similar arrangement in Pompeii where dolia, rather than wooden structures, were used (below, p. 93). For wooden vats used to produce Philippine *patis* see Crisan and Sands, "Microflora," p. 107; for Vietnamese *nuoc-mam* prepared commercially, see Steinkraus et al., *Handbook*, p. 517.

[165] Wright and Hassall, "Roman Britain in 1973," p. 467, no. 44. Writing tablets found in the fort also contained a reference to muria, perhaps forming part of army supplies purchased by

pensive was the Atlantic Sea route, passing through the Strait of Gibraltar and skirting along the western coasts of Spain and Gaul. This was the most direct route and sufficient port facilities existed along the way. The second major route, with variants, utilized the inland waterways of Gaul to arrive at Atlantic ports. For example, one could off-load the cargo from sea-going vessels near Narbo, place it on river craft, and proceed to Burdigala by way of the Garumna (Garonne) River. Or, one could off-load at Fossae Marianae (Fos) onto river craft which could traverse the Rhodanus (Rhone) River to Lugdunum where two options existed. First, one could, after a short trip by land, traverse the Liger (Loire) River to Condevicnum (Nantes). Second, one could transfer to the Arar (Saone) River and farther north transfer again to the Sequana (Seine) River which led directly to the coast at Juliobona (Lillebonne). At Burdigala, Condevicnum, or Juliobona one could transfer back to sea-going ships for the rest of the journey to Britain.[166]

Little evidence exists to indicate that any of these two major western routes or their variants received extensive use to transport salted fish products. One might expect to find a large number of Spanish salt-fish amphorae along the way, particularly in Brittany where the native salteries did not become active until the second century A.D. This is not the case, however. Dressel Forms 7–13, the usual first century A.D. salt-fish types, are quite rare in Armorica.[167] This is also true for the south and southwestern coasts of England which one would expect the Atlantic routes to service extensively. Even when found in Eastern and South-eastern England, though at no time in abundance, salt-fish amphorae of Dressel Forms 7–13 are rare in the land of the Durotriges.[168] That some salt-fish merchants did use the Atlantic routes may be surmised from several scattered finds of Dressel Forms 7–11 and Beltrán Form IIB amphorae near Guernsey, the Channel Islands.[169]

---

a soldier for his private use. See Alan K. Bowman, "Roman Military Records From Vindolanda," *Britannia* 5 (1974): 368–69.

166 For the theoretical costs of the various trade routes from the Mediterranean to Britain see D. P. S. Peacock, "The Rhine and the Problem of Gaulish Wine in Roman Britain," in *Roman Shipping and Trade: Britain and the Rhine Provinces*. Joan du Plat Taylor and Henry Cleere, eds. (London 1978), p. 49 and Table III. For various ports in Lusitania, see Edmondson, *Two Industries*, pp. 152–56; for those in Western Gaul see Galliou, *L'Armorique romaine*, pp. 170–74; for Juliobona, see M. Yvart, "Juliobona," in *Princeton Encyclopedia*, pp. 427–28.

167 Galliou, *L'Armorique romaine*, p. 178. Dressel Form 7–11 amphorae have been found in Narbo and in some of its outer ports, such as La Nautique and l'Étang de Mateille. See Yves Solier, "Les épaves de Gruissan," *Archaeonautica* 3 (1981): 226–27, 255.

168 D. F. Williams, "The Roman Amphora Trade with Late Iron Age Britain," in *Production and Distribution: a Ceramic Viewpoint*. Hilary Howard and Elaine L. Morris, eds. BAR International Series, 120 (Oxford 1981), p. 130. Salt-fish vessels of form Pelichet 46 have been found to the north of Isca (Caerleon). See R. E. M. Wheeler and T. V. Wheeler, "The Roman Amphitheatre at Caerleon, Monmouthshire," *Archaeologia* 78 (1928): 186–88, esp. fig. 23, no. 78.

169 Richard Keen, "Great Britain: Guernsey, Channel Islands: Little Russel Amphora Site A," *IJNA* 8,1 (1979): 87. Ausonius (*Ep.* 25) may confirm use of the Garonne route in the fourth century A.D. when he mentions the gift of a container of Spanish fish sauce sent to him in Burdigala from Barcino. There is no reason, however, to conclude that at this late date the

The third route was without doubt the primary trade route connecting the Mediterranean salteries with markets in the northern provinces and Britain. Transferring from sea-going ships to river craft at Fossae Marianae, salt-fish merchants could ascend the Rhone River to Lugdunum where they had the option first of continuing to Lake Geneva and, after a short hop by land to Vindonissa, of travelling the Rhine River to the Atlantic Coast; or second, of transferring to the Saone and then Doubs Rivers and then travelling overland to the Rhine River at Augusta Raurica (Augst) and thence on to the coast of Germania Inferior near modern Colijnsplaat.[170] It was a short trip from there across the Channel to Britain. Large numbers of salt-fish amphorae and vessels containing other products made their way to the north along this route, bound both for the Rhineland and Britain where legion and auxiliary units manned the frontier and where there were large civilian population centers as well.[171]

A listing of all the places in the northern provinces where Spanish salt-fish amphorae have been found would be long and tedious. A few sites will suffice to illustrate the distribution (Fig. 7): those in Germania Superior include Windisch (Vindonissa) and Hofheim; in Raetia, at Augsberg (Augusta Vindelicum), Breyenze (Brigantium), and Aislingen; and in Germania Inferior, at Oberaden, Haltern, and Nijmegen (Noviomagus).[172] Beltrán Form I amphorae reached Colchester Sheepen in Britain in large numbers in the period A.D. 43–60/61. Other significant finds in Britain in-

---

route extended as well all the way to Britain. For wine amphorae (Dressel Form 1) found along various routes through Armorica, see Patrick Galliou, "Days of Wine and Roses? Early Armorica and the Atlantic Wine Trade," in *Cross-Channel Trade Between Gaul and Britain in the Pre-Roman Iron Age.* Sarah Macready and F. H. Thompson, eds. (London 1984), pp. 24–36.

[170] Geneva: Daniel Paunier, *La céramique gallo-romaine de Genève* (Geneva 1981), pp. 236–38; Vindonissa: Theodora Tomašević *Die Keramik der XIII Legion aus Vindonissa.* Veröffentlichungen der Gesellschaft pro Vindonissa, No. 7 (Vindonissa 1970), pp. 74–75. *Tituli picti* on two amphorae from Augst denote their contents as G(arum) HISP(anum) and MUR(ia) HISP(ana). These probably refer to the Spanish origin of the product since the vessels appear to be of type Dressel Forms 7–11. Oskar Bohn, however, believes that the sauces were possibly made according to a Spanish recipe. A third amphora containing garum made from the mackerel was of form Pelichet 46. See Oskar Bohn, "Pinselschriften," pp. 202–04, esp. Tafel XI, no. 285. The River Scheldt, which empties into the Atlantic near Colijnsplaat, was in antiquity connected by a network of waterways with other major rivers, such as the Rhine, Maas, and Waal. See Piet Stuart, "Nehalennia: Goddess from the Sea," *Delta* 14 (Aug., 1971): 21. See *CIL* XIII.1966 for a Rhodanian sailor (*nauta Rhodanicus*) who was also a *negotiator muriarius* operating on the Saone River.

[171] Peacock, "Gaulish Wine in Roman Britain," p. 50, reaches this conclusion for the wine trade. See also Armand Desbat and Stéfanie Martin-Kilcher, "Les amphores sur l'axe Rhône-Rhin à l'époque d'Auguste," in *Amphores Romaines et Histoire Économique. Dix Ans de Recherche.* Coll. de l'École Française de Rome, 114 (Rome 1989), pp. 339–65.

[172] An extensive list can be found in Berti et al., *Ostia II*, pp. 136–37. See also Carandini and Panella, *Ostia III*, pp. 514–15; Elisabeth Ettlinger, "Aspects of Amphora-Typology, – Seen from the North," in *Méthodes classiques et méthodes formelles dans l'étude des amphores* (Actes du Colloque de Rome, 27–29 Mai 1974). Collection de l'École Française de Rome, 32 (Rome 1977), pp. 9–16, and Desbat and Martin-Kilcher, "Les amphores sur l'axe Rhône-Rhin," esp. pp. 348–52, and Fig. 10.

clude those at London and Canterbury.[173] Amphora finds at several of these places were large enough to form the basis for constructing amphora typologies. These include Vindonissa, Oberaden, Hofheim, and Haltern in the Rhineland and Colchester (Camulodunum) in Britain.[174]

The reason for this concentration of Spanish salt-fish amphorae in Northern Europe close to or along the *limes* is no mystery. The army had to be fed, and salted fish formed part of the soldier's diet. The *Historia Augusta* alludes to this fact and archaeological discoveries at Vindolanda in Britain, Vindonissa in Germania Superior, and elsewhere confirm it. It is significant that the numbers of Spanish salt-fish amphorae decrease in the northern provinces and Britain after the early second century A.D. The reasons for this are unclear. It has been suggested that the ethnic make-up of the legions became less Mediterranean and more Germanic and so soldiers were less inclined to favor fish in their diet.[175] If this suggestion is correct, commerce in Spanish salted fish products, at least to northern markets, may have begun to decline well before the Severan period of the early third century A.D. This does not explain, however, the continued demand for salted fish products in the northern provinces after the second century A.D. *Negotiatores allecarii* (Pl. 6) operated between Colijnsplaat in Germania Inferior and Britain in the late second or early third century A.D., while at roughly the same time the Gallic salteries in Armorica were enjoying their period of greatest activity. Across the Channel, the Peninsular House site, where merchants dealt in preserved herring and sprats, dates to the third century A.D.[176] How much of the salted fish products in Britain or the northern provinces from the third century on were of Spanish origin is uncertain; an

[173] Sealey, *Colchester Sheepen*, pp. 18–19, 77–85; Canterbury: Paul Arthur, "Roman Amphorae from Canterbury," *Britannia* 17 (1986): 244–50; London: Bateman and Locker, "Sauce of the Thames," p. 207; and Milne, *Port of Roman London*, p. 91: "of all the amphoras found in London, some 20 per cent are associated with the Spanish garum trade,. . . ." D. P. S. Peacock has found Spanish fish sauce amphorae at several other sites in Britain, such as in Cornwall, Gloucestershire, Buckinghamshire, and Cambridgeshire. See D. P. S. Peacock, "Roman Amphorae in Pre-Roman Britain," in *The Iron Age and its Hill Forts*. David Hill and Margaret Jesson, eds. (Southampton 1971), pp. 180–84, and *idem*, "Amphorae in Iron Age Britain: a Reassessment," in *Cross-Channel Trade Between Gaul and Britain in the Pre-Roman Iron Age*. Sarah Macready and F. H. Thompson, eds. (London 1984), pp. 37–42.

[174] For references see Ettlinger, "Aspects of Amphora-Typology," p. 12. As an example, Dressel Forms 7–11, primarily of the late first century B.C. to the end of the first century A.D., equate roughly to Haltern 69, Hofheim 72, Vindonissa 586, Oberaden 80/81, and Camulodunum 186A; Pelichet 46, dating from the late first century A.D. into the second century A.D., equates to Beltrán IIB and Vindonissa 587. See Paunier, *La céramique gallo-romaine de Genève*, p. 236.

[175] Parker, "Evidence Provided by Underwater Archaeology," p. 366. For salted fish in the Roman military diet, see *SHA. Elagab.* 29.5 and *Aurel.* 9.6; R. W. Davies, "The Roman Military Diet," *Britannia* 2 (1971): 128–31.

[176] For *negotiatores allecarii* see Bogaers, "Nehalennia en de epigrafische Gegevens," pp. 32–43, Curtis, "*Negotiatores Allecarii*," pp. 147–58, and Piet Stuart, "130 römische Steindenkmäler aus dem Meer," *Archäologisches Korrespondenzblatt* 2 (1972): 299–302. For Gallic salteries see Galliou, *L'Armorique romaine*, pp. 135, 241–42. For the Peninsular House site see above, p. 80.

increasing amount may have been British or Gallic.[177] A Mediterranean shipwreck, Sud-Lavezzi I, carrying a mixed cargo, one-half of which included late Spanish salt-fish vessels (Almagro 50, 51, and 51C), has been found near Corsica, but to my knowledge no amphorae of these types have been reported in Europe north of Trier.[178] Although it cannot be traced in an unbroken succession, the frequency of reference to salt-fish production and commerce in medieval sources implies a continued enjoyment of preserved fish well after Roman occupation.[179]

Spanish products, though they apparently dominated salt-fish imports to Northern Europe until the second century A.D., were not the only ones. A *titulus* on a variant of a Dressel Form 2–4 amphora, datable between the first century B.C. and mid-second century A.D. and found in London, advertises the vessel's contents as "excellent liquamen from Antipolis." This need come as no surprise since literary testimony and archaeological evidence attest to fish preservation installations around this town in Gallia Narbonensis.[180] Little can be said about Gallic export trade in fish products, however, until more is known about Gallic amphorae. African salt-fish products, which apparently overtook Spanish ones in the Western Mediterranean markets from the third century A.D. on, do not seem to have reached Northern European markets in any large numbers.

In the early first century A.D. civil and military populations of Noricum and Pannonia received their Mediterranean imports primarily through the Istrian port of Aquileia (Udine). One route led north by road to Magdalensberg and on up to the Danube River at Lauriacum. Goods might also follow the Amber Route through Poetovio (Ptuj) to military camps along the Danube, such as Aquincum, Carnuntum, and Vindobona. In Noricum Spanish salt-fish amphorae have been found at Emona (Ljubljana) and Magdalensberg, while in Pannonia they have been reported from Poetovio, Salla, Savaria (Szombathely), Vetus Salina, Aquincum, and Gorsium. The *titulus* on an amphora found at Poetovio, G(ari) FLOS/ HISP(anum), recalls a similar one reported from Augst.[181] Magdalensberg enjoyed a particularly prosperous economic life from trade during the early empire. Although most of the

[177] Mark Hassall, "Britain and the Rhine Provinces: Epigraphic Evidence for Roman Trade," in *Roman Shipping and Trade: Britain and the Rhine Provinces.* Joan du Plat Taylor and Henry Cleere, eds. (London 1978), pp. 44–45.

[178] Sud-Lavezzi I: Liou, "Corse du Sud," pp. 437–44. For the distribution of late Roman amphorae, see esp. S. J. Keay, *Late Roman Amphorae in the Western Mediterranean. A Typology and Economic Study: the Catalan Evidence.* 2 vols. BAR International Series, 196 (Oxford 1984), pp. 169–78, 184–212. He declines, however, to identify the contents of Almagro 51C vessels as salt-fish products. Keay (p. 102) notes an example of an Africana I (=Keay Type III) vessel, datable from the third to the fifth century A.D., at Caerleon in Britain.

[179] Curtis, "*Negotiatores Allecarii*," esp. pp. 147–48, 156–58. See below, pp. 184–86.

[180] Hassall and Tomlin, "Roman Britain in 1983," p. 344: LIQUAM(en)/ ANTIPOL(itanum)/ EXC(ellens)/ L(uci) TETTI AFRI/CANI.

[181] Tamás Bezeczky, *Roman Amphorae from the Amber Route in Western Pannonia.* BAR International Series, 386 (Oxford 1987), pp. 22–23, 26. For Augst, see Bohn, "Pinselschriften," pp. 202–04, and above, note 170.

population was native, there were many Romans living there and serving as agents for Italian businessmen.[182] Among goods entering this region of Europe were fish sauce, including perhaps garum from Ostia, and salted fish. From the Domitianic period onward long-distance river-borne trade carried goods, probably including fish sauce, from the western European provinces eastward along the Rhine and Danube Rivers to Pannonia and perhaps Moesia Superior.[183]

Italy

Although Vibo may have operated a fish saltery in the fourth century B.C., literary sources present clear evidence that Italians were actively engaged in the production and commerce of salted fish products by the second century B.C. Tarentum apparently was producing her own preserved fish at this time, while Rome was importing, albeit at great cost, τάριχος from the Black Sea.[184] References to hallec by Plautus and Cato imply the knowledge of garum, although the latter word does not appear in Latin literature until the first century B.C. in the *De lingua Latina* of Varro.[185] There is no reason to assume that at this point Italy was not producing its own brands of fish sauce. Why they do not find more frequent mention prior to the first century B.C. is unknown, but may be related to the increased interest at that time in the more luxurious aspects of pisciculture and in the increased interest in foods among epicures.[186] The flourishing salteries in Spain, Africa, and Gaul would naturally increase the availability of preserved fish products and so create a heavier demand for luxury as well as for less expensive kinds.

Italy was richly blessed with a long coastline which provided many opportunities for fishing. Tunny swam all along the coast of Italy, and a tunny

---

[182] Géza Alföldy, *Noricum*. Anthony Birley, transl. (London 1974), pp. 70–74; and Egger and Görlich, "Der Lebensmittelimport," pp. 410–16.

[183] András Mócsy, *Pannonia and Upper Moesia. A History of the Middle Danube Provinces of the Roman Empire*. Sheppard Frere, transl. (London 1974), pp. 119–31.

[184] Euthydemus *ap*. Athen. 3.116c; Archestratus *ap*. Athen. 7.302a; and Aelian *NA* 15.3. Although fish salting cannot be attested before the fourth century B.C., tunny fishing was apparently practiced in Italy as early as the seventh century, at least in the Adriatic Sea. See Silvio Ferri, "La pesca del tonno nell'Adriatico in una stele garganica," *Magna Graecia* 5 (Nov.-Dec. 1970): 1–3. For Pontic imports see Polybius 31.25.5: καὶ τηλικαύτη τις ἐνεπεπτώκει περὶ τὰ τοιαῦτα τῶν ἔργων ἀκρασία τοῖς νέοις ὥστε πολλοὺς μὲν ἐρώμενον ἠγορακέναι ταλάντου, πολλοὺς δὲ ταρίχου Ποντικοῦ κεράμιον τριακοσίων δραχμῶν.

[185] Plautus *Aul*. fr. 5: *qui mi holera cruda ponunt, hallec adduint*; *Persa* 105: *Ecquid hallecis?*; *Poen*. 1310: *tune hic amator audes esse, hallex viri,/ aut contrectare quod mares homines amant?*; Cato *Agr*. 58: *ubi oleae comesae erunt, hallecem et acetum dato*; and Varro *Ling*. 9.40.66: *item qui reprehendunt, quod non dicatur ut unguentum unguenta vinum vina sic acetum aceta garum gara, faciunt imperite*.

[186] Ludwig Friedländer (*Darstellungen aus der Sittengeschichte Roms*. 10th ed. 4 vols. [Leipzig 1922], 2: 285–86) shows that luxury, particularly in the area of food, did not become pronounced until the first century B.C., when increased commercial activity made foreign imports more readily available. See more recently, Gloria Vivenza, "Gli 'Hedyphagetica' di Ennio e il commercio del pesce in età repubblicana," *E&S* 1 (1981): 5–44. Cf. Cato *ap*. Polybius 31.25.5 and Diodorus 37.3.1–6. For pisciculture see below, note 193.

watch (θυννοσκοπεῖον) operated at Populonia. Aelian states that the people of Italy and Liguria were active in catching tunny, a fish also available near Cosa and Velia, while Strabo adds that due to poor soil conditions the people of Velia abandoned agricultural pursuits and took up fishing. They apparently devoted themselves completely to this endeavor, since, he continues, the Velians established a saltery and "other such industries." Presumably, he meant the manufacture of fish sauce and possibly of purple dye.[187] Cumae possessed a large fishery, Puteoli and Tarentum operated textile factories, while Antium, Pyrgi, and Terracina exported fish to Rome.[188] Italian fishermen caught many fish other than tunny. The lupus entered the Tiber River, and the scarus, at least from the reign of Claudius on, was plentiful off the Italian coast between the Tiber River and Campania. Mullet were apparently available before Juvenal's time, but he complains that by his day Italy had to import them from Sicily.[189] Shellfish were caught near Brundisium and Baiae was the site of large-scale oyster parks.[190]

Even though literary sources show that fishing was a flourishing activity all along Italy's coastline, they provide little help in determining the sites of salteries. Strabo states that Velia possessed a saltery, and Pliny implies that Beneventum did also.[191] Beyond this the sources provide only a hint at saltery locations. Pliny's remark about garum from Pompeii and muria from Thurii implies the presence of fish processing centers at those locations, while references to tunny watches at Cosa and Populonia and to textile factories at Puteoli and Tarentum add a few other possibilities. The fact that the latter exported salt adds further weight to the conjecture that it possessed a saltery.[192]

---

[187] Polybius *ap.* Strabo 1.2.15 (tunny); Strabo 5.2.6 (Populonia) and 5.2.8 (a θυννοσκοπεῖον, also at Cosa); Aelian *NA* 13.16; Strabo 6.1.1. (Velia): ἀναγκάζονται γοῦν διὰ τὴν λυπρότητα τῆς γῆς τὰ πολλὰ θαλαττουργεῖν καὶ ταριχείας συνίστασθαι καὶ ἄλλας τοιαύτας ἐργασίας. Columella (*Rust.* 8.16.6–7) advises people living on the coast where the soil is generally poor to establish a source of revenue from the sea.

[188] Strabo 5.4.4 (Cumae); Pliny *HN* 35.45 (Puteoli), 9.137 (Tarentum); Athen. 6.224c. For vats and piles of murex shells found at Tarentum, see Antonietta dell'Aglio and Enzio Lippolis, "La documentazione anforaria a Taranto," in *Amphores Romaines et Histoire Économique. Dix Ans de Recherche.* Coll. de l'École Française de Rome, 114 (Rome 1989), pp. 542–43. For more on the purple industry of Italy see Blümner *Die gewerbliche Thätigkeit*, pp. 103–24, passim.

[189] Lupus: Horace *Sat.* 2.2.31; Pliny *HN* 9.168–69. Scarus: Martial 13.84; Pliny *HN* 9.62–63. Mullus: Juvenal *Sat.* 5.92–98.

[190] Brundisium and Lake Lucrine: Pliny *HN* 9.168–69; Petronius *Sat.* 119.33; Strabo 5.4.6; Horace *Epod.* 2.49; Martial 6.11.5; 13.82. See also Jerzy Kolendo, "Parces à huîtres et viviers sur un flacon en verre du Musée National de Varsovie," *Études et Travaux IX.*

[Vol] 18 of Travaux du Centre d'archéologie Méditerranéene de l'Académie Polonaise des Sciences (Warsaw 1976), pp. 143–58.

[191] Strabo 6.1.1; Pliny *HN* 32.19: *esse vero illam naturae accidentiam–quod magis miremur–etiam in locis quibusdam, adposito occurret exemplo, siquidem salsamenta omnium generum in Italia Beneventi refici constat.* Although Benventum was situated inland, it did lie near a river.

[192] Pliny *HN* 31.73, 84 (salt). Cumae may also have operated a saltery, but the evidence is ambiguous. See below, p. 130, note 93. Strabo (5.4.4), however, does state that Cumae had the best fisheries for large fish: εἰσὶ δὲ καὶ κητεῖαι παρ' αὐτοῖς ἄρισται.

Archaeology in Italy has not uncovered any salteries unattested in literary sources and has only confirmed three at most.[193] *Tituli picti* on amphorae found in Rome indicate that Pompeii and possibly Antium and Puteoli produced salted fish products.[194] It is interesting to note that of saltery locations explicitly mentioned or hinted at in the literary sources and of those confirmed by archaeological evidence—Populonia, Cosa, Antium, Puteoli, Pompeii, Velia, Thurii, Vibo, Tarentum, and Beneventum—all but Populonia, Cosa and Antium lay in the area of Magna Graecia. It should come as no surprise, however, if in the future salteries are discovered in areas of Central and Northern Italy where fishing also engaged a large number of people.

A case in point is the Roman port of Cosa. Although remains of salting installations are yet to be discovered, the excavators have built a strong prima facie case for their existence, perhaps from as early as the late third century B.C. The reference by Strabo to a tunny watch at Cosa and the excavation of two large commercial fish tanks, reminiscent of those at Punta de l'Arenal in Spain and elsewhere, are suggestive. The fishery-saltery, if it did exist, had its *floruit* from the late second through the first century B.C. and may have been associated with the *gens Sestia* which operated a large amphora factory. Indeed, the family may have produced two types of fish sauce amphora, one of which was modeled on a South Spanish vessel. If the Sestii did export Cosan fish products along with their wine, this would constitute the earliest known instance for the exportation of Italian salt-fish products.[195] Perhaps even Ostia itself should not be excluded as a producer and exporter, since it rested on the banks of the Tiber River in which fish-

---

[193] Archaeology has yielded evidence for fish ponds, though not salting factories as such. Luigi Jacono ("Nettuno: Piscinae in litore constructae," *NSc* 21 [1924]: 333–40) reports evidence for three *piscinae* constructed on the beach between Anzio and Nettuno. All were closely connected with maritime villas nearby. For others in Italy see Giulio Schmiedt, *Il livello antico del Mar Tirreno* (Florence 1972), passim. These maritime piscinae represent evidence only of the Roman penchant for raising all kinds of salt and fresh water fish for pleasure. A few fish ponds were quite large and probably obtained for the owner a profit from selling fresh fish. Many villas may have produced garum domestically, but probably not commercially. See Thomas Corcoran, "Roman Fishponds," *CB* 35 (1959): 37–39, 43. Gareth Schmeling ("Trimalchio's Menu and Wine List," *CPh* 65 [1970]: 249–50) would include garum among the items envisioned by Petronius in his description of foods produced on Trimalchio's estate. For economic interests of maritime villas see also John D'Arms, *Commerce and Social Standing in Ancient Rome* (Cambridge Mass. 1981), pp. 72–96.

[194] *CIL* XV.4686 (Pompeii), 4712 (Antium); 4687–88 (Puteoli). Athenaeus (6.224c) states that Antium exported fish to Rome. In *CIL* XV.4712 Dressel interpreted the letter following the I of ANTI[ ] as an A, and so the sauce as *Liquamen Antiatinum*. If, instead, the letter were a "P", it probably referred to liquamen from Antipolis. In the case of Puteoli the inscriptions probably refer to a merchant, Puteolanus, rather than the point of origin, since the vessels are Spanish (Dressel Form 12). See Zevi, "Appunti," p. 246. Puteoli did, however, operate a textile factory (Pliny *HN* 35.45).

[195] Anna Marguerite McCann, *The Roman Port and Fishery of Cosa* (Princeton, N.J. 1987), esp. pp. 30–43, 137–59, 322–31, with extensive bibliography. For the amphorae, see Elizabeth Lyding Will, in *ibid.*, pp. 169–220, esp. pp. 170–77, 201–04, 208–09, and 213–17.

ermen plied their trade and could easily obtain salt from the nearby *salinae Romanae*.[196]

Cassiodorus, the sixth century A.D. historian and politician, speaks of *garismatia* in the region of Histria.[197] These factories may have also operated much earlier, since amphorae of Dressel Form 6A, a Histrian vessel, may have held garum.[198] If the Histrian factories were operating during the first two centuries A.D., they do not seem to have threatened Spanish imports. Dressel Form 7–11 amphorae have been found in the Po Valley, for example at Verona.[199] As with other Italian salteries, the Histrian producers probably concentrated their efforts in local markets, particularly Aquileia, but may have sent some products into the northern provinces.[200]

Although the evidence is far from clear a few general conclusions on the chronology of Italian salting activity can be drawn. Most of the evidence for Italian salteries or fish sauce production dates between the second century B.C. and the first century A.D. If this represents the period of the flourishing of Italian salteries, then it conforms reasonably well with the evidence from Spain, North Africa, and Gaul. Archaeological remains are extensive only for Pompeii, which perished in A.D. 79. There is no way of ascertaining how long other salteries may have continued to operate. If Juvenal (*Sat.* 5.92–98) is correct when he says that Italian waters were being depleted of fish in his day, then a decline in Italian salteries in the first century A.D. would not be unexpected and the reasons for Spanish dominance of the Italian salt-fish market become clearer. One would not anticipate, however, a complete cessation. The only firm evidence is that in the late empire Tarentum maintained an official textile factory, while fish salteries and a government-owned textile factory operated in Histria.[201]

---

[196] Pliny *HN* 31.89; Livy 1.33.9; 7.19.8. For a contrary opinion see Le Gall, *Le Tibre*, p. 234. For salt resources near Rome see also Forbes, *Technology*, 3: 172–73. For fishermen at Ostia see Suetonius *De rhetoribus* 1, and Testaguzza, *Portus*, pp. 132, 143–44. See also Meiggs, *Roman Ostia*², pp. 267–68 , 348–49 (fishing), and 268–69 (salt). For a possible reference to garum from Ostia, see below, note 206.

[197] Cassiodorus *Variae* 12.22.4: *haec loca et garismatia plura nutriunt et piscium ubertate gloriantur.*

[198] Paolo Baldacci, "Alcuni aspetti dei commerci nei territori Cisalpini," *Atti del Centro Studi e Documentazione sull'Italia Romana* 1 (1967–68): 14–15, 46; Ezio Buchi, "Banchi di anfore romane a Verona. Note sui commerci Cisalpini," in *Il territorio veronese in età romana*. Atti del convegno del 22–23–24 Ottobre 1971 (Verona 1972), pp. 547–50; and Tchernia, *Le vin*, p. 132, note 23.

[199] Zevi, "Appunti," p. 241; and Buchi, "Banchi di anfore," pp. 553–57. Cf. also below, note 204.

[200] Attilio Degrassi, "Aquileia e l'Istria in età romana," in *Studi Aquileiesi* (Aquileia 1953), p. 62. In this context the lead tesserae found at Iulia Concordia may be of interest. The tesserae, dated with uncertainty to the second or third century A.D. and similar to ones found on Africana IIC amphorae found in a shipwreck off the Algerian coast north of Hippo Regius, contained notations identifying either local merchants or owners of the containers. One example indicated the vessel's contents as *allicium*. The type of vessel to which the lead tessera was attached is unknown. See Heikki Solin, "Tabelle plumbee di Concordia," *Aquileia Nostra* 48 (1977): 158. See also *L'AnnEp.* (1977): 85, no. 311. For the shipwreck near Hippo Regius, see Lequément, "Étiquettes de plomb," pp. 667–80.

[201] Histria: Cassiodorus *Variae* 12.22.4; *Not. dign. occ.* 11.67 (Seeck, ed., p. 151); Tarentum: *Not. dign. occ.* 11.65 (Seeck, ed., p. 151). The evidence for a saltery at Antium, if the reading of *CIL* XV.4712 is accurate, may date after the third century A.D. See Zevi, "Appunti," p. 220.

More is known about the salt-fish commerce of Italy than for any other western province except Spain. Polybius speaks of Pontic imports of τάριχος in the second century B.C., and Horace provides evidence that Byzantium sent muria and Spain exported garum to Rome in the following century.[202] Strabo reports that in his day merchants from Turdetania, an area known for its salted fish products, were active at both Ostia and Puteoli, and Aelian in the late second century A.D. describes the problems experienced by Spanish salt-fish merchants at Puteoli.[203] Literary sources and evidence of amphorae at Ostia, Rome, and Pompeii indicate that the major external supplier of salted fish products to Italy between the late first century B.C. and the late second century A.D. was Spain. Although it remains difficult to determine precisely, Spanish products appear to have met with little competition from Italian producers who probably manufactured products primarily for local consumption and expended little effort at competing on a large scale with Spanish merchants, at least in the capitol.[204]

Several areas of Italy did operate export businesses in processed fish. If not merely part of the ship's store for use by captain and crew, the two Pompeian fish sauce vessels of A. Umbricius Scaurus of Pompeii found at Fos-sur-mer in Southern Gaul may be the only clear evidence for the exportation of Italian salt-fish products (Plate 5).[205] The Roman settlement on the

---

[202] Polybius 31.25.5; Horace *Sat*. 2.4.63–66; 2.8.46.

[203] Strabo 3.2.6: τὴν δὲ ἀφθονίαν τῶν ἐκκομιζομένεν ἐκ τῆς Τουρδητανίας ἐμφανίζει τὸ μέγεθος καὶ τὸ πλῆθος τῶν ναυκληρίων˙ ὁλκάδες γὰρ μέγισται παρὰ τούτων πλέουσιν εἰς Δικαιαρχείαν καὶ τὰ Ὦστια, τῆς Ῥώμης ἐπίνειον; Aelian *NA* 13.6: ἀκούω γοῦν ἐν Δικαιαρχίᾳ τῇ Ἰταλικῇ πολύπουν ἐς ὄγκον σώματος ὑπερήφανον προελθόντα τὴν μὲν ἐν τῇ θαλάττῃ τροφὴν καὶ τὰς ἐκεῖθεν νομὰς ἀτιμάσαι καὶ ὑπερφρονῆσαι αὐτῶν. προῄει δὲ ἄρα οὗτος καὶ ἐς τὴν γῆν, καὶ ἐλῄζετο καὶ τῶν χερσαίων ἔπστιν ἅ. οὐκοῦν διά τινος ὑπονόμου κρυπτοῦ ἐκβάλλοντος ἐς τὴν θάλατταν τὰ ἐκ τῆς πόλεως τῆς προειρημένης ῥυπαρὰ ἐσνέων καὶ ἀνιὼν ἐς οἶκόν τινα πάραλον, ἔνθα ἦν ἐμπόρων Ἰβηρικῶν φόρτος καὶ ταρίχη τὰ εκεῖθεν ἐν σκεύεσιν ἁδροῖς, εἶτα τὰς πλεκτάνας περιχέων καὶ σφίγγων τὸν κέραμον ἐρρήγνυ τὰ ἀγγεῖα καὶ κατεδαίνυτο τὰ ταρίχη.

[204] Zevi, "Appunti," p. 241; Carandini and Panella, *Ostia III*, p. 671. For Rome, besides the Spanish salt-fish amphorae discovered in the Praetorian Camp, see Alberto Ciotola, Stefania Picciola, Riccardo Santangeli Valenzani, and Rita Volpe, "Roma: tre contesti. 1. Via Nova-Clivo Palatino. 2. Crypta Balbi. 3. Via Sacra-Via Nova," in *Amphores Romaines et Histoire Économique. Dix Ans de Recherche.* Coll. de l'École Française de Rome, 114 (Rome 1989), pp. 604–09. For Spanish fish sauce vessels found in other parts of Italy, See Baldacci, "Alcuni aspetti dei commerci nei territori Cisalpini," p. 46; D. Gabler, F. Redö, and T. Bezeczky, "Gli scavi nella villa romana a San Potito-di-Ovindoli (l'Aquila) 1983–1984," *AArchHung* 38 (1986): 78–86; Mariavittoria Antico Gallina, "Anfore dei Musei di Alessandria e di Tortona," in *Amphores Romaines et Histoire Économique. Dix Ans de Recherche.* Coll. de l'École Française de Rome, 114 (Rome 1989), pp. 638–41; Emanuele Papi, "Siena: anfore Romane da Castelvecchio," in *ibid.*, pp. 618–19; Giuliano Volpe, " La circolazione delle anfore Romane nella Daunia: dati preliminari," in *ibid.*, pp. 629–32; Matilda Romito, "Il commercio anforario in età Romana sulla costiera Amalfitana," in *ibid.*, pp. 626–28; Dorica Manconi, "Anfore Romane in Umbria alla sinistra del Tevere," in *ibid.*, pp. 590–93; Anselmo Malizia, "Depositi di anfore in Altino," in *ibid.*, pp. 635–37; and Marinella Pasquinucci et al, "Ricerche archeologico-topographiche nella fascia costiera Tirrenica," in *ibid.*, pp. 620–25.

[205] Liou and Marichal, "Les inscriptions," pp. 165–67. As early as the second century B.C. or before, Bruttian and Campanian merchants had participated in the salt-fish trade between Spain and Athens, conveying not only Spanish products but also tunny from Tarentum. See

Magdalensberg in Noricum grew into a large city and in the early imperial period functioned as an important emporion for Italian goods bound for the interior of Europe. Italian merchants, particularly from Aquileia but also from elsewhere, conducted a wholesale trade in bulk quantities, a portion of which was in salted fish products. Archaeologists have found amphorae and dolia bearing *tituli picti* identifying the contents as salsamenta and fish sauce. One amphora may have held garum from Ostia; the origin of the other vessels is unknown.[206] Intraprovincial trade can be attested for Pompeii and possibly Antium who sent their goods to Rome.

The remains of Pompeii's energetic trade in fish sauce provide a unique opportunity for a close look at this industry in Italy. Pompeii was ideally situated for the site of a fish processing center. Fish of many species, especially tunny and mackerel, were abundant in the waters off Campania and provided opportunities for a lucrative fishing industry.[207] Pompeii possessed a ready supply of salt from the nearby salt works, the *Salinae Herculeae,* and fresh water was easily obtained from the Sarno River.[208] Many Pompeians apparently engaged in fishing, as finds of bronze fishhooks, anchors, lead weights and nets attest, and an election notice found in the vicinity of the Triangular Forum indicates that Pompeian fishermen (*piscicapi*) may have even been organized.[209]

As a port city, Pompeii was commercially active as both an import and export market.[210] Although Pompeii's small port was dwarfed in size and importance by those of Ostia and nearby Puteoli, it remained active until its destruction by Mount Vesuvius in A.D. 79. Excavations in the area of the port in 1928 yielded a complex of sheds, warehouses, and other commer-

---

Euthydemus *ap.* Athen. 3.116c: Ἰόνιον δ' ἀνὰ κῦμα φέρων Γαδειρόθεν ἄξει Βρέττιος ἢ Καμπανὸς ἢ ἐκ ζαθέοιο Τάραντος ὀρκύνοιο τρίγωνα, τά τ' ἐν στάμνοισι τεθέντα ἀμφαλλὰξ δείπνοισιν ἐνὶ πρώτοισιν ὀπηδεῖ.

[206] G(arum) OST(iense): Egger and Görlich, "Der Lebensmittelimport," pp. 412, 416. The authors do not identify the amphora shapes.

[207] Athen. 7.302a; Aelian *NA* 13.16; Strabo 5.2.6. Italian fishermen today continue to catch both tunny and mackerel. See *United Nations, Food and Agriculture Organization, Scientific and Common Names Applied to Tunas, Mackerels, and Spear Fishes of the World with Notes on their Geographic Distribution* (Washington, D.C. 1950), pp. 1–4, 78–81.

[208] For the *Salinae Herculeae* see Columella *Rust.* 10.135–36. The exact location of this salt works remains unknown, but it probably lay between Pompeii and Herculaneum. Pompeii's Herculanean Gate was in antiquity called the *Porta Salis* (*CIL* IV.9159), or *veru sarinu* in Oscan, and one of the city's electoral districts was called *Saliniensis* (CIL IV.128, 1611, 4106, 5181). Cf. *CIL* IV.10690, in Herculaneum. See Amedeo Maiuri, "Note di topografia pompeiana," *RAAN* 34 (1959): 79–81; and Paavo Castrén, *Ordo Populusque Pompeianus: Polity and Society in Roman Pompeii.* Acta Instituti Romani Finlandiae, Vol. 8 (Rome 1975), pp. 79–82.

[209] Francesco Fienga, "Esplorazione del pago marittimo pompeiano," *Atti dell'III congresso nazionale di studi romani* 11 (1932–33): 172–76. See also Matteo Della Corte, "Pompei-Borgo Marinaro," *NSc* 6th ser. 4 (1928): 369–72. *CIL* IV.826: POPIDIUM RUFUM AED(ilem) PISCICAPI FAC(iunt). See also Matteo Della Corte, *Case ed abitanti di Pompei.* 3rd ed. (Naples 1965), pp. 259–60.

[210] Strabo (5.4.8) says that by way of the Sarno River Pompeii served as the port city for Nola, Nuceria, and Acerrae.

cial buildings, including finds of produce such as olives and pine cones, which had just come into or were awaiting shipment out of the port.[211]

Laudantur et Clazomenae garo Pompeique et Leptis, sicut muria Antipolis ac Thurii, iam, vero et Delmatia. This simple sentence by which Pliny the Elder (*HN* 31.94) extolls the fish sauces of various places in the empire is the only extant literary evidence which connects Pompeii with the fish salting industry. In a city which possessed all of the requirements for a fish processing center and which had acquired some renown for its garum, one would expect to find archaeological evidence for an elaborate salting installation comparable to those existing in Africa and Spain. This has not been the case, however. Although an uncomplimentary graffito found in the house at Region II.vii.10 confirms the presence of *salsamentarii* at Pompeii, no industrial complex has thus far been discovered, not even basins of the type usually associated with a fish processing installation.[212] This has led some scholars to conclude that fish sauce was imported in its crude form from Spain and then further processed for local distribution or export throughout Italy.[213] Although Pompeian merchants imported pickled fish from Spain to add to their merchandise, nearby fish processing centers, such as at Velia, could more cheaply supply all of the raw garum needed, assuming that it was unavailable at Pompeii itself.[214]

Since the ancient shoreline today lies some distance inland, the Sarno River has shifted from its ancient bed, and modern constructions, such as the Salerno-Pompei highway and private homes, restrict the areas of future excavation, the eventual discovery of Pompeii's salting installations seems highly unlikely. Nevertheless, the available evidence relating to the production and commerce of fish sauce is not insignificant and falls into three groups: containers bearing *tituli picti*, a floor mosaic in the house of Aulus Umbricius Scaurus, and a shop for the preparation and distribution of fish sauce.

Of nearly two hundred inscribed fish sauce vessels found in Pompeii and Herculaneum only thirty-six have been amphorae. Over 140, or approximately 71 per cent of the total, were small vessels called *urcei*, identified in

---

[211] Fienga, "Pago Marittimo pompeiano," pp. 172–76; Della Corte, *Case*³, pp. 444–46. For Pompeii's commercial activity represented in a lararium painting see Amedeo Maiuri, "Navalia pompeiana," *RAAN* 33 (1958): 7–13.

[212] *CIL* IV.10150.

[213] Helen Tanzer, *The Common People of Pompeii: A Study of the Graffiti* (Baltimore 1939), p. 34, followed by Robert Étienne, *La vie quotidienne à Pompéi.* 2nd ed. (Paris 1977), pp. 148–49. Tanzer believes that the initial stages of garum production were not done at Pompeii because the odor was incompatible with a "pleasure resort." Pompeii, however, was a commercial town, not a resort center, and the citizens of a city filled with the smells of the woolen and tanning industries would not object to the smell of fish. The Pompeian was, no doubt, immune to the most rancid smells. In any case, the smell of fish sauce was probably not unbearable. See Grimal and Monod, "Véritable nature," p. 31; and Curtis, "In Defense of Garum," *CJ* 78 (1983): 232–40. But cf. below, p. 189 and note 18. On the odor of modern fish sauces, see above p. 21.

[214] Manacorda, "Anfore spagnole a Pompei," pp. 121–33.

the Mau-Schoene drawings of *CIL* IV as Pompeian Form VI (Pl. 7a). Although these figures include only those vessels bearing a *titulus pictus*, they remain instructive. It seems apparent that at Pompeii this was the vessel which most often held fish sauce. The large number of urcei containing garum and other fish sauces strongly implies that there existed a ready market for this product, and the many different names appearing on the vessels indicate that there were several entrepreneurs who sought to capitalize on this demand.

Aulus Umbricius Scaurus, whose name or the name of one of his slaves, freedmen, or family members appears on over 28 per cent of all fish sauce containers found in Pompeii and Herculaneum, was Pompeii's leading producer of fish sauce.[215] That Scaurus was a Pompeian is proven by the existence of his family tomb located on the Street of Tombs outside the Herculanean Gate. He was obviously a man of wealth and high standing in the community since the sepulchral inscription states that the decuriones honored his son, a former duovir who perhaps died in office, by voting the land and money for the funeral as well as an equestrian statue in the forum.[216]

Scaurus' wealth may be easily seen in his spacious home located at Region VII, *Insula Occidentalis* 12–15 near the Porta Marina, consisting of an upper level of three atria, several cubicula, and a peristyle with fishpond, and a lower level of storerooms, cubicula, and a private bath (Fig. 5).[217] The connection of this residence with Scaurus is assured by the mosaic floor design found in the atrium of Entrance 15. The large black and white mosaic floor is distinguished by having a design of a container located at each of the four corners of the impluvium. The vessel represented is, in each instance, an urceus of Pompeian Form VI and, as in the case with real urcei, each mosaic urceus bears the design of a *titulus pictus* identifying the contents and the producer of the product (Pl. 7a). The products named include liquamen and garum, and the producer was Aulus Umbricius Scaurus.[218]

The final piece of evidence for Pompeii's fish salting industry comes from a modest house located at Region I.xii.8 (Figure 6). This house probably

[215] For a detailed discussion of Scaurus and his fish sauce business see Curtis, "A. Umbricius Scaurus of Pompeii," pp. 19–50. Scaurus' associates in the garum industry included Umbricius Abascantus (*CIL* IV.5671, 5685, 5689, 5724) and Umbricius Agathopus (*CIL* IV.5690–91, 5712, 6921, 7110, 9403–04).

[216] *CIL* X.1024. There is good reason to believe that the elder Scaurus was the one alluded to by Petronius in *Sat.* 77.5. See Amedeo Maiuri, "Petroniana," *PP* 8 (1948): 112, note 1, and Curtis, "A. Umbricius Scaurus," pp. 26–28. For a contrary view see Richard P. Duncan-Jones, "Scaurus at the House of Trimalchio," *Latomus* 32 (1973): 364–67.

[217] Robert I. Curtis, "A Personalized Floor Mosaic from Pompeii," *AJA* 88 (1984): 557–66.

[218] Surprisingly, there is no evidence that Scaurus sold salsamenta. The omission of references to allec and muria in the mosaic is also interesting in light of *tituli* on urcei (*CIL* IV.5723–24, 9410, and possibly 10262) which connect him to these products. For a more detailed discussion of the mosaic, see below pp. 167–69.

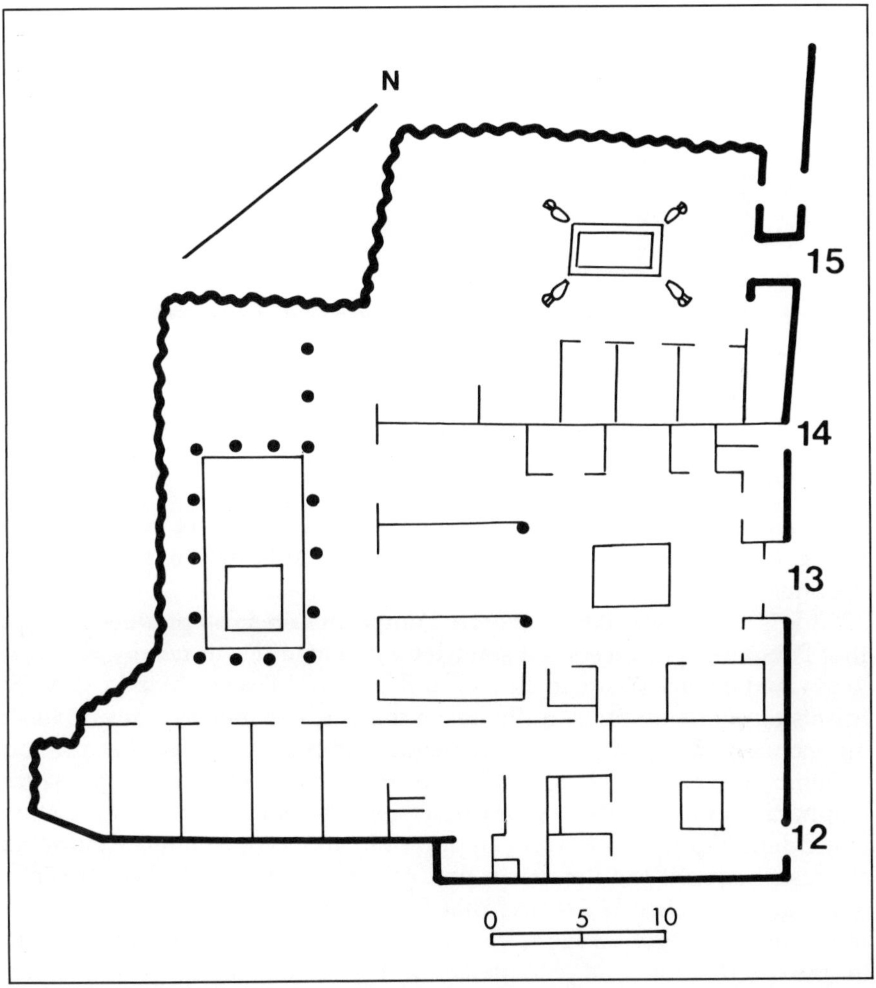

Figure 5: Pompeii: House of A. Umbricius Scaurus (Reg. VII. *Ins. Occ.* 12–15)

served as a central warehouse where raw garum, prepared elsewhere, was further processed in dolia and then transferred to amphorae for distribution.[219] Five of the six dolia in the peristyle, which had been converted for industrial use, contained the dried remains of allec (Pl. 1b). The desiccative material included small lateral bones, vertebrae, and scales of anchovies

[219] Robert I. Curtis, "The Garum Shop of Pompeii (I.12.8)," *Cronache Pompeiane* 5 (1979): 5–23; Amedeo Maiuri, "Dalle anfore esce l'odore della salsa di 2000 anni fa," *Corriere della Sera* (Jan. 26, 1961), p. 3 (="La Bottega del Salsamentario," in *Amedeo Maiuri Mestiere d'Archelologo* [Naples 1978], pp. 635–36).

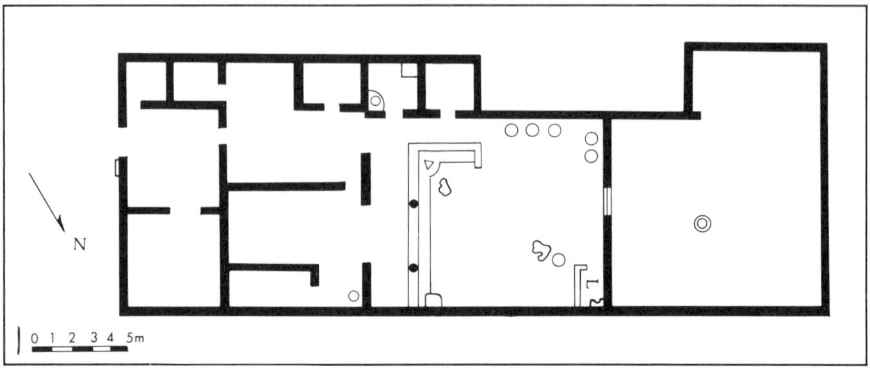

Figure 6: Pompeii: Garum shop (Reg. 1.xii.8)

(*Engraulis encrasicholus*). Although many amphorae were found in the house, none bear inscriptions which permit identification of the owner or operator of the shop.[220]

Little is known about the export of Pompeian salted fish products, except that Pompeian producers did send their commodities to nearby Herculaneum and Stabiae, and to Rome, and possibly Fos-sur-Mer in Gaul.[221] Spanish imports dominated the Italian market, and indeed many Spanish amphorae of the type usually associated with fish sauce have been found at Pompeii.[222] Nevertheless, the paucity of identifiable Pompeian fish sauce amphorae in places outside Campania may be attributable to a combination of accident of preservation and an uncertain knowledge of Italian amphora shapes.[223] Even if the Pompeian product did not rival that from Spain—although Pliny (*HN* 31.94) says that Pompeian garum was well-known—the evidence of urcei of Form VI and of the activity of the Umbricii Scauri in the production and commerce of fish sauce certainly prove that

[220] I wish to thank my colleague Prof. Elizabeth Reitz of the Department of Anthropology and Linguistics for identifying the bones as those of *Engraulis encrasicholus*. I am unaware of any evidence linking this shop to the Umbricii Scauri, an identification first mentioned by Hans Eschebach (*Die städtebauliche Entwicklung des antiken Pompeji*. MDAI[R], Suppl. 17 [Heidelberg 1970], p. 121) and repeated in the archaeological guide to Pompeii, Eugenio La Rocca and Mariette and Arnold De Vos, *Guida archeologica di Pompei* (Milan 1976): 228–29.

[221] *CIL* IV, passim; *CIL* XV.4686 (Rome; the type of vessel is unknown); and Liou and Marichal, "Les inscriptions," pp. 165–67 (Fos-sur-Mer).

[222] Amphorae of Dressel Forms 7–11 are rare at Pompeii, but those of type Beltrán IIB and Pelichet 46 (= Pompeian Form VII) are numerous. See Manacorda, "Anfore spagnole a Pompei," pp. 121–33.

[223] One recent study has suggested that the Umbricii Scauri may themselves have produced fish-sauce amphorae. See Elizabeth Lyding Will, "Ähnlichkeiten zwischen Stempeln auf Amphoren und auf arretinischen Gefässen," *RCRF* 23–24 (1984): 9–11.

a prosperous and active local business thrived in the Vesuvian city up to A.D. 79.[224]

The general organization of Scaurus' fish sauce business is readily apparent from the *tituli picti* of many urcei and amphorae found in Pompeii and Herculaneum. Although these vessels could remain in use for some years, the extant painted inscriptions no doubt referred to people who were active during the last year or final few years of the city. The Pompeian vessels were found most often in business establishments where food was served or in rooms of private homes where eating or cooking took place. The urcei were in use at the time of the eruption, and so the products contained in them probably came from a shop that was still doing business in A.D. 79.

Scaurus owned his own shop and either owned or controlled several other shops located throughout the city. This is evident from the *titulus pictus* of several vessels which advertise the product as coming EX OFFICINA SCAURI, "from the shop of Scaurus."[225] Scaurus had freedmen, slaves, and family members working for him. Two freedmen, Umbricius Abascantus and Umbricius Agathopus, apparently operated separate shops since their names appear in the genitive case following the phrase *ex officina*.[226] Other members of Scaurus' organization worked in these shops and probably signed their names to vessels in their capacity as consignors.[227] All together Scaurus may have controlled six or more shops. That no *titulus pictus* so far discovered records an *officina* belonging to anyone other than a person tied in some way to the *gens Umbricia* may be merely an accident of preservation, but it probably reflects the degree of dominance exercised by this family over the Campanian fish sauce business.

Scaurus apparently engaged both in the importation and exportation of fish sauce. His name in the genitive case appears in the product label on a South Spanish amphora along with the name of the *navicularius* M. Valerius

---

[224] When the industry began at Pompeii is unknown. Strabo, who had firsthand knowledge of the area of Campania, does not list Pompeii among the cities of Southern Italy operating fish salteries. For Strabo's knowledge of the area see Richards, "Strabo," p. 84. Scaurus probably began his business early in the reign of Tiberius. See Curtis, "Personalized Floor Mosaic," pp. 562–64, and *idem*, "A. Umbricius Scaurus," p. 30.

[225] *CIL* IV.2572, 2574, 2577, 5694, 9406. For one other see Wilhelmina Jashemski, "The Excavation of a Shop-House Garden at Pompeii (I.xx.5)," *AJA* 81 (1977): 227. See esp. Curtis, "A. Umbricius Scaurus," p. 31. For the criteria upon which this discussion is based, see Appendix III.

[226] Agathopus (*CIL* IV.5690–91, 9403–04) and Abascantus (*CIL* IV.5689).

[227] Umbricia Fortunata (*CIL* IV.2573(?), 5661, 5674–75) and Eutyches (*CIL* IV.2576). If the single name Umbricia does not also refer to Umbricia Fortunata, then include *CIL* IV.2594(?), 5670, 5688, 5696–97, 5710, 5713(?), 5723, 10262, 10281. See also Fortunata in *CIL* IV.5662. Agathopus appears as consignor in *CIL* IV.5712, 6921, 9394, 9418–19; while Abascantus does so in *CIL* IV.5671, 5685, 5724. Cf. *CIL* IV.9406, where Martialis, an imperial freedman, served as consignor in Scaurus' shop.

Euphemus.[228] Since the vessel and so its contents came from Spain, Scaurus must have purchased the vessel, probably to offer a variety of products, in this case an imported one, to his customers. His export activity can be seen in the urceus of Pompeian Form VI containing garum "from the shop of A. Umbricius Abascantus" and in one of liquamen with Scaurus' name in the genitive case following the product identification which have surfaced in Herculaneum. Two other Type VI urcei, one bearing Scaurus' name, have appeared in Fos-sur-mer in Southern France (Pl. 7b).[229] Admittedly, this is meager evidence upon which to draw any firm conclusions on the scope of Scaurus' import-export business, but it is suggestive.

As active as the Umbricii Scauri were in the production and commerce of fish sauce, they did not possess a monopoly on the industry. *Tituli picti* provide the names of at least fifteen other persons apparently active in the salt-fish industry but not demonstrably connected with Scaurus.[230] These people unfortunately remain for us little more than names. Two Pompeians, M. Arruntius Anteros and Tinnius Restitutus, functioned in the production side of the business as consignors or producers, while perhaps seven others may have as well, but confirmation is lacking. The number of possible producers competing with the Umbricii Scauri, therefore, reaches perhaps nine. One cannot say how many workshops operated in Pompeii and Herculaneum outside of those connected with Scaurus, but there are too many individuals apparently unassociated with the *gens Umbricia* operating in the business to believe that there were no others. The demand for fish sauce and other salted fish products must have been great indeed to support so many competitors.

Sardinia and Corsica

Sardinia and Corsica are best treated as a homogeneous unit, since together they formed a single Roman province from soon after the First Punic

---

[228] Manacorda, "Anfore spagnole a Pompei," p. 131. The name Umbricia in the genitive or dative case also appears on a South Spanish amphora of Pelichet Form 46 in a product label seemingly added at a time later than that of the main *titulus pictus*.

[229] Herculaneum: *CIL* IV.5689 (A. Umbricius Abascantus), 10746 (A. Umbricius Scaurus); Fos-sur-mer: Liou and Marichal, "Les inscriptions," p. 165, no. 69.

[230] *CIL* IV.5695 (Ninnius Agathopus), 5709 (Campanus), 9389 (Marcus Arruntius Anteros), 9411 (Vibia), 9416 (Granius Ter . . .), 9417 (Infantio), 10271 (Tinnius Restitutus), 10281a (Marcus Volusius), Caesia Helpis and M. Acceius Telemachus. The two latter names appear on an unpublished vessel recorded in the Daybook of Excavations at Pompeii for July, 1957. I owe reference to them to the kindness of Wilhelmina Jashemski. Five men, perhaps non-Pompeians since their names appear on amphorae, who may have participated in the Pompeian fish sauce business as merchants, not producers, were Arrius Corinthus, Sal(l)ustius, C. Cornelius Hermeros, and A. A. Atinii, perhaps brothers or father and son known from product labels on amphorae found in Rome. See Curtis, "A. Umbricius Scaurus," pp. 45–46, notes 67–71.

War until sometime in the imperial period. Both had existed under Carthaginian domination from the late sixth century B.C. until the Romans assumed control some 300 years later. Although literary and archaeological evidence for salteries on the two islands is meager, enough exists to give a hint of this activity.

The location of Punic factories in Sardinia remains unknown, as no archaeological evidence for them has been discovered.[231] For that matter, none exists from the Roman period either. This is quite surprising, since in the late second century A.D. Galen declared that Sardinian τάριχος was highly honored.[232] Sardinia was well-suited for fish salting factories, since it had excellent supplies of fish and salt.[233] Purple fish were available near the island of Buccina to the east of Olbia, and mullet were plentiful around Corsica.[234] Year-old tunny were commonly referred to as "Sardinian," perhaps implying the popularity and high quality of salt-fish products from the island.[235] The Roman establishments presumably superseded those of the Carthaginians, and further archaeological work will, perhaps, uncover these installations.[236] Phoenico-Punic settlements in Sardinia concentrated in the southern and western portions of the island.[237]

The only fish salting establishment discovered so far lies near the town of Aleria on Corsica.[238] The installation was situated on the summit of a hill and was connected by a passageway with a bath; an aqueduct probably furnished fresh water. The salting establishment was composed of various rooms, some of which contained several vats of different sizes constructed of tiles. A large number of oyster shells found nearby indicates the type of sea animal prepared here. This installation probably served only the local needs of the inhabitants of the nearby villa. The construction of *opus incertum* found in the saltery dates the factory to the first century B.C.

---

231 Gsell postulates that a Semitic votive inscription found in Carthage (*Corpus Inscriptionum Semiticarum* 351) may have been dedicated by a salt-fish merchant from Sardinia. See Gsell, *L'Afrique du Nord*. Vol. 4, p. 52, note 9.

232 Galen *De alim fac*. 3.30.5. See also Pollux *Onom*. 6.48: ταρίχη Σαρδῷα.

233 Ettore Pais, *Storia della Sardegna e della Corsica durante il dominio romano*. 2 vols. (Rome 1923), 2: 523–24. For tunny and mackerel in Sardinian waters see Diphilus of Siphnos *ap*. Athenaeus 3.120f. For a *societas* of salt merchants in Sardinia see *CIL* X.7856 (= *IGRR* I/II. 511): CLEON SALARI(us) SOC(iorum) S(ervus) AESCOLAPIO MERRE DONUM DEDIT LUBENS MERITO MERENTE.

234 E. S. Bouchier, *Sardinia in Ancient Times* (Oxford 1917), p. 59. See also Juvenal *Sat*. 5.92.

235 Andrews, "Sardinian Fish," p. 184.

236 W. G. St. J. Wilkes indicates that fish tanks may have existed at Nora in the area of a quay. See W. G. St. J. Wilkes, "Underwater Exploration of the Ancient Port of Nora, Sardinia," *PBSR* 35 (1967): 10.

237 Ferrucio Barreca, "The Phoenician and Punic Civilization in Sardinia," in *Studies in Sardinian Archaeology*. Vol. II: *Sardinia in the Mediterranean*. Miriam S. Balmuth, ed. (Ann Arbor 1986), pp. 145–70, esp. Fig. 11.1. Modern tunny fisheries as well lie along the western coast of Sardinia. See Ponsich, *Aceite de Oliva y Salazones de Pescado*, p. 25, Fig. 4.

238 Jean Jehasse, "Les fouilles d'Aléria (Corse): l'acropole et ses problèmes," *Gallia* 21 (1963): 103.

The commercial activity of Sardinian salt-fish merchants has left only an echo, though a strong one, in literary sources. Galen speaks highly of the Sardinian product from personal knowledge and implies its availability in the markets at Rome. In fact, he states that Sardinian salt-fish (ταρίχη σάρδα) was the best preserved fish, and adds the information that in his day salted fish products from Gades in Spain were called σάρδαι. Apparently Sardinian τάριχος, called *sarda* or *sardina*, became a generic term for all salted fish of excellent quality. To acquire such a reputation the Sardinian salteries must have been quite large and Sardinian merchants highly active in foreign markets.[239] Literary evidence for commerce in Corsican salted fish products is nonexistent, and the small saltery found at Aleria apparently produced fish sauce only for local consumption.

In the first two centuries A.D. Sardinia and Corsica must have been at a disadvantage in selling their products in the Italian markets, even though they lay so close to the peninsula. Spanish merchants *en route* to Italian markets passed through the strait of Bonifacio separating the two islands as well as to the south of Sardinia. Several shipwrecks near the île Lavezzi and île Cavallo and in the harbor of Nora in Sardinia yielded Spanish salt-fish amphorae.[240] Shippers of grain from Turris and Carales traded in Ostia, and the latter city maintained an office in the Piazzale delle Corporazioni in the early third century A.D.[241] It seems likely that during the first two centuries Sardinian and probably Corsican salted fish products found their way to the Italian markets along with grain. After the late second century when Spanish fish sauce exports to Ostia began to decline, the products of these two nearby islands, particularly Sardinia whose products had already achieved a high reputation, would naturally find a growing market, much as apparently did the African products.[242] It is unknown if Sardinia and Corsica made their own amphorae or possibly used Italian vessels. Amphora studies cannot as yet offer any help in obtaining a clear picture of the commerce in salted fish products of these two islands.

---

[239] Galen *De alim. fac.* 3.30.4–5; 40.5–6; Andrews, "Sardinian Fish," pp. 171–85; and R. Baltar Veloso, "Una nueva interpretación de Edict. Diocl. 5,12," *HAnt.* 2 (1972): 61–68.

[240] Benoit, "Provence (III)," pp. 174–76; Tchernia, "Direction," pp. 496–99; Bebko, *Les épaves antiques*, pp. 1–6; and Wilkes, "Nora, Sardinia," p. 11. Based upon the evidence of relative numbers of Spanish garum vessels to those of wine and oil from various sites on land as well as in the sea and now stored in the museum of Cagliari in Southern Sardinia and Sassari in the north, Elizabeth Lyding Will suggests that the primary route followed by ships from Spain bound for Italian ports passed by the southern, not the northern, coast of Sardinia. See Elizabeth Lyding Will, "Amphoras and Trade in Roman Sardinia," in *Studies in Sardinian Archaeology.* Vol. II: *Sardinia in the Mediterranean.* Miriam S. Balmuth, ed. (Ann Arbor 1986), pp. 213–15.

[241] Meiggs, *Roman Ostia*², p. 286.

[242] Cf. Baltar Veloso, "Una nueva interpretación," pp. 67–68.

Sicily

Fishing played a major role in the life of ancient Sicily. Sicilian waters were rich in fish of various species, and merchants exported tunny to Athens as early as the late fifth century B.C.[243] Archestratus states that Sicilian tunny excelled in quality that from Byzantium.[244] Coastal towns actively engaged in the preparation and exportation of salted fish.[245] Archestratus mentions Sicilian tunny packed in jars (βίκοι), and Athenaeus relates that Hieron II of Syracuse sent to Ptolemy III Euergetes I (246–221 B.C.) as part of a shipload of gifts ten thousand κεράμιοι of τάριχος.[246] Sicilian exports in the same century reached even to Palestine, where Zenon, the personal secretary of Apollonius, a treasury official of Ptolemy II, probably at the port of Ptolemais (Acre), purchased a jar of Sicilian salt-fish (ταρίχου Σικελικοῦ βικίον).[247]

Sicilian salting installations were apparently active in the Roman period also. Pliny (*HN* 3.91) mentions the inhabitants, *cetarini*, of a city which is probably the same one identified by Ptolemy (3.4.4) on the Gulf of Castellamare as Κεταρία. The name suggests a city of inhabitants active in the salting industry. In the late empire a textile factory operated at Syracuse. Salt for Sicilian fish processing centers probably came from the many salt marshes and lakes located on the island, such as those near Gela, Agrigentum, and Lake Cocanicus.[248]

Archaeological excavation has uncovered salting installations in Western Sicily at Porta Palo, S. Vito (Trapani), Cala Minnola (Levanzo), Isola delle Femmine (Palermo), Tonnara del Cofano (Trapani), and S. Nicola (Favignana).[249] The Sicilian basins in arrangement and construction show characteristics similar to those in Spain, North Africa, and Gaul. At Isola delle

---

[243] Theopompus fr. 51 Edmonds: θύννων τε λευκῶν Σικελικῶν ὑπήτρια. For fish available off Sicily see Vincent M. Scramuzza, *Roman Sicily*. Vol. 3 (1937) of *ESAR*, pp. 283–85. See also Biagio Pace, *Arte e civiltà della Sicilia antica* (Milan 1935), 1: 402–08. For archaeological evidence of fishponds in Eastern Sicily see Schmiedt, *Il livello antico*, esp. pp. 201–14.

[244] Archestratus *ap*. Athen. 7.302a: ἐστὶ δὲ γενναῖος Βυζαντίῳ ἔν τε Καρύστω. ἐν Σικελῶν δὲ κλυτῇ νήσῳ Κεφαλοιδὶς ἀμείνους πολλῷ τῶνδε τρέφει θύννους καὶ Τυνδαρὶς ἀκτή. Cf. Oppian 3.627–28.

[245] Tunny fishing grounds existed at Pachino, on the north coast near Cefalù, and off the promontory of Tindarus. See Athenaeus 7.302; Solinus 5.6; and Pace, *Sicilia antica*. 1: 404. In the fourth and third centuries B.C., Soluntum, a city of Phoenician origin located near Panormus, minted bronze and silver coins bearing on their reverse side the image of a tunny. See Barclay V. Head, *Historia Numorum*. 2nd ed. (Oxford 1911), pp. 170–71.

[246] Archestratus *ap*. Athen. 3.116f: καὶ Σικελοῦ θύννου τέμαχος, φίλε Μόσχε, φαγεῖν χρή, τμηθὲν ὅτ' ἐν βίκοισι ταριχεύεσθαι ἔμελλεν; Athen. 5.209a: Σίτου δὲ ἐνεβάλλοντο εἰς τὴν ναῦν μυριάδας ἕξ, ταρίχων δὲ Σικελικῶν κεράμια μύρια, ἐρεῶν τάλαντα δισμύρια, καὶ ἕτερα δὲ φορτία δισμύρια.

[247] *P.Lond*. 2141_{37} (ca. 258 B.C.).

[248] See esp. Forbes, *Technology*, 3: 173. Gela (Pliny *HN* 31.73, 86); Agrigentum (*ibid*. 31.85). See also Vitruvius *De arch*. 8.3.7. For the textile factory see *Not. dign. occ*. 11.68 (Seeck, ed., p. 151).

[249] Franco Bergonzoni, "Una industria romana nelle isole Egadi," *Antiqua* 7 (1977): 26–31;

Femmine and S. Vito the vats were similar to those at Punta de l'Arenal in Spain; that is, they were not sunk into the ground, but sat upon the hard surface. At Porto Palo, in conjunction with rectangular vats, appear also circular basins similar to some found at Rhode in Hispania Tarraconensis and in the Black Sea at Tyritake and Myrmekeion. Salting activity was modest. Porto Palo, probably to be identified with Pachynum, with at least twelve vats is the largest so far discovered. Tonnara del Cofano had two vats, while those at Isola delle Femmine possessed six, Cala Minnola a minimum of eight, and S. Vito perhaps ten or more. There remains no evidence of any significant permanent structures associated with any of the sites.

Fragments of Punic transport containers of the fourth century B.C., such as type Mañá D, have appeared at salting installations at Isola delle Femmine, Tonnara del Cofano, and S. Vito, and so may reflect Punic salting activity during the pre-Roman period. The salting vats themselves are apparently of Roman date and so offer no information on Punic salting processes. Spanish salt-fish containers of the early imperial period (Dressel Forms 7–11) and finds of fragments of Africana I and II vessels of the third or fourth centuries A.D. may represent importations to be sold along with the local product or were to be re-used for the Sicilian products.

Ancient writers confirm that Sicily exported fresh fish to Rome during the Roman period, but none mention salted fish products specifically.[250] It is unlikely that an industry so active in the fourth and third centuries B.C. would cease altogether to function in the Roman period when the same industry was apparently growing significantly in many other parts of the Western Mediterranean. The Punic and Greek salting installations of Sicily may have suffered heavily during the first and second Punic Wars and did not significantly recover. Its products, apparently like those of other western provinces, were probably dominated by those of Spain and later perhaps of Africa.[251] Future excavations may one day reveal salting installations in Eastern Sicily, and exploration of shipwrecks in Sicilian waters will shed more light on commerce. Since Sicily lay astride two major commer-

---

G. M. Bacci, "Antico stabilimento per la pesca e la lavorazione del tonno presso Portopalo," *Kokalos* 28–29 (1982–83): 345–47; Gianfranco Purpura, "Pesca e stabilimenti antichi per la lavorazione per pesce in Sicilia: I. S. Vito (Trapani), Cala Minnola (Levanzo)," *Sicilia Archeologica* 48 (1982): 45–60; and *idem*, "Pesca e stabilimenti antichi per la lavorazione del pesce in Sicilia: II. Isola delle Femmine (Palermo), Punta Molinazzo (Punta Rais), Tonnara del Cofano (Trapani), S. Nicola (Favignana)," *Sicilia Archeologica* 57–58 (1985): 59–86. Possible sites include Tonnara di Trabia and Punta Molinazzo (Punta Raisi).

[250] Pliny *HN* 9.169; Juvenal *Sat*. 5.93–106. See also Scramuzza, *Roman Sicily*, p. 352.

[251] For Spanish salt-fish amphorae found in Sicilian waters, see Gerhard Kapitän, "I relitti di Capo Graziano (Filicudi): scoperte della spedizione NACSAC nel 1968," *Sicilia archeologica* 34 (1977): 48; *idem*, "Italy: Levanzo and Favignana, Egadi Islands, prov. Trapani, Sicily," *IJNA* 6 (1977): 168–171; for African amphorae, see Gibbins and Parker, "Roman Wreck of c. AD 200," pp. 267–304.

cial routes, for example, it would be surprising if Sicilian merchants did not participate in the commerce of goods between the eastern and western provinces and, particularly in the late empire, between Africa and Italy.[252] The early 4th Century A.D. wreck off Randello (Prov. Ragusa) in Southeastern Sicily, for example, yielded Spanish Almagro 50 amphorae which contained whole sardines (*Sardina pilchardus*).[253]

---

[252] A. J. Parker, "Sicilia e Malta nel commercio marittimo dell'antichità," *Kokalos* 22–23 (1976–77): 622–31; and Gerhard Kapitän, "Le anfore del relitto romano di Capo Ognina (Siracusa)," in *Recherches sur les amphores romaines*. Collection de l'École Française de Rome, 10 (Rome 1972), pp. 243–52.

[253] Alwyne Wheeler and Alison Locker, "The Estimation of Size in Sardines (*Sardina pilchardus*) from Amphorae in a Wreck at Randello, Sicily," *JArchSc* 12 (1985): 97–100; and Anthony J. Parker, "Amphores Almagro 50 de l'épave de Randello (Sicile)," in *Amphores Romaines et Histoire Économique. Dix Ans de Recherche*. Coll. de l'École Française de Rome, 114 (Rome 1989), pp. 650–53.

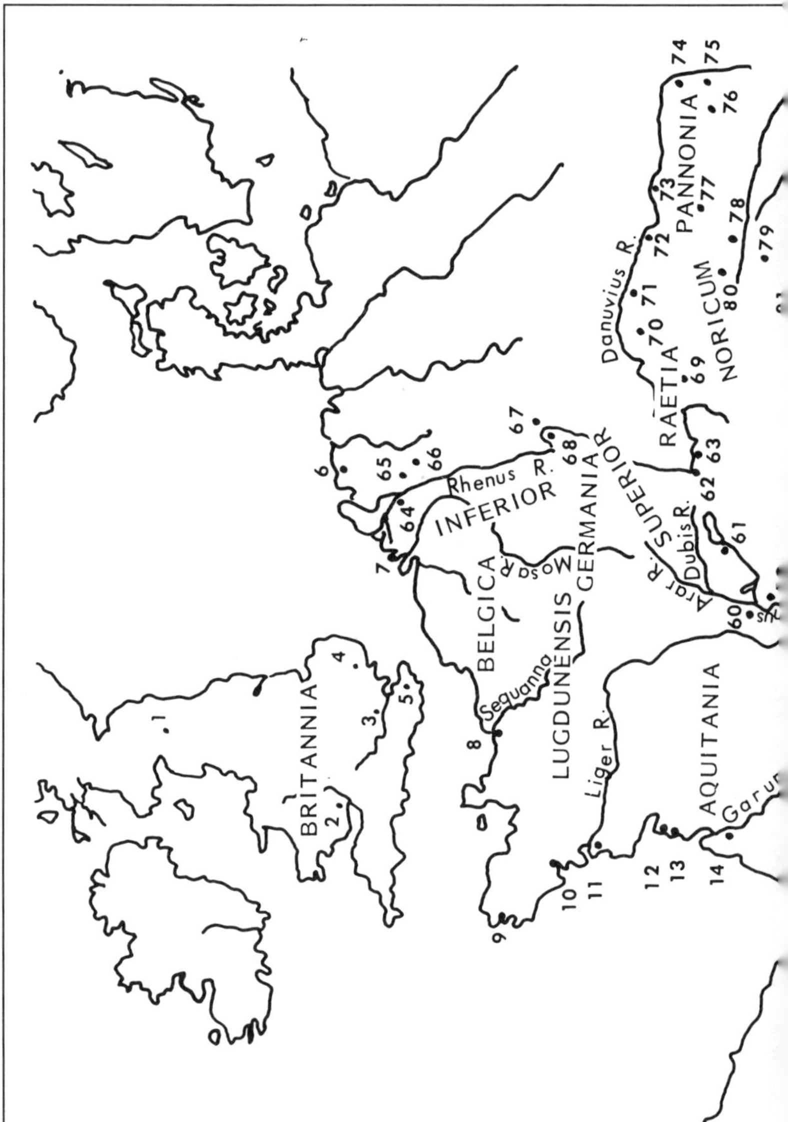
BRITANNIA
BELGICA
LUGDUNENSIS
AQUITANIA
GERMANIA
INFERIOR
SUPERIOR
RAETIA
NORICUM
PANNONIA
Rhenus R.
Mosa R.
Sequana
Liger R.
Garu
Danuvius R.
Dubis R.
Arar R.
N
1
2
3
4
5
6
7
8
9
10
11
12
13
14
60
61
62
63
64
65
66
67
68
69
70
71
72
73
74
75
76
77
78
79
80

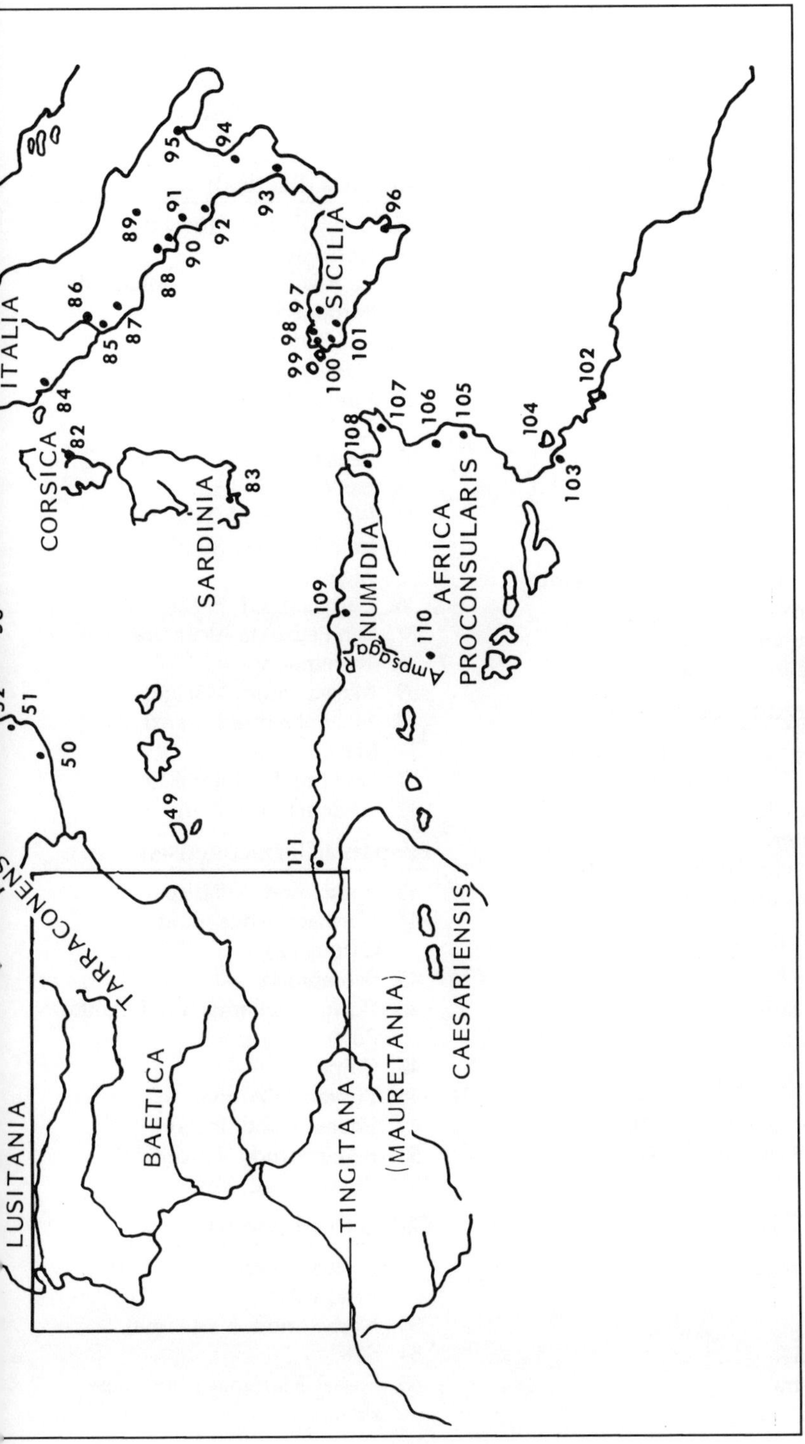

Figure 7: Western Mediterranean
(For inset see Fig. 9)

WESTERN MEDITERRANEAN

Britannia

1. Vindolanda (mod. Chesterholm)
2. Isca (mod. Caerleon)
3. Londinium
4. Camulodunum (mod. Colchester)
5. Durovernum Cantiacorum (mod. Canterbury)

Frisia (Beyond Germania Inferior)

6. Leeuwarden

Germania Inferior

7. Colijnsplaat
64. Noviomagus (mod. Nijmegen)
65. Haltern
66. Oberaden
67. Hofheim

Gallia (Lugdunensis)

8. Juliobona (mod. Lillebonne)
9. Bay of Douarnenez (includes Plomarc'h)
10. Lanester
11. Condevicnum (mod. Nantes)
60. Lugdunum (mod. Lyon)

Gallia (Aquitania)

12. Fief de Chalons
13. Nieul-sur-Mer
14. Burdigala (mod. Bordeaux)

Hispania (Lusitania)

15. Olisipo (mod. Lisbon)
15a. Caetobriga (mod. Tróia de Setúbal)
15b. Ilha do Pessegueiro
16. Boca do Rio
17. Senhora da Luz
18. Paúl
19. Vão
20. Portimão
21. Quateira
22. Olhão
23. Balsa (mod. Torre de Ares)
24. Cacela

Hispania (Baetica)

25. Onuba (mod. Huelva)
26. Cerro del Trigo
27. La Algaida (mod. Sanlúcar de Barrameda)
28. Las Redes
29. Gades (mod. Cadiz)
30. Puerto Real
31. Trafalgar
32. Baesippo (mod. Barbate)
33. Baelo (mod. Belo)
34. Mellaria (mod. Villavieja)
35. Iulia Traducta (mod. Algeciras)
36. Carteia (mod. El Rocadillo)
37. San Pedro de Alcántara
38. Torremolinos
39. Malaca (mod. Málaga)
40. Maenuba (mod. Cerro del Mar)
41. Sexi (mod. Almuñécar)
42. Abdera (mod. Adra)

Hispania (Tarraconensis)

43. Baria (mod. Villaricos)
44. Carthago Nova (mod. Cartagena)
45. Scombraria
46. Portus Illicitanus (mod. Santa Pola)
47. Calpe
48. Punta de l'Arenal
49. Ebusus (mod. Ibiza)
50. Barcino (mod. Barcelona)
51. Rhode (mod. Rosas)

Gallia (Narbonensis)

52. Portus Veneris (mod. Port Vendres)
53. Narbo (mod. Narbonne)
54. Sète
55. Fossae Marianae (mod. Fos-sur-mer)

56. Massilia (mod. Marseilles)
57. Forum Iulii (mod. Fréjus)
58. Antipolis (mod. Antibes)
59. Vienna (mod. Vienne)
61. Geneva

Germania Superior

62. Augusta Raurica (mod. Augst)
63. Vindonissa (mod. Windisch)
68. Moguntiacum (mod. Mainz)

Raetia

69. Brigantium (mod. Bregenz)
70. Augusta Vindelicorum (mod. Augsburg)

Noricum

71. Lauriacum
80. Magdalensberg (near mod. Klagenfurt)

Pannonia

72. Vindobona (mod. Vienna)
73. Carnuntum (near mod. Petronell)
74. Aquincum (mod. Acino)
75. Vetus Salina (mod. Adony)
76. Gorsium (near mod. Székesfehérvár)
77. Savaria (mod. Szombathely)
78. Poetovio (mod. Ptuj)

Italia

79. Emona (mod. Ljubljana)
81. Aquileia (mod. Udine)
84. Cosa (mod. Ansedonia)
85. Ostia
86. Roma
87. Antium (mod. Anzio)
88. Cumae
89. Beneventum
90. Puteoli (mod. Pozzuoli)
91. Pompeii
92. Velia
93. Vibo
94. Thurii
95. Tarentum

Corsica

82. Aleria

Sardinia

83. Nora

Sicilia

96. Syracuse
97. Cetaria
98. Isola delle Femmine
99. Capo S. Vito
100. Egadi Islands
101. Porto Palo

Africa Proconsularis

102. Praesidium Zuchis
103. Tipasa
104. Meninx (mod. El Kantara)
105. Sullecthum (mod. Salacta)
106. Leptis Minor
107. Neapolis
108. Carthage

Numidia

109. Rusicade (mod. Skikda)
110. Zarai
111. Cartennae

Mauretania Tingitana

112. Thamusida (mod. Sidi Ali ben Ahmed)
113. Mogador (off mod. Essaouira)
114. Lixus (mod. Larache)
115. Kouass
116. Tahadart
117. Cotta
118. Sahara
119. Alcazarsegher
120. Sania y Torres

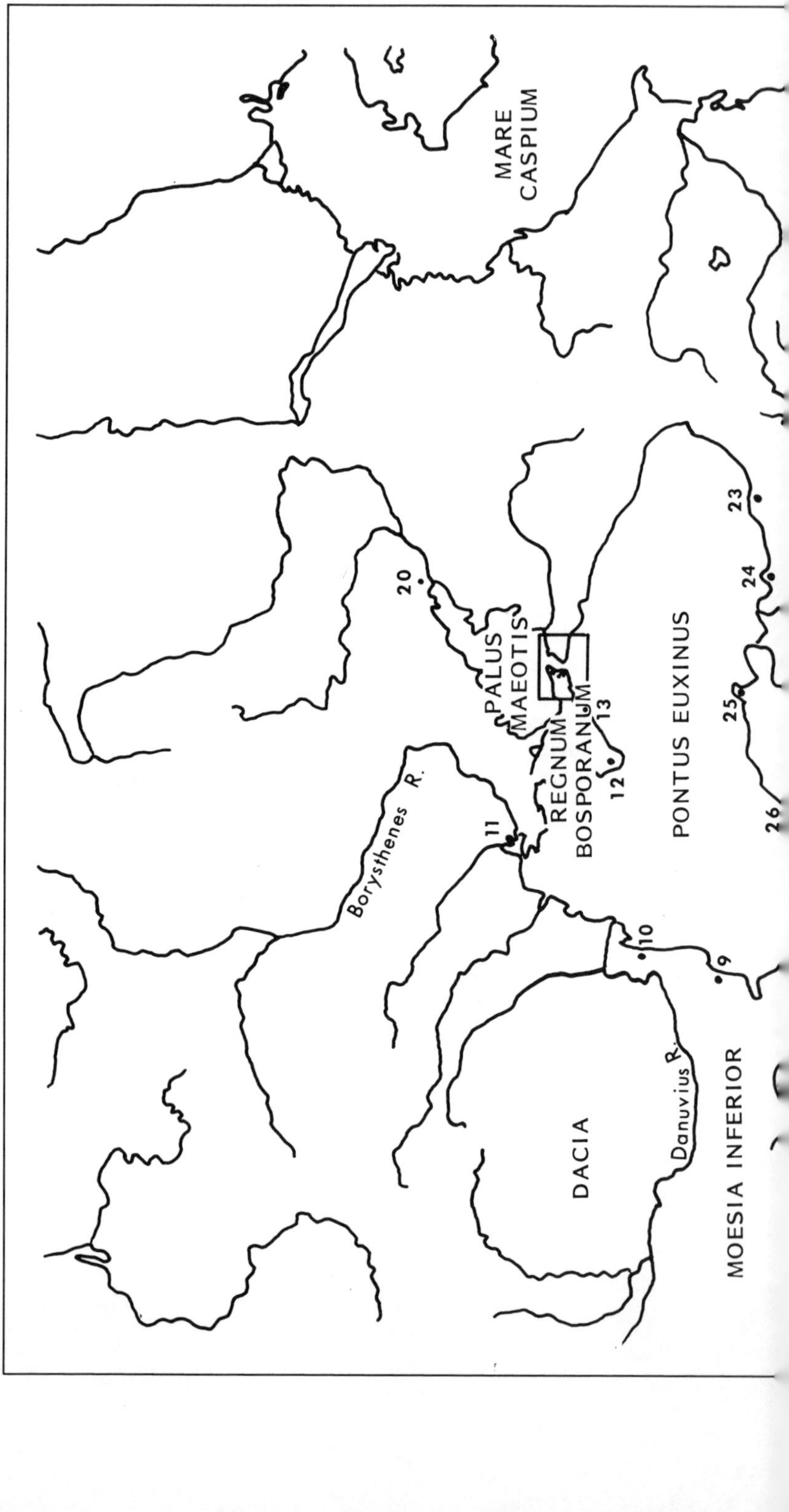
MARE CASPIUM
PALUS MAEOTIS
REGNUM BOSPORANUM
PONTUS EUXINUS
Borysthenes R.
Danuvius R.
DACIA
MOESIA INFERIOR
9
10
11
12
13
20
23
24
25
26

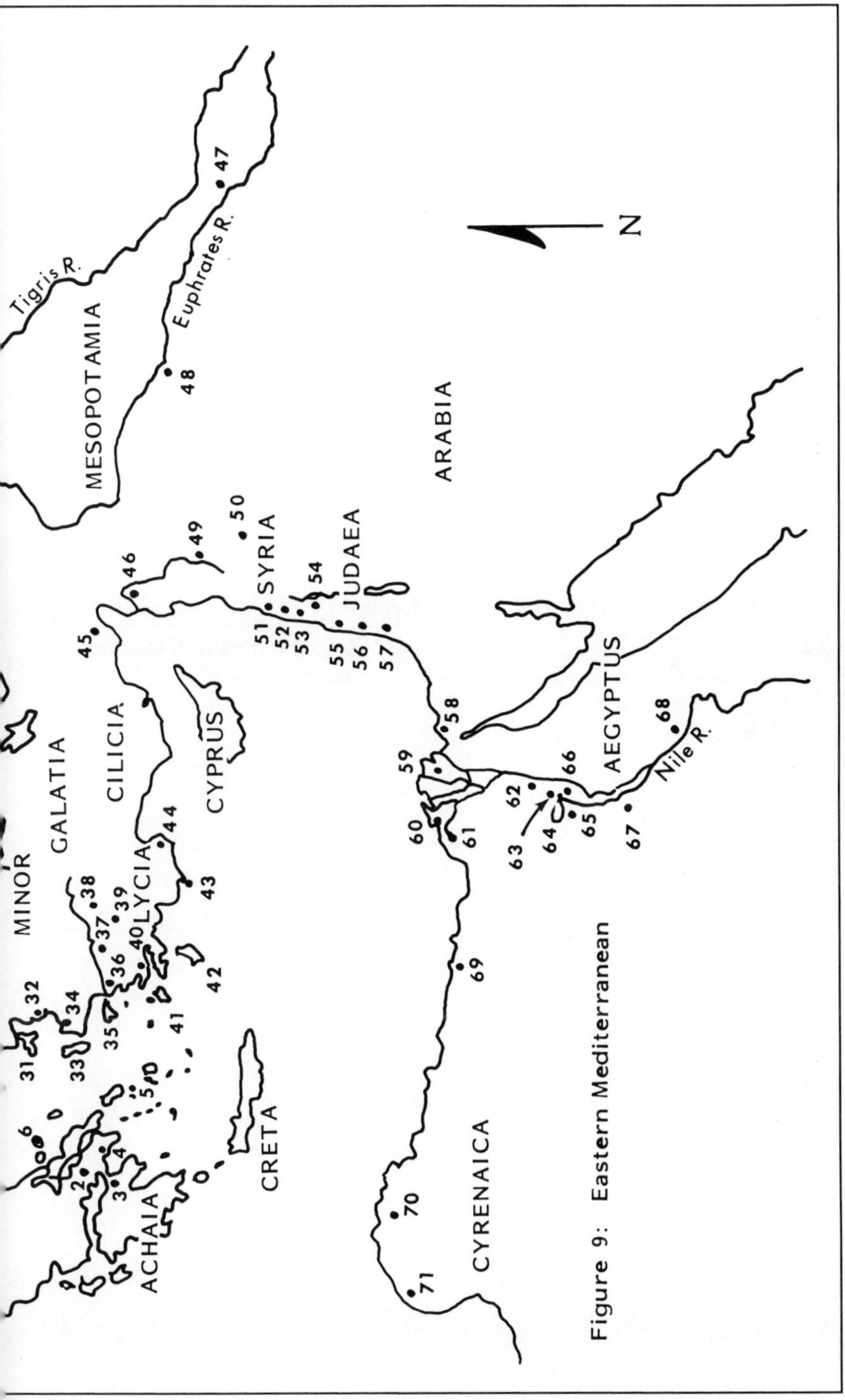

Figure 8: Eastern Mediterranean
(For inset see Fig. 10)

EASTERN MEDITERRANEAN

Macedonia

1. Lychnidus

Greece (Including the N. Aegean Islands)

2. Akraiphia
3. Corinth
4. Athens
5. Delos
6. Peparethus
7. Thasos

Black Sea (including the Bosphoran Kingdom and Lake Maeotis)

8. Byzantium
9. Odyssus
10. Histria
11. Olbia
12. Chersonesos
13. Theodosia
14. Kimmerikon
15. Nymphaion
16. Tyritake
17. Panticapaeum (mod. Kerch)
18. Myrmekeion
19. Parthenion
20. Tanais
21. Phanagoria
22. Gorgippia

Cappadocia

23. Trapezus

Pontus and Bithynia

24. Pharnacia
25. Sinope
26. Tium
27. Heraclea Pontica
28. Chalcedon

Asia Minor (including the Aegean Islands)

29. Cyzicus
30. Parion
31. Lesbos
32. Cyme
33. Chios
34. Clazomenae
35. Samos
36. Miletus
37. Alabanda
38. Hierapolis
39. Aphrodisias
40. Halicarnassus
41. Cos
42. Rhodes

Lycia

43. Megisti (on mod. Castellorizo Island)
44. Phaselis

Cilicia

45. Anazarbus

Mesopotamia

47. Babylon

Syria and Palestine

46. Antioch
48. Dura Europus
49. Apamaea
50. Palmyra
51. Sidon
52. Tyre
53. Akko
54. Taricheia
55. Caesarea
56. Askalon
57. Gaza

Egypt

58. Pelusium
59. Mendes
60. Canopus
61. Alexandria
62. Memphis
63. Bacchias
64. Lake Moeris
65. Theadelphia
66. Arsinoë
67. Oxyrhynchus
68. Panopolis
69. Paratonium

Cyrenaica

70. Cyrene (mod. Shahat)
71. Berenice (mod. Benghazi)

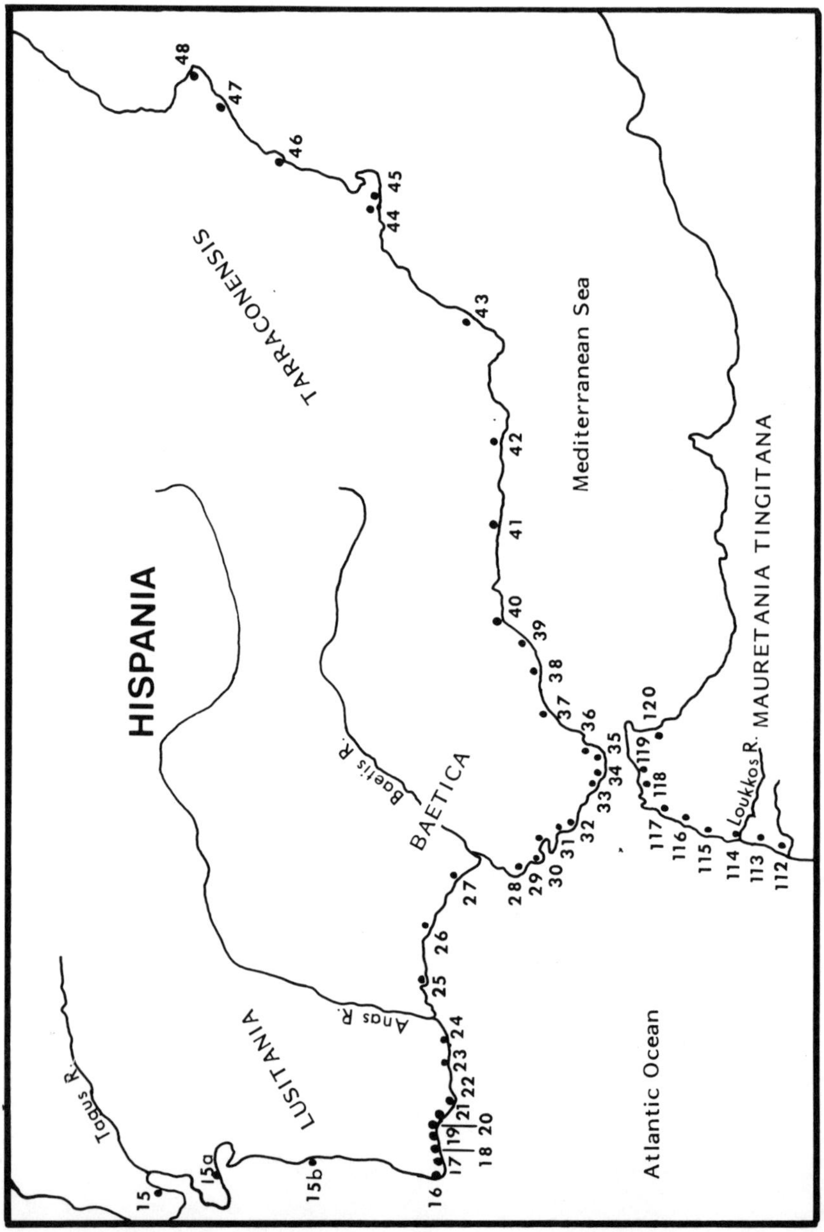

Figure 9: Southern Spain and North Africa

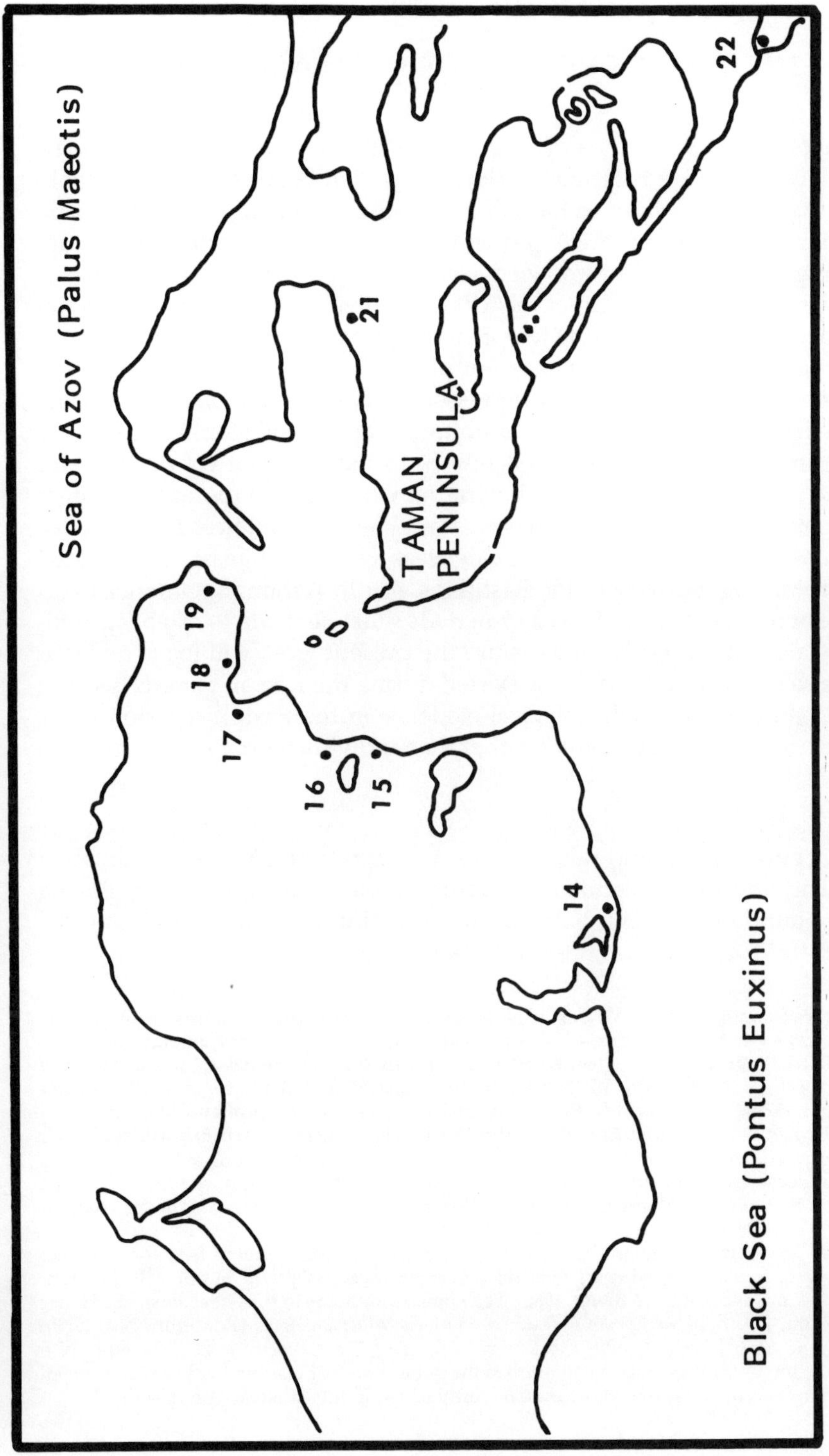

Figure 10: Strait of Kerch

CHAPTER FIVE

THE EASTERN REGIONS OF THE ROMAN EMPIRE

Archaeological excavations of Bronze Age sites in the Eastern Mediterranean have uncovered significant deposits of fish bones.[1] When one looks for archaeological evidence for fish processing centers or for signs of commerce in salted fish products, however, the results are particularly disappointing. The state of our knowledge concerning this activity in the archaic and classical periods of Greek history is negligible, while that for the Roman period is only beginning to register improvement. Except for the Black Sea area, archaeological data are not plentiful. Additionally, classification of Greek amphorae has not progressed sufficiently for one to associate salted fish products with specific amphora shapes, while Roman amphorae found in the East have only recently been made the object of intensive study.[2] This situation is doubly frustrating when one compares the meager archaeological material with the abundant literary references to salted fish products. Nevertheless, enough evidence is available to justify a look at the fish processing industry in the East (Figs. 8, 10). Although reference to literary sources pertaining to earlier periods must be made to establish sufficiently a tradition of fish processing, the present work will focus on what can be said of this industry as it existed during the Roman period. Because of the nature of the archaeological evidence in the East, discussion lends itself better to a survey of areas rather than individual provinces.

The Adriatic Sea

Evidence for fishing and raising fish on *villae rusticae* along the Dalmatian coast and on nearby islands supports the reputation enjoyed by Dalmatia for its abundance of fish. Salt was also plentiful at certain sites along the

[1] See, for example, Richard W. Casteel, *Fish Remains in Archaeology* (New York 1976), passim; John D. Evans and Colin Renfrew, *Excavations at Saliagos Near Antiparos* (London 1968), esp. pp. 78–80, 118–21; and P. H. Greenwood and G. J. Howes, "Fish Remains," in *Excavations in the Neocropolis of Salamis*. Vol. III, Appendix III of *Salamis*. S. V. Karageorghis, ed. (Nicosia 1967), pp. 259–68; and David S. Reese, "Faunal Remains (Osteological and Marine Forms) 1975–1976," in Vol. 3 of *Excavations at Carthage 1976 Conducted by the University of Michigan*. J. H. Humphrey, ed. (Ann Arbor, Mich. 1977), pp. 131–64. I owe these citations to the kindness of David S. Reese who, in a series of correspondences, has graciously apprised me of his own work and that of many others in the study of fish remains from diverse areas of the Mediterranean.

[2] Greek amphora studies are beginning to receive increased attention. See, for example, *Recherches sur les Amphores Grecques. Bulletin de Correspondance Hellénique*, Suppl. XIII. J.-Y. Empereur and Y. Garlan, eds. (Athens, 1986). For Roman amphorae in the Greek East, see Henry S. Robinson, *Pottery of the Roman Period*. Vol. 5 of *The Athenian Agora* (Princeton, N.J. 1959), passim; and Mabel Lang, *Graffiti and Dipinti*. Vol. 21 of *The Athenian Agora* (Princeton, N.J. 1976), passim. One looks with anticipation to the publication of Elizabeth Lyding Will, *Stamped Roman Amphoras in the Eastern Mediterranean*, forthcoming in the Athenian Agora series.

coast as well as from inland salterns, such as at Ad salinas in Bosnia.[3] The Romans were not slow to take advantage of Dalmatia's fish and salt resources. Although it became a Roman province only in A.D. 9, by the middle of the first century Dalmatia had acquired a good reputation for its muria.[4]

Regardless of this salting activity, it is apparent that Spain, at least in the first and second centuries A.D., supplied some of the salted fish products consumed in Dalmatia. Underwater exploration off the Dalmatian coast has brought to light several Spanish salted fish amphorae of Dressel Forms 8 and 11.[5] There exists no evidence to show that Dalmatia exported any of its products, although we can reasonably postulate that enough of it reached Rome for it to acquire a good reputation.[6]

The Aegean Sea[7]

Archaeological excavation in Greece has yielded no trace of fish processing centers, yet salting factories did function in the Aegean, not only during the Roman period but also much earlier. Fish was a staple food for Bronze Age inhabitants and references in Homer show that fishing was practiced in the early Archaic period.[8] The scant notice given to fish as food in the epic poems should probably be attributed to the attitude that fishing as an occupation and the eating of fish implied low social standing. Fish was the food of common men, not of heroes. Nevertheless, Greeks of all social

---

[3] For fishing and salt production in Dalmatia see Marin Zaninović, "The Economy of Roman Dalmatia," in *ANRW* II, 6 (Berlin 1976), pp. 787–90, 795. See also Forbes, *Technology*, 3: 171. Fish hooks are commonly found in graves dating to the late first and early second centuries A.D. See J. J. Wilkes, *Dalmatia* (Cambridge, Mass. 1969), p. 412. Tunny were caught in the Adriatic as early as the seventh century B.C. See Ferri, "La pesca del tonno," pp. 1–3.

[4] Pliny *HN* 31.94. The murex was processed for purple dye, but it is impossible to gauge its role in the Dalmatian economy. See Wilkes, *Dalmatia*, p. 409. In the late empire an imperial textile factory (*bafium*) operated at Salona. *Not. dign. occ.* 11.66 (Seeck, ed., p. 151).

[5] Dasen Vrsalović, *Istraživanja i Zaštita Podmorskih Arheoloških Spomenika u SR Hrvatskoj* (Zagreb 1974), pp. 139–40, nos. 118–20. Spanish trade with Dalmatia also included oil. See Nenad Cambi, "Spanish Amphorae Found Near Split," *Arheološki Vestnik* 26 (1975): 115–24.

[6] Shippers, primarily in wine, who traded in the Adriatic, were active in Ostia in the first and second centuries A.D. See *CIL* VI.9682; XIV.409; Meiggs, *Roman Ostia*², pp. 275–76. Cf. *L'AnnÉp* (1981): 191, no. 732, for a possible dealer in salt-fish, *salmagarius* (= *salgamarius*), who died at Ulpiana, just across the border in Moesia Superior. For σαλγαμάριοςsee also Louis Robert, "Épitaphes ex acclamations Byzantines à Corinthe," *Hellenica* 11–12 (1960): 39–46 (6th cent. A.D.). Cf. Varro *Rust*. 12.46.1. and 12.56.1.

[7] Included in the discussion of the Aegean Sea will be Greece, Crete, the Cyclades Islands, Macedonia, and the North Aegean Islands.

[8] For fish and fishing in the Greek Bronze and Archaic periods see Hans-Günter Buchholtz, Gerhard Jöhrens, and Irmgard Maull, *Jagd und Fischfang*. Archaeologica Homerica. Vol. 1, J (Göttingen 1973), pp. 131–80; H. N. Couch, "Fishing in Homer," *CJ* 31 (1935–36): 303–14; J. A. Scott, "Homeric Heroes and Fish," *CJ* 32 (1936–37): 171–72; Henk Höppener, *Halieutica. Bijdrage tot de Kennis der oud-grieksche Visscherij* (Amsterdam 1931), pp. 1–16; H. Michell, *The Economics of Ancient Greece*. 2nd ed. (Cambridge 1957), pp. 286–87; Radcliffe, *Fishing*, pp. 63–89; and J. Sakellarakis, "Le pêcheur dans l'art préhistorique Égéen," *AAA* 7 (1974): 370–90. For tunny fishing in the Cyclades islands during the Neolithic period see Evans and Renfrew, *Saliagos*, esp. pp. 118–21.

classes in the classical age and later were avid consumers of fresh and processed fish. Greek affection for fish cannot be better illustrated than by observing that the word ὄψον, which designated generally a relish eaten with bread or meat, came to mean "fish."[9] The term γάρον appears in Greek literature in the early fifth century B.C., but was probably in use much earlier.[10]

The demand for fish may have begun as early as the seventh century B.C. when certain Greek cities, perhaps attracted by fishing prospects, began to colonize the north shore of the Black Sea.[11] Fish salting centers in the Euxine were soon sending their products to other Greek markets, particularly to Athens. The Athenian population apparently had an insatiable appetite for processed fish, since literary sources show that salted fish came to Athens from as far away as Byzantium in the East and Spain and Sicily in the West.[12] Indeed, Alexis says that the sons of Chaerephilus were made Athenian citizens because their father, under circumstances not entirely clear, had brought τάριχος to Athens.[13]

The question of who first developed fish salting into a commercial enterprise cannot be answered with certainty. The etymology of the Greek word τάριχος remains obscure.[14] Greeks, having learned the process from inhabitants of the Black Sea, carried this knowledge with them when colonizing the West, or Phoenico-Punic colonists, relying on experience learned perhaps in Phoenicia, spread the knowledge of fish processing in the West, or

---

[9] Athen. 7.276e: εἰκότως, ἄνδρες φίλοι, πάντων τῶν προσοψημάτων ὄψων καλουμένων ἐξενίκησεν ὁ ἰχθὺς διὰ τὴν ἐξαίρετον ἐδωδὴν μόνος οὕτως καλεῖσθαι διὰ τοὺς ἐπιμανῶς ἐσχηκότας πρὸς ταύτην τὴν ἐδωδήν. λέγομεν γοῦν ὀψοφάγους οὐ τοὺς βόεια ἐσθίοντας, οἷος ἦν Ἡρακλῆς, ὃς τοῖς "βοείοις κρέασιν ἐπήσθιε σῦκα χλωρά," οὐδὲ τὸν φιλόσυκον, οἷος ἦν Πλάτων ὁ φιλόσοφος, ὡς ἱστορεῖ Φανόκριτος ἐν τῷ περὶ Εὐδόξου· ἱστορεῖ δ' ὅτι καὶ Ἀρκεσίλας φιλόβοτρυς ἦν, ἀλλὰ τοὺς περὶ τὴν ἰχθυοπωλίαν ἀναστρεφομένους. Cf. Plutarch *Mor.* 667F. Plutarch (*Timoleon* 14) uses the term ὀψόπωλις to refer to the fishmarket. See also Höppener, *Halieutica*, pp. 62–64. I regret that I was unable to consult F. Bourriot, "La consommation du poisson et la pêche maritime dans l'antiquité grecque," *Mer-Outre-Mer. Revue de la ligue maritime et d'Outre-Mer* (Mar., 1972): 14–17.

[10] Γάρον appears in the works of the tragedians Aeschylus (fr. 211 Nauck) and Sophocles (fr. 531 Nauck), the comic writers Plato (fr. 198 Edmonds), Cratinus (fr. 6 Edmonds), and Pherecrates (fr. 173 Edmonds), and the historian Clearchus (Athen. 1.6a).

[11] See Carl Roebuck, *Ionian Trade and Colonization* (New York 1959), p. 127; A. J. Graham, "The Date of the Greek Penetration of the Black Sea," *BICS* 5 (1958): 39; and Vasile Pârvan, "La pénétration hellénique et hellénistique dans la vallée du Danube," *Académie Roumaine. Bulletin de la Section Historique*. Vol. 10 (Bucharest 1923), p. 26. For an opposing view see Robert Drews, "The Earliest Greek Settlements on the Black Sea," *JHS* 96 (1976): 29.

[12] For salted fish products imported from the Black Sea area see Nicostratus frs. 4, 5 Edmonds, Antiphanes fr. 77 Edmonds, and fr. 181 Edmonds: τῆς τε βελτίστης μεσαῖον θυννάδος Βυζαντίας τέμαχος ἐν τεύτλον λακιστοῖς κρύπτεται στεγάσμασιν. For τάριχος from Spain and Sicily see Antiphanes fr. 77 Edmonds, Nicostratus frs. 4, 5 Edmonds, Eupolis fr. 186 Edmonds, and Theopompus fr. 51 Edmonds.

[13] Alexis fr. 77 Edmonds. See also Hyperides ὑπὲρ χαιρεφίλου περὶ τοῦ ταρίχους. Fragments of the speeches of Hyperides are collected in *Oratores Attici*. J. G. Baiter and Hermann Sauppis, eds. (Zürich 1850), 2: 303–04. Cf. David M. Lewis, "Attic Manumissions," *Hesperia* 28 (1959): 219 (lines 510–13), 230.

[14] See Pierre Chantraine, *Dictionnaire étymologique de la langue grecque* (Paris 1977), p. 1094.

a combination of these two theories have all been advanced to explain the salting activity well-established in Spain as early as the fifth century B.C. Recent finds at Gades have suggested to some a western origin of the knowledge, at least for that area of the Mediterranean.[15] More work is needed to resolve this perplexing problem, but excavations in the forum at Corinth have yielded important finds bearing on this question.

Excavators clearing an area of the southwest section of the Roman forum in Corinth discovered a house dating from the early 5th century B.C. In the 460s the house was used partially as a residence and partially as a place of business where wine and salted fish were stored or reprocessed. After renovations in the mid-5th century B.C., the owner devoted the entire house to his business concerns.[16] Inside the building excavators found Punic, Chian, and local Corinthian amphorae in large numbers, along with fewer vessels from other cities, such as Mende. The Punic containers, comprising about 40% of the total, gave the building its modern name, the "Punic Amphora Building." Many of the sherds had adhering to them pieces of preserved bream and tunny. The fish, probably salted or pickled in brine, had been cut into small rectangular segments (τετϱάγωνον) convenient for shipping in amphorae (Pl. 1a).[17] A physico-chemical analysis on examples of Punic vessels determined that the clay content of the amphorae was consistent with the geology of the northwest coast of Morocco to the Strait of Gibraltar and the southern coast of Spain opposite. A more precise localization of origin is not possible at this time, but the suggestion of a connection with Gades seems a strong one. The Punic vessels (Pl. 8), designated Mañá-Pascual A-4a, are common to the area of Cadiz. Another possibility suggested is kouass in Mauretania Tingitana, a conclusion particularly significant, since it has been held for some time that Spanish preserved fish called "Gaditanian" might also include the products of salteries in Northwest Morocco.[18]

---

[15] See above pp. 47–48.

[16] The second phase ended no earlier than the 440s. See Charles K. Williams, II and Joan E. Fisher, "Corinth, 1975: Forum Southwest," *Hesperia* 45 (1976): 104–07; Charles K. Williams, II, "Corinth, 1977: Forum Southwest," *Hesperia* 47 (1978): 15–20; *idem*, "Corinth, 1978: Forum Southwest," *Hesperia* 48 (1979): 107–24; and *idem*, "Corinth Excavations, 1979," *Hesperia* 49 (1980): 108–11. See also Gilles Touchais, "Chronique des fouilles en 1977: Corinthe," *BCH* 102 (1978): 657–60, esp. figs. 37–38.

[17] The amphora fragments were all mixed together, probably having been broken once emptied of their contents. This renders impossible the attribution of the fish to a particular container. The Punic vessels seem the most likely candidates. Williams, "Corinth, 1978," pp. 117–18.

[18] Y. Maniatis et al., "Punic amphoras Found at Corinth, Greece: an Investigation of Their Origin and Technology," *JFA* 11 (1984): 205–22. Mary Lou Zimmerman Munn, in her dissertation "Corinthian Trade with the West in the Fifth and Fourth Centuries B.C." (Bryn Mawr 1982), makes the tentative connection between the Punic vessels at Corinth and Kouass in Mauretania Tingitana. For the suggestion that Punic type Mañá-Pascual A-4 amphorae are indigenous to the area around Gades see Muñoz Vicente et al., "Contribución," pp. 500–02, and esp. Fig. 10–1. I have accepted Muñoz Vicente's classification of the vessels at Corinth. That they may have originated in Motya in Sicily has been discounted. See Maniatis et al., "Punic Amphores," p. 206, note 5.

Since the inhabitants of the Eastern Mediterranean and Black Sea had a long tradition of fishing and processing fish products well before the Romans made their appearance, there is no reason to doubt that these activities continued to operate after 146 B.C.[19] Evidence that the Romans took advantage of fishing resources in the Greek East is provided by discoveries of fish tanks (*piscinae*) in several areas of the Eastern Mediterranean. Eastern Crete alone had three such constructions, at Siteia, Chersonisos, and Mochlos. All are of Roman date and in construction follow closely the suggestions given by Columella and Varro for building fish ponds.[20] Six piscinae of the first century A.D., interconnected and linked with the sea by channels, have been found at Kenchreai, the eastern port of Corinth.[21] Large undivided basins serving as fish tanks have been discovered on the island of Aegina, and similar ones have been found at Lapithos on Cyprus and Caesarea Maritima in Israel. All of these piscinae may have been used either to breed fish or to store live fish between the time when they were caught and eaten. The absence of any evidence for salting facilities raises doubts about their connection with fish processing, a relationship which seems to appertain to piscinae in Spain, for example at Punta de l'Arenal which had a saltery nearby.

Since the Romans had certainly known of the Punic industrial complexes in Spain and North Africa from the period of the Second Punic War at the latest and were themselves importing τάριχος into Italy from Byzantium in the same period or shortly afterwards, they surely would have recognized the value of salting factories in the Aegean and the potential for income which they offered.[22] It is, therefore, strange that we hear no more than we

---

[19] For fishing in Greece see especially Höppener, *Halieutica*, pp. 17–27; Michell, *Economics*², pp. 286–89; H. Bolkestein, *Economic Life in Greece's Golden Age*. 2nd ed. rev. by E. J. Jonkers (Leiden 1958), pp. 36–37; and André Andreades, *Geschichte der griechischen Staatswirtschaft* (Munich 1931), pp. 157–58.

[20] Columella *Rust*. 8.16–17; Varro *Rust*. 3.17. For fish tanks on Crete see John Leatham and Sinclair Hood, "Sub-marine Exploration in Crete, 1955," *ABSA* 53–54 (1958–59): 263–80; and Costis Davaras, "Rock-cut Fish Tanks in Eastern Crete," *ABSA* 69 (1974): 87–93.

[21] Robert Scranton, Joseph W. Shaw and Leila Ibrahim, *Kenchreai, Eastern Port of Corinth*. I. *Topography and Architecture* (Leiden 1978), pp. 25–35.

[22] Epigraphic and archaeological evidence shows that Delos possessed an important purple industry during the Hellenistic and Roman periods. On the eastern shore large deposits of crushed shells of *Murex trunculus* have been found in close proximity to groups of vats used to manufacture the dye. The vats, dating to the first century B.C., have been well preserved, as have also granite "anvils" used to break the shells. The Delian basins were made of granite and allowed for drainage through a hole in the bottom. See especially Philippe Bruneau, "Documents sur l'industrie délienne de la poupre," *BCH* 93 (1969): 759–91; and *idem*, "Deliaca (II): 16: La fabrication de la poupre à Délos," *BCH* 102 (1978): 110–14. There is no evidence, however, that these vats were used for salting fish in addition to preparing purple dye, but the possibility remains. A ταριχοπώλιονhad operated in fourth century B.C. Delos. Dieter Hennig, "Die 'heiligen Häuser' von Delos," *Chiron* 13 (1983): note 12, pp. 413–14. See also *SEG* 33 (1983): 181, no. 624. Cf. also the Roman salting vats at Rhode in Spain and Alcazarsegher in Mauretania Tingitana. Producers of Vietnamese *nuoc-mam* utilize wooden vats with drains near the bottom. See Steinkraus, *Handbook*, p. 517. Roman activity in the purple industry can also be seen in Epirus and in Greece proper at Bulis, Hermione, Isthmus, Lato, Porto-Cheli,

do of the eastern salteries outside those of the Black Sea area. Although a ταριχοπώλιον had operated in fourth century B.C. Delos, and Thasos and Peparethus apparently traded in preserved fish products in the fifth and third centuries B.C. respectively, we can only guess that they continued to operate in the Roman period. Strabo mentions ταριχεῖαι in the vicinity of Lychnidus in Macedonia, which processed fish caught in the surrounding lakes. There were tunny fisheries at places like Corcyra, off the coast of Epirus; Calydon, on the coast of Aetolia; Patrae, Troezen, and perhaps Megara, in the Peloponnesus; and at Carystus, on the island of Euboea, but the sources are silent on processing at these sites.[23] Although literary evidence substantiates some fish processing in the Eastern Mediterranean during the Roman period, it seems apparent that processed fish products did not make their way to the West in any great amount and it seems equally certain that what was produced did not even satisfy the demands of the population in the eastern provinces.

Mainland Greece was always essentially an importer of foodstuffs, such as wine and grain. Although fishing was carried on in many areas, salted fish seems also to have been primarily an import item. This was particularly true for Athens which, as early as the fifth century B.C., imported salted fish from the West and East. In the fourth century B.C. Phaselite merchants contracted to import Bosphoran products, probably including processed fish; and early in the following century Cyprus was sending its salted fish to Athens. Later that same century salted tunny was included among fish whose price was fixed at Akraiphia in Boeotia. The origin of these fish, however, is unknown. Bruttians and Campanians brought ὀρκύνοιο τρίγωνα from Italy and Spain in the second century B.C.[24]

That Greece proper continued to be an importer of salted fish products

---

Corinth and in the area of Laconia. See especially Thompson, *Greek Fishes*, pp. 209–18. See also Pausanias 10.37.3; Pliny *HN* 9.127; and Martial 8.28.9. For Epirus see H. W. Catling, "Archaeology in Greece, 1978–79: Epirus (Nome of Preveza: Kassope)," *Archaeological Reports for 1978–79*. No. 25 (Athens 1979): 26. For salt resources in Greece and Crete see Forbes, *Technology*, 3: 170–71.

[23] Strabo 7.7.8: καταλυθείσης δὲ τῆς Μακεδόνων ἀρχῆς, ὑπὸ Ῥωμαίοις ἔπεσε. διὰ δὲ τούτων ἐστὶ τῶν ἐθνῶν ἡ Ἐγναστία ὁδὸς ἐξ Ἐπιδάμνου καὶ Ἀπολλωνίας· περὶ δὲ τὴν ἐπὶ Κανδαονίας ὁδὸν αἵτε λίμναι εἰσὶν αἱ περὶ Λυχνιδόν, ταριχείας ἰχθύων αὐτάρκεις ἔχουσαι,. . . . Hicesius (*ap*. Athen. 7.298b) mentions salted eels from Macedonia. See also Höppener, *Halieutica*, pp. 17–27; and Rhode, *Thynnorum Captura*, pp. 30–31. For Delos see Hennig, "Die 'heiligen Haüser' von Delos," pp. 413–14; and *SEG* 33 (1983): 181, no. 624.

[24] Black Sea: Demosthenes *In Lacritum* 933–34, the story of Phaselite merchants who borrow money for a voyage from Athens to Pontus where they were to purchase a cargo and return it to Athens. The cargo obtained at Panticapaeum included jars of τάριχος and Coan wine. This cargo was conveyed to Theodosia in the Crimea and formed part of the object of charges brought against the Phaselites who had contracted to return to Athens with a Pontic cargo. Cf. Diogenes Laertius *De vita Antisthenis* 9. For Cyprus see Poseidippus fr. 17 Edmonds. Salted tunny (θουννόκειτος, οὔπο[γ]άστρια, and θουννίδια) and other fish were included among sea fish listed in the inscription (224–210 B.C.) found at Akraiphia in Boeotia. See Fr. Salviat and Cl. Vatin, "Le tarif des poissons d'Akraiphia," in *Inscriptions de Grèce centrale* (Paris 1971), pp. 95–109, and Paul Roesch, "Sur le tarif des poissons d'Akraiphia," *ZPE* 14 (1974): 5–9. Bruttians and Campanians: Euthydemus *ap*. Athenaeus 3.116c.

in the Roman period is evidenced by finds of Spanish salted fish vessels in the Athenian Agora, Corinth, and on the islands of Crete and Delos.[25] Although this is meager evidence upon which to base a conclusion, it seems that Spain was a major supplier of salted fish products to the Athenian and Corinthian markets in the first century A.D., as it had been in the fifth century B.C. Exportation of salted fish products by producers among the Greek islands is attested only for the fifth century B.C. when the North Aegean island of Thasos sent its ἅλμη to Athens and in the third century B.C. when both Thasos and Peparethus, located just north of Euboea, were apparently sending their τάριχος to Egypt.[26] Evidence for the Roman period is totally absent.

The Black Sea

We are better informed of the production and commerce of salted fish products of the Black Sea region than for any of the eastern provinces of the Roman Empire (Figs. 8, 10).[27] This happy state of affairs is due both to the wealth of ancient literary sources which comment on various aspects of the fishing industry in the Pontus Euxinus and to important excavation work carried out there by Russian, Bulgarian, Romanian, and Polish archaeologists.[28]

That the Black Sea was an ἰχθυοέσσα χῶρα did not go unnoticed by the Greeks of the fifth century and, as noted earlier, may have played an im-

[25] Lang, *Graffiti and Dipinti*, p. 74, no. Hd 8. Cf. *ibid.*, no. Hd 3 and p. 93, no. L 47. Cf. Lucian *Navigium* 22: τάριχος μὲν ἐξ Ἰβηρίας. See also Beverly Adamsheck, *Kenchreai, Eastern Port of Corinth*. Vol. IV: *The Pottery* (Leiden 1979), p. 108, and Will, *Stamped Roman Amphoras in the Eastern Mediterranean* (forthcoming). Will designates Spanish amphorae as Type 16. Cf. Libanius *Or*. 62.46–48, who speaks of ἄνθρωπος δέ τις γάρου κάπηλος, named Heliodorus, at Corinth in the fourth century A.D. For Crete, see J. W. Hayes, "The Villa Dionysos Excavations, Knossos: the Pottery," *ABSA* 78 (1983): 146–47.

[26] Peparethos: *PSI* V.535$_{37}$: κυβίων πεπονηκὸς Πεπαρή(θιον) κερ(άμιον) α; Thasos: *PSI* V.535$_{44-45}$: ταρίχου ὡραίων ἀπολέ/κτων πεπονηκὸς Θάσι(ον) κερ(άμιον) α. For ἀπόλεκτον see Xenocrates *ap*. Orib.2.58.141; Pliny *HN* 9.48; 32.150. See also Cratinus fr. 6 Edmonds and Aristophanes *Acharnae* 671. Pollux (*Onom*. 6.63) mentions Θασία ἅλμη.

[27] Included in the discussion will be the lands bordering both sides of the Hellespont and Propontus, the Thracian Bosphorus, and regions surrounding the Pontus Euxinus and Palus Maeotis (Sea of Azov). This area included portions of the provinces of Thrace, Moesia Inferior, Asia, Pontus, Bithynia, and Cappadocia, as well as the Crimea (Tauric Chersonese) and the semi-independent client kingdom of the Bosphorus, centered in the Cimmerian Bosphorus and the Taman Peninsula.

[28] Unfortunately most of the published material has appeared in languages little read by western scholars, and so is imperfectly known outside Eastern Europe. The works of Christo M. Danov and Viktor F. Gajdukevič are major exceptions. Christo M. Danov, "Pontos Euxeinos," *RE*, Suppl. IX (1962): cols. 866–1175, especially sections dealing with fish and fishing (cols. 955–72), fish preserves (cols. 972–79), and the organization for production and commerce (cols. 979–85), with bibliography; Viktor F. Gajdukevič, *Das Bosporanische Reich* (Berlin 1971), esp. pp. 185–86, 376–78, 406–08, and the lengthy bibliography on pp. 538–72. Noteworthy also is the book on Russian archaeology by Alexander Mongait, *Archaeology in the U.S.S.R.* David Skivirsky, transl. (Moscow 1959), esp. pp. 187–217; and the old, but still useful work by Ellis H. Minns, *Scythians and Greeks* (Cambridge 1913), esp. pp. 436–49.

portant role in Greek colonization of the area in the seventh century B.C.[29] Pre-Roman literary references to fish, fishing, and fish processing are quite numerous, and the epigraphic and numismatic evidence tends to bear out this economic picture. Tunny appear on the coins of Sinope, on the southern shore of the Black Sea, and of Cyzicus, lying on the southwest coast of the Propontus. A tunny was still being used on coins of Byzantium in the reign of Tiberius.[30] Herodotus praises the fish of the Borysthenes (Dneiper) River, especially the sturgeon, which, he adds, was salted. Epigraphic evidence of the third century B.C. shows that Olbia, the great emporion at the mouth of the Borysthenes River on the north shore of the Pontus Euxinus, had a fishmarket.[31] Fishing was a much practiced and lucrative livelihood throughout the Black Sea area, especially with regard to the tunny or pelamys, whose migration route was such that all areas of the Pontus Euxinus, Lake Maeotis, the Propontus, and Hellespont took advantage of fishery resources.[32]

Fish preservation formed a substantial portion of fishing activity in the pre-Roman period. Euthydemus, states that the Bosphorus was rich in salted fish and that the inhabitants cut the fish into squares and pickled them. Whether he refers to the Thracian or Cimmerian Bosphorus is unknown; he may merely be using the expression generically, referring in general to salted fish from the Black Sea.[33] Cratinus, for example, uses the

---

[29] *Inscriptiones Graecae Metricae* (T. Preger, ed. Leipzig 1891) 7: ἀμφί τε Βυζάντειον ὅσοι θάνον, ἰχθυόεσσαν ῥυόμενοι χώραν ἄνδρες ἀρηίθοοι. For fishing as a motive for Greek colonization in the Black Sea area see above page 114.

[30] Sinope: Bohlen, *Fischerei*, p. 17; Cyzicus: *ibid.*; Head, *Historia Numorum*, pp. 523–25, esp. figs. 269–74. For epigraphic evidence on fishermen see below, p. 120. For coins of Byzantium see Jacques Dumont, "La pêche du thon à Byzance à l'époque hellénistique," *REA* 78–79 (1976–77): 114, note 111.

[31] Herodotus 4.53; Ditt. *Syll.*³ I, 495. 101 (ἰχθυοπώλιον). Cf. Ditt. *Syll.*³ 1039 (ca. 230 B.C.), as amended in *SEG* 3 (1929): 587. Olbia issued coins in the shape of a fish which have as legend ΘY, possibly a reference to θύ(ννος), and APIX, which may indicate salted fish, (τ)άριχ(ος). See Köhler, Τάριχος, pp. 82–88, and Bohlen, *Fischerei*, p. 18. Minns (*Scythians and Greeks*, pp. 483–84), however, argues that the legends refer to magistrates' names and the coin shape is that of a dolphin, not a tunny. The father of the Philosopher Bion, a native of Olbia, traded in τάριχος. See Diog. Laert. 4.46. Cf. also Pomponius Mela *De chorographia* 2.1.6.

[32] For fish and fishing in the Black Sea area see esp. Danov, "Pontos Euxeinos," col. 955–72; S. Semenov-Zuser, "Rybnyj Rynok v Xersonese," *VDI* 2 (1947): 237–46; Erik Gren, *Kleinasien und der Ostbalkan in der wirtschaftlichen Entwicklung der römischen Kaiserzeit* (Uppsala 1941), pp. 77–79; D'Arcy W. Thompson, "'Byzantios olent lacertos' (Stat. *S.* 4, 9, 13)," *CR* 46 (1932): 246–48; and Dumont, "La pêche du thon à Byzance," pp. 96–117.

[33] Euthydemus *ap.* Athen. 3.116b: οἷς ὁ ταριχόπωλεως ἅδε Βόσπορος, οἵ θ' ὑπόγαστρα τμήγοντες τετράγωνα ταρίχια τεκταίνονται.The Greeks imported salted fish from both the Thracian and Cimmerian Bosphorus. Dorion (Athen. 3.118b), in his treatise περὶ ἰχθύων, for example, discusses the κορακῖνος from Lake Maeotis, a fish which he says was salted. The description by Demosthenes (*In Lacritum* 934) of salted fish being transported from Panticapaeum, in the Cimmerian Bosphorus (Strait of Kerch), to Theodosia in the Crimea in an Athenian ship is equally appropriate. Exportation of salted fish from Byzantium, in the Thracian Bosphorus, is a well-known fact. See Archestratus *ap.* Athen. 7.284e, who also refers ambiguously περὶ τῶν ἐν Βοσπόρῳ ταρίχων.

term τάριχος Ποντικός, and ταρίχη Ποντικά is found in Pollux.[34] Several cities of the region, however, drew specific mention and sometimes even praise for their fish products. These include Sinope, which was known for its mullets; Parion, on the southern coast of the Hellespont, for its salted mackerel; and especially Byzantium, in the Thracian Bosphorus, which Euthydemus calls "the mother of salted tunny."[35]

Fishing continued to play an important role in the economy of the Black Sea region during the Roman period, or approximately from the late second century B.C., when its products were being sent to Rome.[36] Parion, a Roman colony from the time of Caesar and refounded by Hadrian, had an association of fishermen, and Xenocrates, writing in the first century A.D. praises its salted mackerel.[37] Evidence for an active fishing industry continuing at Cyzicus comes from a dedication to Poseidon by an association of fishermen of a cylindrical base having carved figures of tunny and dolphins.[38] There was an association of tunny fishermen (θυνεῖται) at Odyssus (Varna) on the western shore of the Black Sea in Moesia Inferior; and a Dionysiac thiase of fishermen living near Byzantium set up a votive inscription to Dionysus Parabolos.[39] There were tunny watches (πηλαμυδεῖα) operating at Sinope, Trapezus, and Pharnacia, and the Clazomenians maintained σκοπαί on the Cimmerian Bosphorus.[40]

That the Black Sea inhabitants continued to produce salted fish products during the Roman period can be seen from references to ταριχεῖαι at the

---

[34] Cratinus fr. 40 Edmonds. Cf. Sopater of Paphos (*ap.* Athen. 3.119a) speaking of partially salted fish from the Danube River: ἐδέξατ' ἀντακαῖον, ὃν τρέφει μέγας Ἴστρος Σκύθαισιν ἡμίνηρον ἡδονήν. For fishing at Histria, located at the mouth of the Danube River, see Pârvan, "La pénétration hellénique," pp. 26–27. For ταρίχη Φρύγια see Pollux *Onom.* 6.48 and Eupolis fr. 186 Edmonds.

[35] Sinope: Dorion *ap.* Athen. 3.118c; Parion: Euthydemus *ap.* Athen. 3.116c. Cf. Hermippus fr. 63 Edmonds for salted mackerel from the Hellespont: ἐκ δ' Ἑλλησπόντου σκόμβρους καὶ πάντα ταρίχη; Byzantium: Euthydemus *ap.* Athen. 3.116b (θύννων δ' ὡραίων Βυζάντιον ἔπλετο μήτηρ). For other references to processed fish products from Byzantium see Nicostratus frs. 4,5 Edmonds (Βυζάντιον τέμαχος); Diphilus *ap.* Athen. 3.120f and 4.132c-d; Antiphanes *ap.* Athen. 3.118b; 7.303f; and Archestrates *ap.* Athen. 3. 117a; 7. 303e, 314e-f. Euthydemus (*ap.* Athen. 3.118d) notes that fish caught in the Delcon River near Byzantium were salted.

[36] Cato *ap.* Polybius 31.25.5. Ovid wrote his *Halieutica*, a poem in praise of the many fish of the area, from Tomis on the Black Sea.

[37] Association of fishermen: Louis Robert, "Pêcheurs de Parion," *Hellenica* 9 (1950): 80–97, and *idem*, "La pêche à Parion,"*Hellencia* 10 (1955): 272–74. See also Xenocrates *ap.* Orib. 2.58.143.

[38] Louis Robert, "Dédicace de Cyzique," pp. 122–25. The monument was found near the temple of Hadrian.

[39] *L'AnnÉp.* (1928): 146 (Odessus). For another inscription see Milko Mirčev, "Novi epigrafski pametnici ot Černomorieto," *Arxeologičesko Družestvo* (Varna), *Izvestija* 12 (1961): 7–8 (θοινεῖται). I regret that I could not consult N. S. A. Minčev, "Ribolovut v Odesos prez antičosfta," *Phar* (1976): 104–11. For the thiase of fishermen of Byzantium see Louis Robert, "Documents d'Asie-Mineure: XVI. Du Bosphore à l'Eubée avec une inscription errante," *BCH* 102 (1978): 522–34.

[40] Πηλαμυδεῖα: Strabo 7.6.2 (Trapezus); 7.6.2, 12. 3.11 (Sinope); 12.3.19(Pharnacia); σκοπαί: Strabo 11.2.4.

mouth of the Rhombites River, south of Tanais in Lake Maeotis, and in the Tauric Chersonese, fronting on the same body of water.[41] A first century A.D. inscription from Histria in Moesia Inferior indicates that much of the city's revenue came from fishing and salted fish.[42] Perhaps the best evidence comes from the *Geoponica*, which describes the Bithynian process for making garum.[43] Other cities in the Roman period which received praise for their fish products include Trapezus and Chalcedon, for their pelamydes; Tium, Heraclea Pontica, and especially Byzantium, for their tunny; and Panticapaeum, for its sturgeon.[44]

Although many different kinds of fish were caught and processed in salting establishments of the Black Sea area, the tunny, particularly the pelamys, was the most important commercially.[45] Archaeologists have in recent years uncovered the bones of many of these fish as well as those of anchovies, herring, sturgeon, sea roach, flounder, and mackerel.[46] Some of these fish bones have been found in salting vats discovered by Soviet archaeologists in the strait of Kerch at Tyritake and Myrmekeion and in the Crimea (Tauric Chersonese) at Chersonesos.

Soviet excavations at Tyritake and Myrmekeion, two cities lying in the strait of Kerch (Cimmerian Bosphorus) opposite the Taman Peninsula, uncovered salting installations with well-preserved vats (Fig. 10). The saltery at Tyritake, which contained fifty-nine vats, had a capacity of almost 460 cubic meters, while the smaller one at Myrmekeion (eight vats) had a volume of ca. 130 cubic meters. Together these two cities, located near one another, could process about 160 crude tons of fish.[47] The source of salt for these factories may have come from the Tauric Chersonese (Crimea).[48] A brief discussion of Tyritake will furnish a good idea of the characteristics of

[41] Rhombites River (Strabo 11.2.4); Chersonesos (*ibid*. 7.4.6).

[42] James H. Oliver, "Texts A and B of the Horothesia Dossier at Istros," *GRBS* 6 (1975): 143–56. See below, p. 128.

[43] *Geoponica* 20.46.3 (Appendix I-8).

[44] Black Sea in general: Strabo 7.6.2; Pliny *HN* 9.47–54; 32.149. For Trapezus: Strabo 7.6.2. Chalcedon: Varro *ap*. Aul. Gell. 6.16.5. Tium, Heraclea Pontica, and Amastris: Aelian *NA* 15.5. Byzantium: Strabo 7.6.2. Panticapaeum: Strabo 7.3.18. For general statements on Pontic salted fish products during the Roman period see Pliny *HN* 32.146, and Galen *De alim. fac*. 3.40.6.

[45] Thompson, *Greek Fishes*, s.v. Ἀμία (p. 13), θύννος (pp. 79–90), and πηλαμύς (pp. 197–99); *idem*, "Byzantios olent lacertos," pp. 246–48; Rhode, *Thynnorum Captura*, esp. pp. 7–8, 31–36; Dumont, "La pêche du thon à Byzance," pp. 96–117; and Semenov-Zuser, "Rybnyj Rynok v Xersonese," pp. 237–46.

[46] See esp. Casteel, *Fish Remains*, pp. 124–30 (Crimea); and V. D. Lebedev and Ju. E. Lapin, "K voprosu o rybolovstve v Bosporskom carstve," *MIA*, No. 33 (Moscow 1954), pp. 197–214 (Cimmerian Bosphorus).

[47] Danov, "Pontos Euxeinos," cols. 973–74; Gajdukevič, *Das Bosphoranische Reich*, pp. 376–78.

[48] Gajdukevič, *Das Bosphoranische Reich*, p. 378. Dio Chrysostom (*Orat*. 36.3), the first century A.D. orator and philosopher who was born in Prusa in Bithynia, says that the Greeks and Scythians of the Tauric Chersonese bought salt from Olbia, which possessed salt works near the mouth of the Borsythenes River. Dioscurias apparently was also noted for its salt. See Strabo 11.5.6, and Bohlen, *Fischerei*, p. 18.

fish salting installations of the Bosphoran kingdom during the Roman period.

Tyritake, which lies on the coast a few miles south of Panticapaeum (Kerch), was a commercial and agricultural city founded in the sixth century B.C. Its two major industries were wine making and fish processing, activities which existed side-by-side concentrated in the eastern and southern part of the city. Tyritake's salting and wine making installations were usually placed behind or between dwelling houses essentially arranged on either side of a central street.[49] It is significant that fish processing occurred within the walls of the city itself, not outside as was predominantly the case in the Western Mediterranean. Most of the houses in Tyritake in the first and second centuries A.D., however, were rather modest in size.[50]

The salting vats vary in size but are essentially rectangular or square in shape, having dimensions ranging between ca. 2.00 x 1.40 x 1.80 meters and 2.50 x 1.50 x 2.87 meters.[51] They are usually grouped together; for example, one group of six vats is arranged in three rows of two pairs, another has four vats in a single row, and two groups have four vats in two rows of two pairs.[52] The vats were sunk into the ground and had walls made of limestone slabs of between 0.15 to 0.27 meters in thickness. The exterior of the vats was unfinished, but the interior (sides and bottom) was coated with several layers of mortar made of lime and finely crushed ceramic (*opus signinum*). The ceramic dust gave the vats a reddish appearance and ensured that they would be water-tight.[53] There was no provision for drainage. Roof tile fragments found in the vats indicate that they were covered for protection against the rain. Many of the vats also contained large limestone slabs which were used during processing to press the fish down into the salt solution.[54]

In close proximity to many of the large vats were smaller ones or, more

[49] Gajdukevič, *Das Bosporanische Reich*, p. 186, and esp. Figs. 95–97; Mongait, *Archaeology*, p. 205.

[50] Gajdukevič, *Das Bosporanische Reich*, pp. 185–86. Gajdukevič postulates that the wealthy owners probably lived in nearby Panticapaeum, while the workers lived near the vats. He briefly describes, however, an elaborate house in Tyritake which he dates to the third or fourth century A.D., a period of apparent decline for the fish processing industry (*ibid.*, pp. 407–08). See also *idem*, "Raskopki Tiritaki i Mirmekija v 1946–1952 gg.," *MIA*, No. 85 (Moscow 1958), pp. 149–218.

[51] Gajdukevič, "Raskopki Tiritaki v 1935–1940 gg.," *MIA*, No. 25 (Moscow 1952), pp. 30–32, 46–49, 55–62; esp. Plan 62, p. 56.

[52] *Ibid.*, pp. 56–60, and Plan 62, Plot XIII, Groups A–D, respectively. In Plot X (*ibid.*, p. 48) there are six vats arranged as in Group A of Plot XIII; and in Plots V–VI there is a group of five vats, four of which are arranged in pairs with a single vat attached to the north side of the group of four. For Plot XIII, see also *idem*, *Das Bosporanische Reich*, Fig. 97.

[53] *Idem*, *Das Bosporanische Reich*, pp. 376–77.

[54] *Idem*, "Raskopki Tiritaki v 1935–1940 gg.," p. 31. These slabs were also found in Plots V–VI at Tyritake and in vats uncovered at Myrmekeion. For Myrmekeion see *idem*, "Raskopki Mirmekija v 1935–1938 gg.," *MIA*, No 25 (Moscow 1952), p. 207. The tiles, including some covered with a white cement, found in vats in Armorica may have played a similar role. See Sanquer and Galliou, "Garum," p. 219.

frequently, groups of pithoi, or dolia, buried in the ground.[55] The precise use of these small vats and pithoi is uncertain, but they obviously had a connection with the fish processed in the large vats. It has been suggested that the small vats may have served to store the brine or to wash the fish before placing them in the large vats, and the pithoi may have been used to store the processed fish transferred from the large vats. It seems more likely, however, that the pithoi, and probably the small vats as well, were used to prepare garum. The analogy of the small vats in Spanish salteries comes immediately to mind, but it should be remembered that their use for garum is only a conjecture. The dolia used at Pompeii may also provide a parallel, but in that instance it is unlikely that the complete maturation process took place in the house. It is not insignificant that literary sources which describe the production process for fish sauce always specify small or relatively small containers. More to the point is the description of garum production found in the *Geoponica*. To retrieve the fish sauce a fine-meshed basket is dipped into the container and when lifted up the garum is strained through the holes.[56] At Myrmekeion inside one of the pithoi located near the salting vats was found a near-cylindrical vessel which had provisions at the top for attaching a rope and along the body and probably in the bottom (not extant) perforations to allow drainage of the brine.[57]

There is no doubt that the large vats were used for salting fish, since inside many of them excavators have found dried fish bones. At Tyritake the fish were primarily herring and mullet, while at Myrmekeion the remains were mainly of xamsa, a small fish similar to the anchovy. Large quantities of mussel and crab shells were found nearby.[58] Frequently found in or near the vats were fishhooks, lead weights, and bone needles. Many groups of vats had associated with them a hearth or stove in which ceramic vessels were probably made.[59]

Fish processing probably operated in the following manner. The fish and salt were brought into town and taken directly to the salteries. In a work

---

[55] Gajdukevič, "Raskopki Tiritaki v 1935–1940 gg.," pp. 57–59; *idem*, *Das Bosporanische Reich*, Fig. 97. Group C of Plot XIII had small vats, while pithoi were found near Group A. Pithoi were also discovered near the vats uncovered at Myrmekeion and at Chersonesos. For Myrmekeion see *idem*, "Raskopki Mirmekija v 1935–1938 gg.," p. 207. For Chersonesos consult G. D. Belov, "Raskopki Xersonesa v 1961 g.," *Soobščenija Xersonesskogo Muzeya* 3 (1963): 56–57; Vladimir I. Kadeev, *Očerki Istorii 'Ekonomiki Xersonesa Tavričeskogo v I-IV vekax n.è.* (Xar'kov 1970), p. 17; and Mongait, *Archaeology*, p. 199.

[56] *Geoponica* 20.46.1–6. The use of a strainer of some kind to extract fish sauce is also mentioned by Ps-Rufius Festus and Ps-Gargilius Martialis. See Appendix I–4,5, and 8.

[57] Gajdukevič, "Raskopki Tiritaki v 1935–1940 gg.," pp. 57–59; *idem*, *Das Bosporanische Reich*, p. 378; and *idem*, "Raskopki Mirmekija v 1935–1938 gg.," p. 207, esp. Fig. 126.

[58] Danov, "Pontos Euxeinos," col. 974 (shellfish). For Tyritake see Gajdukevič, "Raskopki Tiritaki v 1935–1940 gg.," pp. 59–60. For Myrmekeion see *idem*, "Raskopki Mirmekija v 1935–1938 gg.," p. 207. The vats in Chersonese processed primarily anchovies, with some herring and xamsa. See Kadeev, "Očerki," p. 14

[59] Gajdukevič, "Raskopki Tiritaki v 1935–1940 gg.," pp. 32, 60. The 3rd–4th century house in Tyritake had many weights and net needles in nearly all rooms. Fishing instruments have been found in many places in the Bosphoran kingdom, including private homes. Fishing was

area located next to the vats the fish were cut up, cleaned, washed, and those pieces suitable for salting were placed into the large vats. They were probably arranged in alternating layers of fish and salt up to the top of the vats where large slabs of limestone were placed on top to press down the fish during the maturation process. Small fish and fish innards to be made into fish sauce were placed into the small vats and pithoi located nearby. One can easily imagine that frequently wine was added to the garum to make a special recipe, a process which the author of the *Geoponica* ascribes to the Bithynians. This step would be a logical one for the producers at Tyritake, since wine making was an important industry in the city and many of the wine presses found there were lying next to and were contemporary with the salting vats.[60] Once prepared, the processed fish was transferred either to pithoi for further aging or processing or, as was probably the case with ἡμιτάριχος ("half-salted"), placed directly into amphorae for immediate shipment. The garum could be transferred to commercial vessels as needed.

The determination of a chronology for the salteries at Tyritake and Myrmekeion is based primarily on finds of dated coins and of pottery and tiles whose styles can be assigned certain chronological limits. The salteries seem to date from the first to the third centuries A.D., although some, for example those at Tyritake, may have functioned into the fifth or sixth century, albeit at a much reduced level of activity.[61] The zenith of the salteries was apparently during the first and second centuries A.D., and its end probably came as a result of the Hun invasions of the late fourth century A.D. Evidence of violent destruction has been found in both cities.[62]

Before discussing commerce in salted fish products in the Black Sea area, a few words should be said concerning Chersonesos, near Sevastopol, the only other place where salting vats have been found and which displays some unique characteristics. The saltery here is much larger (over 90 vats)

---

a primary occupation of many people in the area and fish was an important element in their diet. For the house at Tyritake see Gajdukevič, *Das Bosporanische Reich*, p. 408. For the kilns see *idem*, "Raskopki Tiritaki v 1935–1940 gg.," p. 59. For fishing see Lebedev and Lapin, "K voprosu," pp. 197–99.

[60] For the wine industry in the Cimmerian Bosphorus, particularly at Tyritake, see Gajdukevič, "Raskopki Tiritaki v 1935–1940 gg.," p. 49; *idem*, *Das Bosporanische Reich*, passim; and Mongait, *Archeology*, p. 205. For Myrmekeion see also Kazimierz Michalowski, "Fouilles polonaises à Mirmeki en Crimée," *Atti del settimo congresso internazionale di archeologia classica* (Rome 1961) 3: 68–69; Viktor F. Gajdukevič, "Vinodelie na Bospore," *MIA*, Vol. 85 (Moscow 1958), pp. 352–457; and Zofia Sztetyllo, "Production et commerce du vin à Mirmekion à l'époque hellénistique," *Études et Travaux* IV, Vol. 10 of Travaux de Centre d'Archéologie Méditerranéenne du l'Académie Polonaise des Sciences (Warsaw 1970), pp. 96–112.

[61] Gajdukevič, "Raskopki Tiritaki v 1935–1940 gg.," pp. 30–32, 49, 58–60.

[62] *Idem*, *Das Bosporanische Reich*, pp. 185–86. A recent study questions Gajdukevič's chronology, preferring to date the Hun invasions to the second quarter of the sixth century A.D. If this new dating bears scrutiny, then salt-fish production may have actively continued well past the fourth century. See A.V. Sazanov and Ju. F. Ivanščenko, "K voprosu o datipovkax pozdneantičnyx sloev gorodov Bospora," *Sovetskaja Arxeologija*. no. 1 (1989): 84–102, and A. V. Sazanov, "O xronologii Bospora rannevizantijskogo vremeni," *Sovetskaja Aarxeologija*. no. 4 (1989): 41–60.

than that at Tyritake, and the vats are scattered over a wider area. Some are constructed in a manner similar to and are roughly contemporary with those in the strait of Kerch. They are, however, not usually grouped together in a series, but dispersed individually or at most in groups of two or three basins. Most vats are rectangular or square, but a few are pear-shaped and cut into the rock.[63] The vats of Chersonesos are generally quite large and, if one considers all the basins of every period together, have a volume of approximately 2000 cubic meters. Small vats, but of considerable depth, were probably used for fish sauces. The annual production of preserved anchovies alone may have approached 3000–3500 metric tons of fish, enough to make the Crimea one of the largest centers of salted fish.[64] Pithoi have been reported closely associated with the vats at Chersonesos. There was apparently a salt-work nearby, and the fish remains found in most abundance are those of the anchovy. The salting installations at Chersonesos date mostly to the first century A.D., but a few seem to date to the fourth through the sixth centuries A.D.

One cannot help but be struck by the similarities of the salting installations in the Crimea and the strait of Kerch with those of Spain, North Africa, and Gaul. First, the same characteristics seem to have determined the location of salteries; that is, the availability of fish, salt, and fresh water. Second, the salting vats were constructed in an almost identical manner, particularly with respect to being sunk into the ground or cut into the rock and being coated on the inside with a waterproof mortar of lime and crushed ceramic (*opus signinum*). The reddish color of vats at Tyritake immediately recalls similar shading of vats in Gaul in the Department of Charente-Maritime and in the Bay of Douarnenez. The major difference between vats in the Black Sea and those in the Western Mediterranean is that the former ones lack a hole in the bottom as well as the ovolo in the corners, or at least I have been unable to find references to them in sources available to me. The pear-shape of vats in Chersonesos also show a marked difference from vats in the western provinces. Third, the vats within the saltery are, with the exception of those at Chersonesos, grouped in rows by pairs. Fourth, the chronological limits of the salting installations, which range from the first to the third or fourth century A.D., with a few extending to the fifth or sixth century but operating at a reduced capacity, correspond closely to those of western salteries.

There apparently occurred in the first century A.D. throughout the Roman Empire a remarkable increase in the fishing industry and its various

[63] For fish processing at Chersonesos see Kadeev, *Očerki*, esp. pp. 5–26; Vladimir I. Kadeev and S. G. Rižov, "Nova ribozasoljuval'na cisterna u Xersonesi," *Arxeologia* 12 (1973): 76–80; I. B. Brašinskij, "Recherches soviétiques sur les monuments antiques des régions de la Mer Noire," *Eirene* 7 (1968): 96–97; Mongait, *Archaeology*, p. 199; Danov, "Pontos Euxeinos," col. 975; and Belov, "Raskopki Xersonesa," pp. 56–57. For pear-shaped vats see Mongait, *Archaeology*, p. 199.

[64] Kadeev, *Očerki*, p. 15. Kadeev gives a figure for anchovies of over 30,000 tsentners. One tsentner equals about 100 kg.

subsidiary activities, particularly the manufacture of salted fish products. This upsurge of industrial activity in the Bosphoran kingdom was probably related to the establishment of Roman garrisons in the area of the Black Sea and Asia Minor.[65] This expansion could not have been due to an increased demand for luxury fish products alone, as has been suggested, but probably resulted from a need to supply the Roman armies stationed in Moesia, to which the Bosphoran kingdom was tied militarily, and the soldiers manning the frontiers with Armenia in the provinces of Pontus, Bithynia and Cappadocia. In effect, whereas the salteries of Spain supplied the legions stationed in Europe along the limes and in Britain, those of the Bosphoran kingdom were probably the major suppliers of the armies of the lower Danube and in the East. Salt-fish and fish sauce also supplied the growing civilian populations and might also serve as reserves in case of food shortages and famine. The salteries of Pontus, for example, furnished preserved fish to the inhabitants of Cappadocia during a food shortage in A.D. 369.[66] This increased demand for salted fish products was met by the Bosphoran engineers who in adopting Roman construction techniques probably obliterated evidence for earlier facilities used during the Hellenistic period.[67]

Commerce in salted fish products from the Black Sea area in the pre-Roman period was not inconsiderable. Athens imported salted fish from the Hellespont and other areas of the Pontus Euxinus and Bosphorus.[68] Pontic processed fish was not unknown to the Romans at this time since Italy was importing it from as early as the second century B.C., when Cato the Elder decried the expense of τάριχος. Its expense may indicate that commerce in the Western Mediterranean in salted fish from the Black Sea was not fully developed or that only the most expensive kinds came from this region.[69] Polybius says that salted fish was among the luxury products

---

[65] Danov, "Pontos Euxeinos," col. 975, who cites a work by J. J. Marti; Kadeev, "Očerki," p. 19.

[66] Gajdukevič, *Das Bosporanische Reich*, p. 377. See also Michael Rostovtzeff, "Pontus, Bithynia and the Bosporus," *ABSA* 22 (1916–18): 1–22, and *idem*, *SEHRE*², pp. 259–61. Among amphorae of wine, grain, and other food items found in a store-room of the Roman military garrison in Olbia, dated to the 2nd or 3rd century A. D., were vessels containing fish. See Aleksandra Wąsowicz, *Olbia pontique et son territoire. L'aménagement de l'espace* (Paris 1975), p. 121. For famine in Cappadocia see St. Gregory Nazianzen, *Funerary Oration In Honor of Basil the Great, Bishop of Caesarea of Cappadocia* 35.4: Συναγαγὼν γὰρ ἐν ταὐτῷ τοὺς λιμοῦ τραυματίας, ἔστι δὲ οὓς καὶ μικρὸν ἀναπνέοντας, ἄνδρας καὶ γυναῖκας, νηπίους, γέροντας, πᾶσαν ἡλικίαν ἐλεεινήν, πᾶν ἔδος τροφῆς ἐρανίζων, ὅση τυγχάνει λιμοῦ βοήθεια, ἔτνους τε πλήρεις προθεὶς λέβητας καὶ τοῦ ταριχευτοῦ παρ' ἡμῖν ὄψου καὶ πένητας τρέφοντος; and Ramon Teja, *Organizacion economica y social de Capadocia en el siglo IV, segun los padres capadocios* (Salamanca 1974), p. 147. For the text of St. Gregory Nazianzen I have used *Grégoire de Nazianze Discours Funèbres en l'Honneur de son Frère Césaire et de Basile de Césarée*. Fernand Boulenger, ed. (Paris 1908), p. 134.

[67] Gajdukevič, *Das Bosporanische Reich*, p. 377.

[68] Hermippus fr. 63 Edmonds; Demosthenes *In Lacritum* 934. For the popularity of salted fish products from the Black Sea in the Hellenic and Hellenistic East see Rostovtzeff, *SEHRE*², passim; Danov, "Pontos Euxeinos," passim; and Dumont, "La pêche du thon à Byzance," pp. 96–117.

[69] Cato *ap*. Polybius 31.25.5. Cf. Plutarch *Mor*. 668B-C. See also F. W. Walbank, *A Historical Commentary on Polybius*. 3 vols. (Oxford 1957–79), 3: 500–01.

the region furnished Greece.[70] Horace, who mentions muria from Byzantium, provides the only evidence for a specific city exporting processed fish to the Western Mediterranean. Usually the authors refer merely to Pontic salt-fish, leaving in doubt the specific point of origin. There is too little evidence to be certain, but the possibility remains that Byzantium may have served as a middleman for most Pontic fish exported to the West.[71] Italy continued to import Pontic salted fish products, but the western salteries, particularly those of Spain, could and apparently did provide the bulk of the basic needs of Italy and other western provinces between the first century B.C. and the third century A.D. It seems certain that, although Pontic salteries continued to be active during this period, they did not effectively compete in western markets with Spanish producers.[72]

The salteries of the Black Sea region concentrated in and, although the evidence is far from clear, may have dominated commerce in salted fish products in the Greek East during the Roman period.[73] The best evidence comes from Strabo, whose references to Pontic salteries give some idea of the salting activity in the Augustan period. He notes that since the time of Mithridates Eupator (120–63 B.C.) the Bosphorus had been subject to the Romans, but remarks that prior to that time the salteries of Lake Maeotis had sent salted fish to the Greeks.[74] Pontic salt-fish was also sent to Egypt in the first century B.C., if one can credit the humorous story told by Plutarch concerning Antony and Cleopatra.[75]

The paucity of evidence, both literary and archaeological, inhibits any clear understanding of the organization for production and commerce in salted fish products of the Black Sea region. Evidence for production comes

[70] Polybius 4.38.4: Πρὸς μὲν γὰρ τὰς ἀναγκαίας τοῦ βίου χρείας τά τε θρέμματα καὶ τὸ τῶν εἰς τὰς δουλείας ἀγομένων σωμάτων πλῆθος οἱ κατὰ τὸν Πόντον ἡμῖν τόποι παρασκευάζουσι δαψιλέστατον καὶ χρησιμώτατον ὁμολογουμένως, πρὸς δὲ περιουσίανμέλι κηρὸν τάριχος ἀφθόνως ἡμῖν χορηγοῦσιν.

[71] Horace *Sat.* 2.4.63–66: *est operae pretium duplicis pernoscere iuris/ naturam. simplex e dulci constat olivo,/ quod pingui miscere mero muriaque decebit/ non alia quam qua Byzantia putuit orca.* For Byzantium as middleman in the exportation of Pontic products, see Dumont, "La pêche du thon à Byzance," pp. 97–110. Rostovtzeff (*SEHRE*², p. 261) points out the importance of Panticapaeum in this trade and adds that, "Merchants from the Greek cities ultimately secured the produce and exported great quantities of salted and dried fish to the Greek and Roman markets, including those of the Western provinces."

[72] Galen, in the second century A.D., refers to Pontic salted fish products but indicates that they were inferior to those of Spain and Sardinia. See Galen *De alim. fac.* 3.30.5; 3.40.6.

[73] This was probably also true in the pre-Roman period, but Danov's strong statement in this regard may have to be modified in light of recent excavations at Corinth in the Punic Amphora Building. See Danov, "Pontos Euxeinos," cols. 983–85. For the Punic Amphora Building, see above, p. 115.

[74] Strabo 7.4.6: φόρον τε ἐτέλουν ὀκτωκαίδεκα μυριάδας μεδίμνων Μιθριδάτῃ, τάλαντα δ' ἀργυρίου διακόσια σὺν τοῖς 'Ασιανοῖς χωρίοις τοῖς περὶ τὴν Σινδικήν. κἀν τοῖς πρόσθεν χρόνοις ἐντεῦθεν ἦν τὰ σιτοπομπεῖα τοῖς Ἕλλησι, καθάπερ ἐκ τῆς λίμνης αἱ ταριχεῖαι. Cf. Polybius 4.38.4.

[75] Plutarch *Ant.* 29.3–4. Danov ("Pontos Euxeinos," col. 978) cites the reference to salted sturgeon (ἀντακαῖον) in *PSI* V.535$_{35}$ as evidence for Pontic exports to Egypt in the third century B.C. See also Georgacas, *Ichthyological Terms*, pp. 111–12, 164.

only from the three salteries excavated in the strait of Kerch and in the Tauric Chersonese. Danov, following Gajdukevič, notes that the majority of workers in these fish salting establishments were, to all appearances, slaves and the owners probably the Bosphoran kings.[76] There is no clear evidence for this assertion other than the tradition of monopolistic control exercised by the Bosphoran kings prior to incorporation into the Roman sphere of influence. What organization appertained elsewhere is even less certain. Strabo says that the tunny catch provided the citizens of Byzantium and the Roman people a considerable revenue.[77] Apparently the Romans exercised some kind of control, if not in direct ownership, since the Byzantines derived a profit as well, at least in the form of taxation. Roman taxation of the municipal profits from fishing and fish salting is strongly implied for the first century A.D. at Histria in Moesia Inferior, where imperial legates on several occasions granted an exemption from taxes of their fishery products, including τάριχος.[78] The question of the extent of municipal control over fishing and fish salting cannot be ascertained either. At Histria apparently the city did not completely control the fishing rights of its inhabitants. A tax was probably paid by fishermen to the city.[79] Fishermen, such as at Parion and Byzantium, probably paid a tax, but *societates* of fish salters have not been attested. If they did exist, as seems likely, we do not know whether they acted on their own behalf and merely paid a tax to the city on their products or else leased the fishing and salting rights from the city.[80]

The commerce of salted fish products was apparently not controlled by the state, at least not before the fourth century A.D. In the fourth century B.C., Phaselite merchants had contracted with a private businessman to import Pontic products, including probably τάριχος, to Athens from Panticapaeum. This practice apparently continued to prevail in the Roman period, since Lucian describes how Phoenician ταριχοπῶλαι sailed the Pontus Euxinus as far as Lake Maeotis and the Cimmerian Bosphorus, as well as other Greek waters, before returning home in late autumn.[81] There is also no evidence for a state monopoly of *negotiatores* dominating traffic in salted fish products. In fact, we have no evidence from *tituli picti* on amphorae, epigraphy, or elsewhere of even private organizations in salted fish prod-

---

[76] Danov, "Pontos Euxeinos," cols. 974 (owners), 982–83 (workers). See also Gajdukevič, *Das Bosporanische Reich*, pp. 185–86.

[77] Strabo 7.6.2: παραλαβὼν δ᾽ ὁ ἐνταῦθα ῥοῦς, ἅμα καὶ τῶν τόπων εὐφυῶν ὄντων πρὸς τὸ τὸν ἐκεῖ ῥοῦν τῆς θαλάττης ἐπὶ τὸ Βυζάντιον καὶ τὸ πρὸς αὐτῷ Κέρας τετράφθαι, φυσικῶς συνελαύνεται δεῦρο καὶ παρέχει τοῖς Βυζαντίοις καὶ τῷ δήμῳ τῶν Ῥωμαίων πρόσοδον ἀξιόλογον.

[78] Oliver, "Texts A and B," pp. 143–56. See also Pârvan, "La pénétration," p. 27.

[79] Corcoran, "Roman Fishing Industry," p. 115; Bohlen, *Fischerei*, pp. 49–50.

[80] On the question of state monopolies at Byzantium in the Hellenistic period see Dumont, "La pêche du thon à Byzance," pp. 114–15.

[81] Demosthenes *In Lacritum* 934; Lucian *Tox*. 4. For state interference in trade, see below, note 13, p. 152.

ucts. Our sources say that it was transported from the Pontic regions to other places, they do not indicate who did it.

Asia Minor[82]

The fishing resources of Asia Minor were significant and had been tapped long before the Romans acquired hegemony over the region.[83] Tunny fisheries operated along the coast of the mainland and around the offshore islands. In the fifth century B.C. a fishery for large tunny (ὀρκυνεῖον) operated at Halicarnassus, and in the following century Lesbos was maintaining tunny watches.[84] Tunny figured prominently on the coins of Methymna on Lesbos, the island cities of Chios and Samos, and the mainland cities of Clazomenae and Teos.[85] Likewise, tunny served as emblems on the coins of the provinces of Lycia and Cilicia.[86] Fish processing formed an integral part of this activity, particularly on the islands of Samos, Cyprus, and possibly Rhodes.[87] The city to receive most notice in this respect was a Lycian city, Phaselis. Philostephanus and Heropythus both relate the story of the founding of the city at which the founder purchased the territory for the colony with τάριχος. From this fact, the story goes, the Phaselites annually made a sacrifice with salted fish to Cylabras, the shepherd from whom the land was purchased.[88] This association of Phaselis with salted fish occurs again in the oration of Demosthenes in which is related the story of Phaselite merchants contracting to transport to Athens some salt-fish from the Black Sea region.[89]

The Romans also drew advantage from the fishery resources of Asia Minor. Cos operated public and private σκοπαί and purple factories.[90] The

[82] This section will include all areas of modern Turkey and its offshore islands not previously discussed; that is, those areas which at one time or another formed the Roman provinces of Asia, Lycia, Galatia, Cilicia, and the islands of Rhodes and Cyprus.

[83] For fishing in Asia Minor see Bohlen, *Fischerei*, passim; Corcoran, "Roman Fishing Industry," pp. 101–02.

[84] Alciphron 1.20.1 (Lesbos): ὁ σκοπιωρὸς ὁ Λέσβιος; Ditt. *Syll.*[3] 46a 43 (Halicarnassus): ὀρκυνεῖον.

[85] Rhode, *Thynnorum Captura*, p. 37.

[86] Lycia: Rhode, *Thynnorum Captura*, p. 37; Keller, *Antike Tierwelt*, 2: 385; Cilicia: Rhode, *Thynnorum Captura*, p. 37 (Tarsus).

[87] Samos: Crates *ap*. Athen. 3.117b-c; Cyprus: Posidippus fr. 17 Edmonds. Theocritus of Chios mentions a salt-fish market, ταριχόπωλις· ὁ αὐτὸς (sc. Theocritus) τῶν Χίων οὐκ ἐώντων αὐτὸν στῆσαι τὴν εἰκόνα αὐτοῦ πρὸς τῇ στοᾷ, ἀλλὰ φασκόντων τοὺς ὀλυμπιονίκας ἐκεῖ δεῖν ἵστασθαι, ἔφη. "ἐὰν Ὀλύμπιά τις ὑμῶν νικήσῃ, μετάθετέ μου τὴν εἰκόνα εἰς τὴν ταριχόπωλιν." See Leo Sternbach, "De Gnomologio Vaticano inedito," *WS* 11 (1889): 44, no. 340. Rhodes: Chion *Ep*. 6. Rhodes did have purple factories.

[88] Philostephanus (*FHG* III.29); Heropythus (*FHG* IV.428). Cf. Suidas s.v. Φάσηλις: Φασηλίτας γὰρ τάριχον τῷ Καλαβρῷ θύειν φησὶ Καλλίμαχος ἐν βαρβαρικοῖς ὀμίμοις.

[89] Demosthenes *In Lacritum* 933–34.

[90] Ditt. *Syll.*[3] 1000. The dating of this inscription is uncertain, but is perhaps of the late second or early first century B.C. See Susan M. Sherwin-White, *Ancient Cos* (Göttingen 1978), pp. 229–34. Cf. Rostovtzeff, *SEHRE*[2], pp. 241–42. For Coan purple see Horace *Od*. 4.13.13 and Juvenal *Sat*. 8.101.

latter enterprise also engaged the inhabitants of Rhodes, Cyprus, and the mainland city of Miletus.[91] Concerning fish processing specifically, literary sources substantiate at least three locations for the Roman period.[92] Pliny praises the garum manufactured at Clazomenae and relates that fish processing centers (*cetariae*) operated on Cyprus. Julius Africanus (fl. early 3rd cent. A.D.), writing probably from Jerusalem, notes that, although Lydia produced excellent γάρος, it did not surpass that of Spain.[93] Archaeological evidence in support of these references, however, has not been forthcoming. Fish tanks and deposits of fish bones found on Cyprus give some indication of the fishing industry on the island, but salting vats have not been discovered.[94] The only archaeological evidence for fish salting comes from Megisti (the modern island of Castellorizo), off the southern coast of Lycia. Two submerged rectangular vats lying in the shallow Mandraki basin may have been salting basins dating perhaps to the late imperial period.[95]

Evidence for commerce in salted fish products of Asia Minor is meager indeed. Posidippus (fl. 3rd cent. B.C.) says that some τάριχος was called Κύπριον, perhaps implying a measure of commercial transport of salted fish products from that island.[96] For the Roman period, however, literary sources are silent. Xenocrates, Pliny, and Julius Africanus leave no doubt that production continued, but the extent to which salted fish products formed part of Roman commerce cannot be ascertained. Archaeology pro-

---

[91] Rhodes: Vitruvius *De Arch.* 7.13.2; Cyprus: Isidore *Orig.* 19.28.3; Miletus: *Edict. Diocl.* XXIV.6–7. See also Peter Herrmann, "Milesischer Purpur," *MDAI(I)* 25 (1975): 141–47, for a first century A.D. inscription concerning the purple industry of Miletus. For the purple factories (πορφυράβαφα) of Hierapolis see *IGRR* IV.816, 822.

[92] Cos should probably be included, since the second-first century B.C. inscription (Ditt. *Syll.*[3] 1000) also includes apparently locally produced τάριχος (line 15). The evidence of σκοπαί on Lesbos offered by Alciphron (1.20.1), purportedly for the fourth century B.C., might equally apply to his own lifetime, ca. A.D. 200.

[93] Pliny *HN* 31.94 (Clazomenae), 37.66 (Cyprus); Julius Africanus Κεστοί 7.19: Ἀπὸ Λυδίας ὁ σπουδαῖος γίνεται. ὁ δὲ "σόκκιος" ὀνομαζόμενος ὃν μᾶλλον ἁπάντων γάρων ἐπαινοῦσι. For the text of the *Cestes*, see Jean-René Vieillefond, *Les 'Cestes' de Julius Africanus* (Florence 1970), p. 181. Xenocrates (*ap.* Orib. 2.58.144) says that the best ὠμοτάριχος comes from Cyme: αὐχὴν μὲν γὰρ αὐτῶν γίνεται ὠμοτάριχος, ἐστὶ δ' εὔστομος, δύσφθαρτος διὰ τὸ ἀπίμελον· κράτιστος δ' ὁ Κυμαῖος. Höppener (*Halieutica*, p. 51) identifies this city as Cumae in Italy, and certainly Strabo (5.4.4) does say that Cumae had fisheries for large fish (κητεῖαι). Since Xenocrates came from Aphrodisias in Caria, he would probably have been personally aware of the fishery products of Asia Minor and could very well here be referring to Cyme in Lydia. Rhode (*Thynnorum Captura*, p. 37) believes that Cyme of Lydia is referred to in this citation. For salt resources in Asia see Forbes, *Technology*, 3: 169–70.

[94] Fish tanks: K. Nicolaou and Alexander Flinder, "Ancient Fish-Tanks at Lapithos, Cyprus," *IJNA* 5 (1976): 133–41, esp. pp. 136–41; fish bones: Marie José Chavane, *Les Petits Objects*. Vol. VI of *Salamine de Chypre* (Paris 1975), pp. 189–90.

[95] The basins measure 2.8 x 1.5 to 1.6 m. and 2.2 x 1.2 m. Their depth is undetermined at present. See Paolo Antonio Pirazzoli, "Submerged Remains of Ancient Megisti in Castellorizo Island (Greece): A Preliminary Survey," *IJNA* 16,1 (1987): 59 and Fig. 5, p. 61.

[96] Posidippus fr. 17 Edmonds: Κύπριον. Τὸ τάριχον.That Rhodes also exported salted fish may perhaps be inferred from Chion (4th cent. B.C.) who, in a letter to his mother, remarks that Phaidimos had sent to him a Rhodian container of salt-fish. See Chion *Ep.* 6 (Hercher, ed., p. 198): Ἐκόμισέ μοι Φαίδιμος ταρίχου ῥοδιὰν καὶ μέλιτος ἀμφορέας πέντε καὶ τοῦ μερσίτου οἴνου κεράμια εἴκοσι καὶ πρὸς τούτοις τρία ἀργυρίου τάλαντα.

vides no clues, but two inscriptions offer some hope that the state of our knowledge may in time improve. At Alabanda, a city in Caria, lying some thirty-five kilometers from the sea, excavators have discovered a sarcophagus with an epitaph perhaps identifying the occupant as a merchant in salted fish (ταρειχοπώλης).[97] If the inscription has been correctly interpreted—and some doubt does exist—the merchant must have imported his product from the coast, perhaps from Miletus, a large emporion for goods of all kinds. If so, did Miletus produce its own salted fish along with its purple, or did it serve as a distribution point for commercial traffic inland of goods produced elsewhere, such as from Clazomenae, Rhodes, or even from as far away as the Black Sea region? Little can be said for certain at present. The second example is a tariff inscription found at Anazarbus in Cilicia and dated to the fifth or sixth century A.D.[98] Included among a list of mostly food items (only a small part of the inscription is extant) is γάρον taxed at one keration for an undisclosed amount. The fish sauce may have been a product of coastal Cilicia or an import, probably from an Eastern source, perhaps as far away as the Black Sea or as close as Syria or Gaza. At this late date, it is unlikely to have come from Spain or North Africa.

Egypt

There has been no study devoted to fish processing in Graeco-Roman Egypt, although it has received brief attention in studies aimed largely at the fishing industry.[99] Archaeology has yet to yield any significant artifacts relating to the Egyptian fish processing industry, but it has brought to light an invaluable source of information which augments the meager literary evidence and provides a unique look at an important part of Egyptian life. Papyri are a mine of information which, like underwater archaeology, has hardly been tapped.[100] Non-literary papyri yield the best information on and impart a certain charm to the study of daily life. Numerous references to processed fish products indicate that production and commerce of these commodities were integral parts of that life.[101] Many papyri merely record

[97] George F. Bean, "Epitaphs at Alabanda," *Anadolu Araştirmalari* 1 (1955): 52–55. Bean records the epitaph as ΟΤΟΣΤΑΡΕΙΛΟ, and states, "The latter part of this appears to be a tradename formed from τάριχος, such as ταρειχοπώλης, or possibly, and more interestingly, ταρειχώτης" (p. 53).

[98] Gilbert Dagron and Denis Feissel, *Inscriptions de Cilicie*. Travaux et Mémoires de Centre de Recherche d'Histoire et Civilisation de Byzance, 4 (Paris 1987), pp. 170–85.

[99] Theodor Reil, *Beiträge zur Kenntnis des Gewerbes im hellenistischen Ägypten* (Borna-Leipzig 1913): 162–64; Maria Carlotta Besta, "Pesca e pescatori nell'Egitto greco-romano," *Aegyptus* 2 (1921): 67–74; Bohlen, *Fischerei*, pp. 25–28; and Jacques Dumont, "La pêche dans le Fayoum hellénistique: traditions et nouveautés d'après le Papyrus Tebtynis 701," *CE* 52 (1977): 125–42.

[100] R. Zahn, for example, in his discussion of garum in *RE* 7 (1912), cols. 842–49, draws upon a wide variety of literary sources and some archaeological evidence, but does not make use of the wealth of information found in papyri.

[101] See, for example, Friedrich Preisigke, *Wörterbuch der griechischen Papyrusurkunden*. 3 vols. (Berlin 1925), passim. Many other examples have appeared in papyri collections published

processed fish products among other food items in a sort of grocery list, but others provide significant details on fish preservation, not only on its role in the Egyptian economy but also on the part it played in meeting family needs. Some papyrus fragments refer to products imported into or exported from Egypt and so throw light on commerce in other parts of the Mediterranean.

Used in conjunction with literary sources papyrological evidence enables one to form a good, but uneven picture of the processed fish industry in Egypt from the third century B.C. to the Arab conquests. Of the one hundred and eighteen published papyri consulted for this study almost one-half can be dated to the second and third centuries A.D.[102] This may be due more to the exigencies of preservation than to any particular period of increased activity in the processed fish industry, but its chronological agreement with the phenomenon in the Western Mediterranean and the Black Sea area may not be entirely coincidental. Since the remaining papyri are scattered throughout the other centuries, the task of discerning any trends in the growth and decline of the industry, made difficult by the lack of archaeological information, becomes even more formidable. For this reason the following discussion, although at times drawing upon evidence of the Ptolemaic and Byzantine periods, will of necessity focus on Roman Egypt.

The Nile River provided the inhabitants of Egypt with more than just land. Fishing and fish consumption formed an integral part of daily life as early as the Pre-Dynastic and Pharonic periods.[103] There is some evidence that the early Egyptians salted fish, perhaps even producing a product similar to caviar, called today botargo.[104] Herodotus (2.77), in the fifth century B.C., says that Egyptians ate fish either raw, sun-dried, or preserved in brine (ἐξ ἅλμης τεταριχεύμενους), while Diodorus provides evidence for

since 1925. The papyrological sources, and indeed also the literary evidence, are many times unhelpful in distinguishing sun-dried or smoked fish from those which have been salted.

[102] Of 118 papyri used in this study, 51 or 43.2 per cent, have been dated to the second and third centuries A.D. If papyri of the first and fourth centuries A.D. are included, the figure jumps to 69, or 58.5 per cent. Seventeen, or 14.4 per cent, come from the third century B.C.; and 27, or 22.9 per cent, can be dated between the fifth and eighth centuries A.D. The remaining examples are undatable.

[103] See, for example, Oric Bates, "Ancient Egyptian Fishing," *Harvard African Studies* 1 (1917): 199–271; Radcliffe, *Fishing*, pp. 301–45; Pierre Montet, *Everyday Life in Egypt in the Days of Ramesses the Great*. A. R. Maxwell-Hyslip and Margaret S. Drower, transl. (Reprint, Westport, Conn. 1958), pp. 79–80; F. Danelius and H. Steinitz, "The Fishes and Other Aquatic Animals in the Punt Reliefs at Deir El-Bahri," *JEA* 53 (1967): 15–24; and Ingrid Gamer-Wallert, *Fische und Fischkulte im alten Ägypten*. Ägyptologische Abhandlungen, XXI (Wiesbaden 1970), passim. For the Papyrus Harris, a lengthy document of the reign of Ramses III (1198–1166 B.C.), in which preserved fish forms a part of the king's gifts to the gods and of a list of offerings for a feast, see J. H. Breasted, *Ancient Records of Egypt*. Vol. 4 (Chicago 1906), nos. 243, 380, 394. I regret that I was unable to consult F. R. Schiemenz, "Fischerei vor 4500 Jahren im Reiche der Aegypten," *Deutsche Angler Zeitung* 34 (1933): 95–101.

[104] Thompson, *Greek Fishes*, p. 145; for botargo see L. Keimer, "La boutargue dans l'Égypte ancienne," *Bulletin de l'Institut d'Égypte* 21 (1938–39): 215–43; John P. Hughes and R. Gordon Wasson, "The Etymology of Botargo," *AJPh* 68 (1947): 414–18; and Georgacas, *Ichthyological Terms*, pp. 146–48, 179–87.

continuity into the Hellenistic period when he says that the Nile River and Lake Moeris contain a wide variety of fish in unbelievable numbers, many of which were processed in salteries (ταριχεῖα). Xenocrates confirms that Egypt continued to exploit her fishery resources, including fish processing, during the Roman period.[105] The most important Egyptian fish included the κορακῖνος, φάγρος, τύφλη, λάτος, θρίσσα, and βωρεύς.[106] Some salted fish products acquired specific names derived from these fish; for example, κορακίδια, βωρίδια, and τυφλινίδια.[107]

Salt to preserve fish was readily available from lakes near Memphis, Mt. Casius, and Paraetonium, from salt pans or deposits, and from mines located between Egypt and Mt. Sinai.[108] Evidence is scanty, but it seems probable that the Roman government maintained a monopoly on salt production, and it is almost certain that it did so on the retail salt trade. Specially licensed dealers could lease from the state the right to sell salt in certain districts at a fixed price and would pay a rent (φόρος) for this privilege. Private salt dealers apparently operated in other areas of Egypt, but they had to sell at the price fixed by the government and to pay a trade-tax to the state. Since evidence is lacking, one can only speculate on the arrangement used by fish salters. Individual fish salters could purchase the necessary salt from either state or private dealers. Large salting complexes requiring huge quantities of salt probably dealt directly with the state, paying a rent for the salt as well as a tax on the processed fish products.[109]

The ancient Egyptian method of preparing dried salt-fish was probably similar to that used in modern Egypt.[110] The fish are cleaned, washed, and

[105] Diodorus 1.36.1 (Nile River): τοῖς γὰρ ἐγχωρίοις οὐ μόνον ἐκ τῶν προσφάτως ἁλισκομένων παρέχεται δαψιλῆ τὴν ἀπόλαυσιν, ἀλλὰ καὶ πλῆθος εἰς ταριχείαν ἀνίησιν ἀνέκλειπτον; 1.52.6 (Lake Moeris): εἴκοσι γὰρ καὶ δύο γένη τῶν κατ᾽ αὐτήν φασιν ἰχθύων εἶναι, καὶ τοσοῦτον αὐτῶν ἁλίσκεσθαι πλῆθος ὥστε τοὺς προσκαρτεροῦντας ταῖς ταριχείαις ὄντας παμπληθεῖς δυσχερῶς περιγίνεσθαι τῶν ἔργων; Xenocrates *ap*. Orib. 2.58.148–50. Cf. Aelian *NA* 10.43.

[106] See Thompson, *Greek Fishes, op. cit*; Corcoran, "Roman Fishing Industry," pp. 102–03; Athen. 3.118f–119a; 7.311f–312b; Strabo 17.2.4; Pliny *HN* 32.95, 125; Martial 13.85. Shellfish were also caught in Egyptian waters and even exported. See Xenocrates *ap*. Orib. 2.58.54, 59, 96, 115, 117, 121. See also Allen Chester Johnson, *Roman Egypt* (1936), Vol. II of *ESAR*, pp. 374–75, and David S. Reese, Henk K. Mienis and Fred R. Woodward, "On the Trade of Shells and Fish from the Nile River," *BASO* 264 (1986): 79–84.

[107] Xenocrates *ap*. Orib. 2.58.152. Other examples listed by Xenocrates include κολίδια and ἀβραμίδια. Βορίδια (= βωρίδια) is found in *P.Ryl*. IV.629_{88} (ca. A.D. 317–23), while βωρειδεῖον can be read in *P.Coll.Youtie* II.84 (4th cent. A.D.). *PSI* III.206_{21} (3rd cent. A.D.) has κορακινίδια, while *P.Cair.Zen*. 59680_{31} (ca. 259 B.C.) has listed under τάριχος a product called οἀραγναθίδον.The ἀντακαῖον (salted sturgeon) mentioned in *P.Cair.Zen*. 59682_{6} and *PSI* V.535_{35}, both of the third century B.C., may be salted fish imported from the Black Sea area. So Danov, "Pontos Euxeinos," col. 978. Cf. Thompson, *Greek Fishes*, s.v. ἀντακαῖος, pp. 16–17.

[108] Vitruvius *De arch*. 8.3.7. For the salt resources of Egypt see Forbes, *Technology*, 3: 157–74, passim. For state control of salt production see Raphael Taubenschlag, *The Law of Greco-Roman Egypt in the Light of the Papyri, 332 B.C.–640 A.D.* 2nd ed. (Warsaw 1955), pp. 666–67; Sherman Leroy Wallace, *Taxation in Egypt from Augustus to Diocletian* (Princeton 1938), pp. 183–84; and Johnson, *Roman Egypt*, pp. 240, 325–26.

[109] Cf. P. J. Sijpesteijn, *Customs Duties in Graeco-Roman Egypt*. Studia Amstelodamensia ad Epigraphicam Ius Antiquum et Papyrologicam Pertinentia, 17 (Zutphen 1987), p. 58.

[110] Forbes, *Technology*, 3: 186–87.

rubbed-down with salt. They are then stacked in alternating layers of salt and fish. These stacks are covered by dry matting and exposed to the sun for three to five days. Following this they are turned over and allowed to stand another three to five days, sometimes longer. This process is variously depicted in Pharonic Egyptian reliefs and probably appertained to Ptolemaic and Roman Egypt as well. Sometimes the fish were sliced and hung up on racks to dry or merely laid out on the ground exposed to the sun. These processes obviously would result in a product of low keeping quality in the hot climate. That fish were salted in vats, as in other areas of the Mediterranean, is probable but not verifiable owing to a lack of archaeological evidence.

Little is known of commercial fish processing installations beyond the fact of their existence. Pelusium and Canopus maintained factories in the fifth century B.C., while the reputation enjoyed outside Egypt by the salted fish of Mendes implies salting activity there on a significant scale during the Roman period.[111] Diodorus mentions the presence of other Egyptian salteries but does not specify their locations. Pollux provides perhaps an indirect reference to large scale fish salting when he lists ταρίχη Αἰγύπτια alongside the products of other areas (Phrygia, Gades, Sardinia, and Pontus) famous for their salteries.[112] The identification of salting activity can sometimes be inferred from papyri when one finds mention of the fish pickler, or ταριχευτής. All too frequently, however, the context does not permit a distinction between the fish pickler and the mummifier, both of whom answered to the same name.[113]

Preserved fish was a staple in the diet of Egyptians of all classes. A few papyri indicate that salted fish products were destined for the table of the upper classes, such as that of the Prefect of Egypt or of his staff, and, in one example, that of the emperor Caracalla, who made an official visit to Alexandria in A.D. 215–16.[114] Preserved fish also played a role in provisioning

[111] Herodotus 2.15 (Pelusium), 113 (Canopus); Xenocrates *ap*. Orib. 2.58.150; and Athen. 3.118f–119a (Mendes). Athenaeus, a citizen of Naucratis in the Nile Delta, would be familiar with the food products of Egypt. Stephanus of Byzantium (s.v. Ταριχέαι) also lists Mendes, Senos, and Canopus under the rubric ταριχέαι, indicating their association with fish salting: Ταριχέαι πόλεις παλλαί, αἱ μὲν Μενδήσιαι αἱ δὲ Σηνικαὶ αἱ δὲ Κανωβικαί. οἱ πολῖται ταριχευταί. παρὰ τὸ ταριχεύω.

[112] Diodorus 1.52.6; Pollux *Onom*. 6.48; Cf. *P.Strassb*. 73_2 (3rd cent. A.D.).

[113] *P.Fay*. 13_4 (2nd cent. B.C.) and commentary on ταριχευταῖς. Cf. *P.Fay*. 15_4 and editor's note. For other papyri see Preisigke, *Wörterbuch*, s.v. ταριχευτής. See also Caspar John Kraemer, Jr. and Floyd Albert Spencer, "New Light on the Ταριχευτῆς in Augustan Egypt," *TAPhA* 65 (1934): xlv. Study of the processed fish industry in Egypt is further complicated by the fact that the word τάριχος can refer either to preserved fish or to a mummy.

[114] Prefect of Egypt: *P.Lond*. III.1159 (A.D. 145–47). For salted fish listed among provisions of governor's staffs see *P.Ryl*. IV.627, 629, 630, 639, (A.D. 317–23), memoranda and accounts of Theophanes, a financial official for the Prefect of Egypt. Cf. from the third century B.C. *BGU* VI.$1495_{11,\ 41}$ and the accounts of Zenon, secretary to the treasurer of Ptolemy II (*P.Cair.Zen*. 59012, 59680, 59082, 59206, 59682, 59684, 59705). For the imperial consumption of salted fish products in Egypt see *P.Got*. 3, wherein a fisherman stands as guarantor for a companion who is to provide garum and salted and fresh fish to the imperial table on the occasion of Caracalla's

the army stationed in Egypt. Many soldiers coming from areas of the Roman world where processed fish was an important element of their diet would naturally have a penchant for it, but more importantly the army needed a food which would better withstand the hot Egyptian climate.[115] The annona of Theadelphia furnished fish sauce along with other goods to feed the army of the emperor Probus.[116] Another papyrus (*P.Oxy.* 1657) of the same period includes among a list of utensils contained in a sort of military chest, κυβιά[ϱ]ιον, a vessel apparently designed to hold salted fish.

Rivers and lakes furnished an abundant supply of fresh fish, but their expense in the market place probably put them beyond reach of the majority of poor inhabitants. This was no doubt due to the fact that the hot, dry climate made the transportation of fresh fish over even short distances risky at best. Preserved fish (sun-dried or salted, the distinction is rarely apparent), to judge from the frequency of their mention in papyri, were readily available at an easily affordable price.[117] Sea fish, such as tunny, rarely receive mention in papyri, and so apparently did not play an important part in the diet of the lower classes.[118] The preservation of fish from

---

visit (lines 4–15): ὁμολογῶ ἑκουσίως καὶ αὐθεραίτως/ ἐνγυᾶσθαι Ψάις Ψάιτος μητ(ϱὸς) Σεκῶτος/ ἁλιέα καὶ εἰσδοθέντα ἐπὶ τῆς ἑτοιμα/σίας γάϱου τε καὶ ταϱείχου λεπτοῦ καὶ/ ἰχθύος πϱὸς εἰς τῆν εὐκλẹιṣτά̣την/ ἐπι̣[δ]ημίαν τοῦ κυϱίου ἡμῶν Αὐτοκϱά(τοϱος)/ Καίσαϱος Μάϱκ[ο]υ Αὐϱηλ̣ίου Σ[εου]ήϱου/ Ἀντωνίνου [Παϱ]θικοῦ Μ[εγί]στοὺ/ Βϱεντανι̣κ̣ο[ῦ Μ]εγίσ[τ]ο̣υ Γẹ[ϱμ]ανικοῦ/ Μεγίστου Εὐ[σεβ]ο̣ῦ̣ς [Σε]βα̣σ̣[τοῦ], καὶ ὀμνύω/ τὴν του κυϱί̣[ου τύχην παϱασ]τ̣ησειν τὸν/ πϱοκ(είμενον). See *SHA. Carac.* 6; Dio Cass. 78.22–24; Herodian 4.8–9. Cf. *P.Apoll.* 93 (A.D. 703–15), where fish sauce appears among goods requisitioned for Arab Sailors and members of the governor's staff and those of other governmental bodies.

[115] The inclusion of preserved fish in the military diet can be traced back to Pharonic times when it was included in provisions for the army of Seti I (ca. 1318–1301 B.C.). See Breasted, *Ancient Records*, Vol. 3, no. 207.

[116] *SB* VI.9614 (A.D. 283). See Roger Rémondon, "Un nouveau document concernant Probus," *RPh* 28 (1954): 199–210.

[117] Salted fish and garum figure prominently in accounts, inventories, and grocery lists. The following examples are not exhaustive. From the third and second centuries B.C.: *UPZ* I.89, II.158; *PSI* IV.428; *BGU* VI.1495; *P.Tebt.* III.889; and *P.Sakkakini*. For the latter see Ulrich Wilcken, *Griechische Ostraka aus Aegypten und Nubien* (Leipzig and Berlin 1899), p. 139, note 3. From the first century B.C. and first century A.D.: *BGU* III.781; *P.Lond.* III.1171. From the second to the fourth centuries A.D.: *P.Oxy.* III.520, XIV.1727, XIX.2240; *BGU* I.14, XIII.2357; *P.Corn.* 35; *SB* I.1974, VI.9095, 9614; *P.Mich.* XI.619; *O.Mich.* I.3; *P.Wisc.* II.80; *P.Amst.* I.39, 99; *P.Herm.* 23. From the post-fourth century A.D.: *P.Oxy.* XIV.1656, XVI.1924; *P.Lond.* I.113; *P.Osl.* III.147; *SB* I.1960 (= *O.Petr.* 452); *P.Erl.* 16; *BGU* II.377; *P.Apollo* 85, 93, 96; *P.Amst.* I.44, II.156. Papyri record fish sauce as γάϱος, or in a varied form of this word, such as γαϱηϱόν. Ἄλιξ (allec) appears only in *P.Got.* 17 (ca. 6–7th cent. A.D.) and possibly as ἁλική in *P.Apollo* 93 (A.D. 703–15); in each case the meaning of "fish sauce" is open to question. Λικουάμεν (liquamen), found in *Geoponica* 20.46.1, appears not at all in papyri, and the rare references to ἅλμη (muria) are too ambiguous to associate with fish sauce. For γαϱηϱόν see *P.Wisc.* I.6 (A.D. 210–11), *P.Oxy.* X.1299 (4th cent. A.D.), and possibly *SB* VI.9614 (A.D. 283). For ὀξάλμη see *UPZ* I.89$_{14}$ (160–159 B.C.).

[118] *P.Amst.* inv. no. 44$_2$ (6th cent. A.D.) lists among items in a receipt γαϱο 'υ' αἱματίτου λακύναιον ἕν, "Bloody garum, 5 keratia of gold." The *Geoponica* (20.46.6), which perhaps dates ultimately to the same period, indicates that the best garum, called τὸ γάϱος αἱμάτιον, was made from the tunny. It is unknown if tunny is meant in the papyrus or if any garum prepared in a certain way could be described as haimation. For this papyrus see K. A. Worp, "Deux

the Nile River and its surrounding lakes formed an important part of the home economy and may explain the infrequent references in papyri to professional salters.[119] Private letters frequently contain the request that the recipient make fish preserves. In one particularly charming letter a mother assures her son that a new batch of fish sauce will be ready for him when he returns home.[120]

Many letters present a picture of salt-fish and fish sauce production in the hands of private individuals, a family activity for family members. If a purchase were necessary, there was no dearth of merchants, termed variously γαροπώλης, ταριχοπώλης, or τεμαχοπώλης, ready to satisfy that demand.[121] In fact, in third century A.D. Arsinoë (Crocodilopolis), there was an entire street set aside for selling preserved fish, ταριχοπώλων-street.[122] Although not attested to in papyri, salt-fish shops probably went by the name of ταριχοπώλεια, but a "general merchandise store" (παντοπώλιον) might also sell this commodity.[123]

Papyri provide a glimpse at intraprovincial trade. *P.Tebt.* 701 (235 B.C.), a

papyrus byzantins d'Amsterdam," *CE* 49 (1974): 132–34; and John Shelton, "Garum rouge Sang," *ZPE* 17 (1975): 156. References to salted tunny slices, such as ὑπογάστρια, κύβιον and ὡραῖον, appear in papyri, but in regard to provisions (some obviously imports) for the upper class, specifically goods listed by Zenon in the mid-third century B.C. See *PSI* V.535, *P.Cair.Zen.* 59012 (= *SB* III.6779), 59680, 59682. The κυβιάριον of *P.Oxy.* XIV.1657$_9$ (late 3rd cent. A.D.) may refer to a vessel of κύβιον forming part of military supplies. A farm account of the Augustan period lists among its incidental expenses a tax on τέμαχος. That a slice of salted fish (tunny?) would appear in a farm account may be doubted, but it is not impossible. See *P.Lond.* III.1171 (8 B.C.). Cf. Wallace, *Taxation*, pp. 223–24.

119 Reil, *Beiträge*, p. 163.

120 Request that salted fish be made: *PSI* III.206 (3rd cent. A.D.), *P.Oxy.* VI.928 (2nd or 3rd cent. A.D.); fish sauce for a son's homecoming: *P.Oxy.* X.1299 (4th cent. A.D.). St. Jerome (*Ep.* 108.17) in A.D. 404 wrote a letter to Eustochium in which he praises the almost excessive moderation of her mother Paula, who hardly put oil on her food except on feast days and spurned wine, liquamen, and other savory foods judged by others to be normal fare. References to salted fish products in the *Regulae* of St. Pachomius (ca. A.D. 292–346) provide other examples of widespread use of these commodities in Egypt. See above, note 29, p. 35. For the text of St. Jerome's letter I have used *Sancti Eusebii Hieronymi Epistulae*. Isidor Hilberg, ed. *Corpus Scriptorum Ecclesiasticorum Latinorum*, 55, pars II (Leipzig 1912), pp. 328–29.

121 Γαροπώλης: *P.Bad.* II.42 (2nd cent. A.D.); τεμαχοπώλ[: *P.Genov.* inv. no. 1386$_{14}$ (4th cent. A.D.?). For the latter term see Augusto Traversa, "Spunti sociologici nel papiro inedito genovese (PUG inv. n. 1386)," *Atti dell'XI Congresso Internazionale di Papirologia, Milano 2–8 Settembre 1965* (Milan 1966), pp. 260–71. For a ταριχοπράτισσα, a female salt-fish dealer of the sixth century A.D., see *P.Cair.Masp.* I.67023$_8$ (A.D. 569). The ὡραιοπώλ[ης] mentioned in *P.Lond.* III.1028 (7th cent. A.D.) may be, as the editor suggests, a seller of fruit, but might it also refer to a seller of salted tunny (ὡραῖον)? But cf. P. J. Sijpesteijn, "Varia Papyrologica," *ZPE* 73 (1988): 57. Some of these terms are found in literary sources as well; for example, ὡραιοπώλης (Hesychius, s.v. ὡραιοπώλης); γαροπώλης (*CGL* III. 470, 48); ταριχοπώλης (Nicostratus frs. 4, 5 Edmonds; Alexis frs. 15 and 77 Edmonds; Plutarch *Mor.* 631D; and Pollux *Onom.* 7.27). Cf. Alexis fr. 218 Edmonds for ταριχηγός. Preisigke (*Wörterbuch*, loc. cit.) mentions, but I did not have access to, papyri in which other terms are used for salt-fish dealers: τεμαχίτης in *P.Flor.* III.338$_{24}$ (2nd cent. a.D.) and ταριχᾶς in *Stud.Pal.* X.113$_6$ (2nd cent. A.D.).

122 Ulrich Wilcken, "Zusätze zu dem Aufsatz: Zur Topographie der Ruinenstätte des alten Schet (Krokodilopolis-Arsinoë)," *Zeitschrift der Gesellschaft für Erdkunde zu Berlin* 22 (1887): 81.

123 For παντοπώλιον see *P.Oxy.* III.520 (A.D. 143). For the identification of a παντοπώλης, or merchant of general merchandise, with a ἁλμαιοπώλης, or *salgamarius*, a seller of muria, see

papyrus particularly important for understanding the Ptolemaic fishing industry, provides information on the movements of preserved and fresh fish within the Arsinoite nome and between the Fayum and Alexandria in the Delta.[124] The administrative correspondences collected in this document speak of sending rather large consignments of fish, such as shad, carp, and mullet, to a certain Alexander (II. 60–67), and of selling fish in the nome, throughout the surrounding area, and at Alexandria (II. 195–218). The latter section, as well as line 221, speaks also of cargoes of salted fish sent to Alexandria and the amount of tax levied on them there. The quantity of fish concerned indicates that this particular operation was quite large and may have been a state enterprise or one managed by a holder of a gift-estate.[125]

The Roman government also kept a firm control on commerce within Egypt. Customs stations exacted tolls for goods traveling on the Nile River and over the few good roads. Processed fish formed part of this trade and appears in customs house registries of the Roman period. *P.Wisc.* II.80, dating to September, A.D. 114 and recording tolls on overland shipments of various products, especially oil, bound for Memphis, listed among goods passing through the customs house at Bacchias in the Fayum during the month one donkey-load of τάριχος taxed at a rate of seven drachmae, one obol.[126] Salted fish (ταριχηρὰ ἰχθύα) also appears in *P.Coll.Youtie* I.31, a registry from Arsinoë dated to September, A.D. 199. Since most fishing in Egypt occurred during the autumn and winter months, it is not unusual that both customs house registries date to September.[127]

Numerous private letters of the Roman period announce the dispatch or receipt of garum or τάριχος or request their dispatch.[128] These missives elicit a picture of easily obtained processed fish products commonly found among goods transported throughout Egypt.[129] Transport containers for these commodities varied between baskets of various types, probably for dried or smoked fish, and earthenware vessels, for garum and salted or pickled fish.[130] Some vessels seem from their name to be containers partic-

---

Robert, "Épitaphes," pp. 44–45. Cf. *P.Tebt.* III.841 (114 B.C.). The scholiast to Aristophanes *Eq.* 1247 uses the spelling ταριχοπωλεῖον, and the form ταριχόπωλις (sc. ἀγορά) is found in *Gnomol. Vat.* 340. Antiphanes (fr. 128 Edmonds) calls a salt-fish shop a τεμαχοπώλη.

[124] Dumont, "La pêche dans le Fayoum," pp. 125–42.

[125] Rostovtzeff, *SEHHW*, pp. 296–97.

[126] N. Y. Clauson ("A Customs House Registry from Roman Egypt [P.Wisconsin 16]," *Aegyptus* 9 [1928]: 260) is unsure whether to include the salted fish as an export.

[127] Sijpesteijn, *Customs Duties in Graeco-Roman Egypt*, p. 62.

[128] Requests for a salted fish product: *P.Stras.* I.73; *P.Meyer* 65; *P.Bas.* 16; *P.Oxy.* VI.928, 937, VIII.1158, XIV.1759–60, XXXIV.2729; *BGU* IV.1095. Notice of dispatch: *P.Iand.* II.8; *SB* V.7600 (= W. Aly, "Privatbrief aus der Freiburger Papyrusammlung, P.Frib. 39," *Aegyptus* 13 [1933]: 487–92), 7662; *P.Oxy.* XXXIII.2680, XLI.2983; *P.Col.* inv. no. 318 (= Clinton W. Keys, "Four Private Letters from the Columbia Papyri," *CPh* 30 [1935]: 143–47). Notice of receipt: *P.Oxy.* XXXI.2596, XLII.3060; *P.Osl.* III.161.

[129] For processed fish sent by boat see *P.Coll.Youtie* II.84 (4th cent. A.D.), and *P.Oxy.* XVI.1924 (5th-6th cent. A.D.).

ularly associated with salted fish products. A list of provisions among the Zenon papyri, for example, includes a garum jar termed βῖχος γαριτικός, while a list of vessels of the first century A.D. includes a container called a γαράριον.[131] A private letter of the fourth century A.D. refers to something described as γαρηρόν, a term which refers either to the jar of garum or to the garum itself. One large container of the third century A.D., called a κυβιά[ρ]ιον, apparently carried salted tunny slices (κύβια).[132]

With both fresh and preserved fish so abundant within the borders of Egypt one might expect some level of exportation of these products and little need for importation. The former assumption, though not the latter, appears justified. If Sophocles refers to salt-fish when he says νεκρὸς τάριχος εἰσορᾶν Αἰγύπτιος, then at least as early as the fifth century B.C. Egypt may have sent some of its products to Greece.[133] In 259 B.C., Zenon, the private secretary to Apollonios a treasury official (*dioiketes*) of Ptolemy II, preserved the report and inventory of a four-camel caravan carrying salted fish and other items from Egypt to Galilee.[134]

Egyptian exportation of preserved fish may have fared even better under the Romans, at least there exists better evidence for it. Xenocrates of

---

[130] Baskets: σπυρίς (*PSI* IV.428), σφυρίδιν (*SB* V.7662), χλίβιον (*P.Wisc.* II.80). Vessels: κεράμιον (*P.Wisc.* I.6; *P.Oxy.* VI.937, XXXIII.2680, XXXIV.2729; *P.Stras.* I.73; *PSI* III.206, IV.428; *P.Fay.* 104). Cf. Aristotle *HA* 534^{a}21. Other containers of unknown or doubtful nature include the ὀμφοκερᾶς (*P.Oxy.* XVI.1924$_6$), ἀμφόριτον (*PSI* V.535$_{31}$), μαῦρα (*P.Lond.* II.239; *P.Coll.Youtie* II.84), χύτρα (*PSI* IV.428), κοῦρι (*O.Petr.* 452 = SB I.1960), and κυτίνιον (*P.Amst.* II.1563). Salt-fish vessels might also be put to other uses. See the interesting Demotic papyrus *P.Leid.* II.V$_{16}$ (3rd cent. A.D.), which states that a magic formula should be written on a τῆς ταρείχου ὄστρακον. See also Wilcken, *Ostraka*, Vol. I, p. 7.

[131] Βῖχος γαριτικός: *PSI* V.535$_{36}$ (3rd cent. B.C.); γαράριον: *BGU* III.781. III$_7$ (1st cent. A.D.). The latter papyrus is fragmentary and reads γα[·]αια β̄ which Liddell and Scott (*Greek-English Lexicon*^{9}, s.v. γαράριον) expand to γαράριον and identify as a small garum jar. For γαράρια see also *Stud.Pal.* XX.151$_{6/16}$ (6th cent. A.D.). It is interesting that the scholiast to Nicander *Theriaca* 526 says that the common expression for the ὀξύβαφον was γαργάριον. *Scholia in Theriaca.* Heinrich Keil, ed. in *Nicandrea. Theriaca et Alexipharmaca.* Otto Schneider, ed. (Leipzig 1856), p. 41. When this association became common is unknown. The ὀξύβαφον was, according to Athenaeus (3.67e), the vessel used to store ὀξύγαρον, a mixture of garum and vinegar. *BGU* III.781 also has listed two lines previous ὀξόβαφα. Phrynicus (*Praep. soph.* s.v. ὀξύβαφον) condemns this spelling, citing an analogy with ὀξύγαρον. Neither γαργάριον nor γαράριον appear in the glossaries.

[132] Γαρηρόν: *P.Oxy.* X.1299. Cf. *P.Wisc.* I.6 (A.D. 210–11) and *SB* VI.9614 (A.D. 283). J. R. Rea ("P.Wisc. 6 Revised," *ZPE* 12 [1973]: 262–64) suggests that it may refer to pickled fish. For κυβιάριον see *P.Oxy.* XIV.1657.

[133] Sophocles *ap.* Athen. 3.119c. Although νεκρὸς τάριχος may refer to a mummy, as translated in the Loeb edition, the context within which Athenaeus quotes from Sophocles *Phineus* is a discussion of salt-fish.

[134] *P.Col.* III. 2$_{17}$: τῶν ταριχηγησάντων. Cf. ταριχηγός (a seller of salted fish) in Alexis fr. 218 Edmonds. For Zenon and his archive, see M. I. Rostovtzeff, *A Large Estate in Egypt in the Third Century B.C.* (Madison, Wisc. 1922), Campbell F. Edgar, *Zenon Papyri in the University of Michigan Collection* (Ann Arbor 1931), esp. pp. 1–55, and P. W. Pestman, *A Guide to the Zenon Archive.* 2 vols. (Leiden 1981). Egypt was apparently shipping its preserved fish eastward as early as approximately 1100 B.C. Wenamon, an official of the Temple of Amon at Karnak, lists preserved fish in his report of items transported to Syria. See Breasted, *Ancient Records*, Vol. 4, No. 582.

Aphrodisias, writing from Rome in the first century A.D., in discussing preserved fish from lakes and rivers speaks primarily of Egyptian fish.[135] In the following century Lucian, in his satire *Navigium*, alludes to commerce between Alexandria and Athens in which merchant ships from Egypt brought pickled fish from the Nile River in the same cargo with perfume from Canopus.[136] Evidence from the Talmud (*BT. Makshirin* 6.3) indicates that Egyptian fish, probably dried, made its way to Syria during the Roman period. Egypt was still exporting her products to Africa as late as the fifth century A.D. Educated at Alexandria, Synesius of Cyrene was apparently so partial to Egyptian salt-fish that he had it sent to him at his rural estate in Southern Cyrenaica far from the coast.[137] Writing in ca. A.D. 408 to his Syrian friend Olympius, he said that villagers near his estate were so ignorant of fish that to show them proof of their existence he broke open before their eyes a jar of salted fish from Egypt.

Egypt imported salted fish products from both East and West, but the evidence is too spotty or uncertain to obtain a clear picture of this activity. What evidence does exist falls primarily into the Ptolemaic period. Hieron of Syracuse in the late third century B.C. sent a ship loaded with ten thousand jars of τάριχος as a gift to Ptolemy.[138] The Zenon papyri lists salted fish from Byzantium, Syria, and the Greek islands of Peparethos and Thasos.[139] Importation of Pontic salt-fish (Ποντικὸν τάριχος) is proven by reference to it in the amusing story which Plutarch (*Ant*. 29) relates of a jest played on Antony by Cleopatra in Egypt. The Roman period provides little evidence beyond one possible reference to Spanish fish sauce.[140] Increased production during the Roman period may have significantly reduced the need to import salted fish products.[141] Further study of papyri and transport containers found in Egypt may someday provide more information.[142]

Evidence for the commercial organization of fish salters is sparse and ambiguous. They do not seem to be differentiated from fishermen, and so

---

135 Xenocrates *ap*. Orib. 2.58.148–52.

136 Lucian *Navig*. 15: ἀλλ' ὤγαθέ, πρὸς τῆς Ἴσιδος κἂν τὰ Νειλῷα ταῦτα ταρίχη τὰ λεπτὰ μέμνησο ἡμῖν ἄγειν ἀπ' Αἰγύπτου.

137 Synesius *Ep*. 148 (Hercher, ed., p. 732): ἐγὼ δέ ποτε αὐτοῖς ἀνανεύουσι πρὸς τὰ περὶ τῶν ἰχθύων, ἀναλαβὼν τινὰ κέραμον καὶ προσαράξας πέτρᾳ ἔδειξα τῶν ἀπ' Αἰγύπτου ταρίχη συχνά. See also Augustine Fitzgerald, *The Letters of Synesius of Cyrene* (London 1926), esp. p. 43.

138 Athen. 5.209a.

139 Byzantium: *P.Cair.Zen*. 59682; *PSI* IV.413, V.535. Syria: *P.Cair.Zen*. 59012, 59013. See also Giuseppina Vaggi, "Siria e Siri nei documenti dell'Egitto greco-romano," *Aegyptus* 17 (1937): 40. For Peparathos and Thasos see *PSI* V.535.

140 *P.Herm*. 23_6: [γάρου] μέλανọ[ς] (4th cent. A.D.). For the identification of "black garum" with garum sociorum, see Jardin, "Garum," p. 78.

141 "Foreign garum" (γάρου ξενικοῦ) mentioned in one papyrus of the late third century A.D. (*P.Fay*. 104_{28}) may refer to non-Egyptian, that is imported, fish sauce. The next line lists γάρου κεραμίω[ν], as if to distinguish an imported (foreign) sauce from a vessel of garum of no particular distinction (local?). Cf. *PSI* IV.428_{69} (3rd cent. B.C.): ταρίχου ξενικοῦ.

142 Elizabeth Lyding Will has identified some Spanish fish sauce vessels among those she has studied at Alexandria.

probably fell under the same organization and controls. Fishing in public waters, such as in Lake Moeris, was a state monopoly under the Ptolemies. The right to fish was leased to tax gatherers (τελῶναι), who then contracted out to professional fishermen the actual catching of the fish. The latter group paid to the state a tax in kind of twenty-five per cent of their catch, an impost called the τετάρτη ἁλιείων (or ἰχθυικῶν), in addition to other minor taxes.[143] They could then do as they pleased with the remainder of the catch, either consuming it or selling it (under the auspices of the state) to fish dealers.[144] That part of their catch which was made into processed fish may also have been taxed in a similar fashion (τετάρτη τοῦ ταρίχου).[145] In the Roman period fishing remained a state monopoly (at least in certain areas), and the fishing rights continued to be leased as before. The τετάρτη, however, seems to have disappeared in this period.[146] In one second century A.D. papyrus from Oxyrhynchus a fisherman leases the right to fish in private waters for six years in exchange for a fixed sum of 240 drachmas plus a special payment in kind of 30 jars (κεράμια) of fish sauce, two jars of shad, two jars of Spanish mackerel, one jar of mullet, and one jar of catfish. The fish were probably salted by the fisherman himself, except possibly for the Spanish mackerel, a sea fish, which may have been purchased as an import from the coastal areas of Egypt or from abroad. In another lease of fishing rights from Oxyrhynchus, dating to A.D. 210–11, a fisherman agrees that in return for the right to fish in certain waters for two years he will pay as a rent a fixed sum of money plus two jars of shad and six jars of garum (γαρῆρω[ν] κεραμίων ἕξ).[147]

Under Roman rule fishing and fish preservation occasionally became a liturgy. In *P.Got.* 3 (A.D. 215–16), from Panopolis in Upper Egypt, a fisherman swears that he will stand as surety for another fisherman who has been given the responsibility of providing fresh and salted fish and fish sauce for the imminent visit to Alexandria of the emperor Caracalla.[148]

---

[143] Private ownership of fishing rights did apply to those owning certain waters. See Taubenschlag, *Law of Greco-Roman Egypt*, pp. 665–66, and the bibliography cited therein; and more recently, Dumont, "La pêche dans le Fayoum," pp. 125–42.

[144] Rostovtzeff, *SEHHW*, pp. 296–97, and p. 1387, note 101.

[145] Wilcken, *Griechische Ostraka*, pp. 396–97. Wilcken believes that the τετάρτη τοῦ ταρίχου of *P.Petr.* I.28 concerned pickled foods (Pökelwäre) in general, rather than specifically salted or dried fish (Pökelfische). See Preisigke, *Wörterbuch*, s.v. τετάρτη, for other citations to this tax, all of the third century B.C.

[146] Wallace, *Taxation*, p. 219. For a discussion of the economic differences between the Ptolemaic and Roman periods, see Naphtali Lewis, "Greco-Roman Egypt: Fact or Fiction?" in *Proceedings of the 12th International Congress of Papyrology*. Deborah H. Samuel, ed. American Studies in Papyrology, 7 (Toronto 1970), pp. 3–14.

[147] Second century A.D.: *P.Lond.* inv. 2143 (= G. M. Parássoglou, "A Lease of Fishing Rights," *Aegyptus* 67 [1987]: 89–93). The mullet (ἀβράμιδος), shad (θρίσσα), and catfish (συνοδοντίς) are Nile fish. See Thompson, *Greek Fishes*, pp. 1–2, 77–78, and 254, respectively. The Spanish mackerel (κόλλιος) inhabits the Mediterranean Sea. See *ibid.*, pp. 120–21 (κολίας). A.D. 210–11: *P.Wisc.* I.6. Cf. Rea ("P.Wisc. 6 Revised," pp. 262–64) who reads the fixed sum as 100 drachmas, whereas Sijpesteijn (*The Wisconsin Papyri I*. P. J. Sijpesteijn, ed. [Lyon 1967], pp. 22–24) reads 77 drachmas.

[148] Cf. *P.Lond.* III.1159 (A.D. 145–47).

Here, as above in the cases of the lease of fishing rights, the fisherman was seen as both fisherman and fish salter. This may be a second reason why ταριχευταί appear so rarely in papyri. There is some evidence that, as a profession, fish salters did not fare well. Ps-Manetho, writing probably in the second century A.D., indicates that they lived a "mournful life with loathsome skills," a situation they apparently shared with embalmers.[149]

Fishermen formed organizations, or guilds; fish salters *per se* probably did not.[150] Whether this is true and whether it continued into the Roman period cannot be learned. Sellers of processed fish, on the other hand, apparently did form professional organizations and, as in third century A.D. Arsinoë, congregated in specific areas of town to ply their trade. Beyond this little can be said.

Syria, Palestine, and the Near East[151]

The Eastern Mediterranean washes the shores of the provinces of Syria and Judaea. Fish of many kinds were abundant along the coast, and the inhabitants took advantage of this fact centuries before the Romans appeared on the scene. The most obvious example is the Phoenician purple dye industry, whose products derived from the murex and dominated markets throughout antiquity. Piles of murex shells have been found along the coast between Akko (modern Acre) in Judaea and Latakia in Syria, but especially near Tyre and Sidon.[152] This important activity continued into the Roman period. Strabo remarks that the large number of dyeing factories at Tyre renders the city unpleasant in which to live, but quite wealthy. Tyrian coins of the second century A.D. bore the emblem of the murex.[153] The Tyrians

---

[149] Ps-Manetho *Apotelesmata* 456–64 Koechly:

> εἰ δὲ μέσον κέντρον Πυρόεις Φαίνων τ᾽ ἐφέποιεν,
> μοίραις δ᾽, ἅς κε θέωσ᾽ αὐτοί, ἑτέροιο τύχοιεν,
> μηδέ τις εὐ ἐργῶν κείνων χῶρον καθορῷ η,
> τέχνῃσιν μυσαραῖς λυγρὸν βίον ἐξανύουσιν˙
> ἤτοι γὰρ νέκυας μαλερῇ πνείοντας ὑπ᾽ ὀδμῇ
> γαστέρας ἀμπτύξαντες ἰδ᾽ ἔγκατα πάντ᾽ ἀφύσαντες
> χρίουσιν κέδρου κυαναυγέος ἔνδοθι πίσσῃ,
> ἢ τοίγ᾽ εὐχανδεῖ χαλκῷ ποιλοις τε λέβησιν
> πυθομένοις μέλδουσιν ἅμ᾽ ἰχθύσιν οὖλοδν ἅλμην.

For the date of Ps-Manetho see R. Garnett, "On the Date of the ᾽Αποτελεσματικά of Manetho," *Journal of Philology* 23 (1895): 238–40.

[150] *P.Fay.* 13 (2nd. cent. B.C.) may refer to an organization of fish salters of the Ptolemaic period, since the letter is addressed to "Psais and partners" (Ψάιτι καὶ μετόχοις ταριχευταῖς). Although the context is obscure, fish-salter seems a strong possibility. See editor's note to ταριχευταῖς in *P.Fay.* 13_4. Cf. *P.Tebt.* III.841 (114 B.C.) and Rostovtzeff, *SEHHW*, p. 1590, note 25.

[151] In this section I shall discuss the provinces of Syria and Judaea as a single unit and shall also consider Mesopotamia and other areas of the Near East where evidence of fish preservation has been found.

[152] Sabatino Moscati, *The World of the Phoenicians*. Alastair Hamilton, transl. (New York 1968), pp. 82–83; and Georges Contenau, *La civilisation phénicienne* (Paris 1928), pp. 302–04.

[153] Strabo 16.2.23. On Tyrian purple see Jean-Paul Rey-Coquais, *Inscriptions grecques et latines découvertes dans les fouilles de Tyr (1963–1974)*: I. *Inscriptions de la nécropole*. Bulletin du Musée de

also processed tunny fish in their installations.[154] Lucian informs us that Phoenician merchants, to whom he refers as mainly salt-fish merchants (ταριχοπώλαι), sailed into the Black Sea region and elsewhere to ply their trade, and the tombstone of a fish sauce merchant (γαροπώλης) has been found in the necropolis of Tyre.[155] The name Sidon refers to fish, and farther down the coast in Judaea the city of Akko was among those cities famous for their fish.[156]

The inland waters of Syria and Palestine also supplied an abundance of fish. A common saying expressed the point that it made no sense to send fish to Akko or muries to Aspamia (=Apamaea). Apamaea, usually taken to be a Spanish city, may have been the Syrian city located some forty-five kilometers east of Laodicea.[157] If this is the case, Apamaea probably obtained its fish from Lake Apamaea and the Orontes River. The Lake of Galilee, the Valley of the Huleh, and other inland waters in Judaea teemed with many varieties of fish and offered a steady livelihood to many inhabitants of the area. The most noted salting installation was at Mejdel, the Talmudic Migdal Nunaiyya, located just north of Tiberias on the Sea of Galilee. Strabo confirms that a large fish salting industry operated there and calls the city Ταριχέαι. Archaeological finds of net-sinkers and anchors support the references to fishing activity.[158]

Although archaeological evidence for fish processing installations in Syria and Palestine is almost totally lacking, the picture of an active salting industry, hinted at in Greek and Latin authors and in a few papyri, is con-

---

Beyrouth, 29 (Paris 1977): 158–60, esp. p. 159, note 2; and Arye Ben-David, *Talmudische Ökonomie* (Hildesheim 1974), pp. 157–60; and *Edict. Diocl.* XXIV.4.

[154] Pollux *Onom.* 6.63: θύννος Τύριος.

[155] Lucian *Toxaris* 4: λέγοις ἂν ἤδη ὅ τι τὸ σεμνὸν καὶ θεῖον ἄλλο ἐξειργάσαντο˙ ἐπεὶ ὅσον ἐπὶ τῷ πλῷ καὶ τῇ ἀποδημίᾳ πολλοὺς ἂν σοι θειοτέρους ἐκείνων ἀποδεῖξαιμι τοὺς ἐμπόρους, καὶ μάλιστα τοὺς Φοίνικας αυτῶν, οὐκ εἰς τὸν Πόντον οὐδὲ ἄχρι τῆς Μαιώτιδος καὶ τοῦ Βοσπόρου μόνον ἐσπλέοντας, ἀλλὰ πανταχοῦ τῆς Ἑλληνικῆς καὶ βαρβαρικῆς θαλάττης ναυτιλλομένους˙ ἅπασαν γὰρ αὖτοι ἀκτὴν καὶ πάντα αἰγιαλόν, ὡς εἰπεῖν, διερευνησάμενοι καθ ᾽ ἕκαστον ἔτος ὀψὲ τοῦ μετοπώρου εἰς τὴν αὐτῶν ἐπανίασιν. οὓς κατὰ τὸν αὐτὸν λόγον θεοὺς νόμιζε, καὶ ταῦτα καπήλους καὶ ταριχοπώλας, εἰ τύχοι, τοὺς πολλοὺς αύτῶν ὄντας. See also Rey-Coquais, *Inscriptions de la nécropole*, p. 154.

[156] Sidon: Rhode, *Thynnorum Captura*, p. 38; Akko: *Gen. Rab.* 5.8 and *Exod. Rab.* 9.6 (translated in Sperber, "Fish and Fisheries," p. 265).

[157] *Exod. Rab.* 9.6. Sperber ("On Social and Economic Conditions in Third Century Palestine," *ArchOrient* 38 [1970]: 13–14) argues that Apamaea should be identified with the Syrian city. For the identification with the Spanish city see Ben-David, *Talmudische Ökonomie*, pp. 225–26; and S. Applebaum, "Economic Life in Palestine," in *The Jewish People in the First Century.* Section One of Compendia Rerum Iudaicarum ad Novum Testamentum (Philadelphia 1966), 2: 670. Cf. Aelian *NA* 12.29.

[158] Strabo 16.2.45: ἐν δὲ ταῖς καλουμέναις Ταριχέαις ἡ λίμνη μὲν ταριχείας ἰχθύων ἀστείας παρέχει, φύει δὲ δένδρα καρποφόρα, μηλέαις ἐμφερῆ. For the location of Tarichaeae see *Greek and Latin Authors on Jews and Judaism*. Menahem Stern, ed. (Jerusalem 1974), 1: 309. See also Applebaum, "Economic Life," p. 683; Ben-David, *Talmudische Ökonomie*, p. 156; and E. W. G. Masterman, "The Fisheries of Galilee," *Palestine Exploration Fund* (1908): 40–51. Cf. Stephanus of Byzantium s.v. Ταριχέαι: ἔστι καὶ Ταριχέα καὶ ἑνικῶς καὶ πληθυντικῶς λεγομένη πόλις τῆς Ἰουδαίας, ὡς Ἰώσηπος.

firmed by many references to processed fish products in the Jewish Talmud, a valuable historical source frequently neglected by Roman historians. A collection of opinions and teachings concerning Jewish traditional law, it is a mine of information on Jewish social and economic life during the Hellenistic and Roman periods. This body of writings is formed of two parts. The Mishna, or teaching, is a collection of rules which, originally mostly oral, were written down in the early third century A.D. The second part, or Gemara, is in essence a commentary on each Mishna composed by Jewish scholars in schools in Palestine and Babylonia between the third and fifth centuries A.D.[159] Because of the nature of the material, exact dating of specific references contained in the Talmud can frequently be difficult to ascertain, even by those expert in Talmudic studies. Nevertheless, information contained in the Talmud can be taken to represent conditions in the Near East between the first and fifth centuries A.D.

Jewish and non-Jewish inhabitants of the Near East during the Graeco-Roman period consumed large amounts of fish, both fresh and processed.[160] There is no reason to think that this was a newly acquired taste. Egypt sent processed fish to Syria as early as the eighteenth dynasty, and the Zenon Papyri show evidence that Palestine imported salt-fish from Egypt and Sicily in the third century B.C.[161] That Syrian imports from Egypt continued into the Roman period can be seen from *P.Meyer* 65, a letter of the third century A.D. from a Syrian requesting that two Kolophonian measures of salt-fish be sent to him. Egyptian fish, probably dried since they were packed in baskets, and Spanish tunny were declared by Rabbi Judah (fl. 2nd cent. A.D.) to be presumed clean.[162] What he meant by the "tunny of the Spaniards" is not entirely clear, but there is no reason to dismiss the

[159] My discussion of the Talmud is of necessity an over-simplification of a complex body of writings, but I hope not seriously misleading. My lack of a reading knowledge of Hebrew constrains me to use translations, the problems of which I am all too cognizant. I have consulted *The Babylonian Talmud*. Rabbi Dr. Isidore Epstein, ed. 18 vols. (London 1961). No effort has been made to be exhaustive in citing from the Talmud. I did not have access to the Palestinian Talmud, but little will be lost, I believe, since the Mishnah of the Babylonian and Palestinian Talmuds are almost identical and the Gemara of the former is fuller. In any case, I have relied heavily on scholars at home in Talmudic literature, particularly Samuel Krauss, whose work *Talmudische Archäologie* (3 vols. Leipzig 1910), is still indispensible, and Daniel Sperber. My debt to these two scholars will be all too noticeable in the text and notes, although I dare to disagree with them on some minor points. I wish also to thank my colleague Jared Klein for his translation of particularly troublesome Hebrew texts and in sharing his ideas on their interpretation. Responsibility for all statements, as always, remains with me.

[160] See esp. Krauss, *Talmudische Archäologie*, 1: 110–12; 2: 145–46.

[161] For Egyptian exports to Syria in the 18th dynasty see above note 134. For the Zenon Papyri see *P.Col.* III.2_{17} (Egypt) and *P.Lond.* VII.2141_{37} (Sicily). The former papyrus (259 B.C.) describes a four-camel caravan which departed Pelusium enroute to Galilee via Gaza and Sidon. The latter document (258 B.C.) lists goods purchased by Zenon in Palestine, probably at Ptolemais (Akko), among which was a ταρίχου Σικελικοῦ βικίον.

[162] *BT. Makshirin* 6.3 (Epstein, p. 494). Cf. *BT. Shabbath* 39a (Epstein, pp. 180–81) and *BM. Shabbath* 145b (Epstein, pp. 735–36).

possibility of a genuine Spanish import since third century A.D. South Spanish amphorae have been found in Palestine.[163] Syrian merchants trading in Spain and Italy could easily have brought Spanish processed fish back to the Near East.[164] One need not assume that cost of transportation would have precluded imports from the West, nor indeed to justify the appearance of imported products must one postulate that a cheaper work force in the exporting area was necessary to compete in the foreign market.[165] Even if the latter situation were true, another explanation is at hand. There was a Roman army in the area whose soldiers, like those in the western provinces and in Asia Minor, must have preferred, at least occasionally, to enjoy the well-known and highly touted Spanish products.[166] In addition, the wealthier families, Roman and non-Roman, could afford the (presumably) more expensive Spanish products and would no doubt desire the best. An enterprising merchant would cater to the latter clientele and surely the Roman government would not disappoint the former. Nevertheless, the majority of inhabitants no doubt consumed the local products which were probably more abundant and cheaper.

Amphora studies and underwater archaeology hold out the best chance to learn more about eastern trade in processed fish products. Some success has already been registered. Many amphorae found in shipwrecks off the coast of Israel as well as in storehouses inland have received classification. Four, identified as Zemer Forms 39 (1st cent. A.D.), 49 (3rd–4th cent. A.D.), and 50–51 (5th–6th cent. A.D.), may have carried processed fish products. Examples of Zemer Forms 49–51, which may have originated in Gaza and were found at Kassarwit, contained traces of fish.[167]

Although there is no clear evidence for Syrian or Palestinian exports of salt-fish products (with the possible exception of the Tyrians), we can form

---

[163] Sperber, "Fish and Fisheries," pp. 265–69. But cf. Emil Schürer, *Geschichte des Jüdischen Volkes im Zeitalter Jesu Christi*. 4th ed. (Leipzig 1907), 2: 78–79. South Spanish amphorae of the third century A.D. (Keay XVI = Almagro 50) have been found in Samaria in Palestine. See Keay, *Late Roman Amphorae*, p. 151.

[164] For Syrian merchants in Malaca in Spain see *IGRR* I/II. 26; for Tyrian merchants in Italy see *OGIS* 595. See also Charlesworth, *Trade Routes*, pp. 36–56.

[165] So Sperber, "Fish and Fisheries," p. 267.

[166] For fish in the diet of Roman soldiers see, in general, Davies, "The Roman Military Diet," pp. 128–31. In the northwest section of the wall at Masada, in a storeroom dated to the period preceding the revolt of A. D. 66 and so doubtless used by the Roman army garrison, excavators found among many "pseudo-Rhodian"amphorae some inscribed with Latin letters. One of these still contained the remains of fish. Although the origin of the fish is unknown, but was probably not Spanish, the find does reveal an element in the military diet common to the Roman army both of the eastern and western provinces. See Y. Yadin, "The Excavation at Masada–1963/64: Preliminary Report," IEJ 15 (1965): 76.

[167] Avshalom Zemer, *Storage Jars in Ancient Sea Trade* (Haifa 1977), pp. 49 (Form 39), 61 (Forms 49–51), 113 (Kassarwit). Zemer Type 37, identified as having held fish products, seems to correspond to the Tripolitanian II type vessel and so most probably held olive oil. See Peacock and Williams, *Amphorae and the Roman Economy*, pp. 169–70. Peacock and Williams (*ibid.*, pp. 198–99) identify Zemer Forms 49–51 with Almagro Form 54 and mention only wine and olive oil or sesame oil as possible contents.

some idea of the intraprovincial trade.[168] The Talmud has numerous references to processed fish.[169] Most references concern whether or not this or that food product is considered clean or unclean; that is, permitted to Jews (kosher) or denied to them (non-kosher). This dietary concern was so dominant a theme in Jewish life (hence its prominence in Talmudic literature) that it was known, at least imperfectly, even to Romans. Pliny the Elder comments on this specifically, but incorrectly, when he says that a special fish sauce, called *castimoniarum*, was required by Jews since they could eat only scaleless(!) fish.[170] There had to be, therefore, some way of determining the permissibility of processed fish products whose kind of fish or process could be in doubt. This is probably the purpose of amphora inscriptions with the adjective *casta* or *castum*, modifying the product designation, found on vessels in Pompeii and perhaps in Rome.[171]

Since Talmudic sources frequently make a distinction between muries made by Jewish producers and that produced by non-Jews, apparently both groups produced and sold salted fish products in Palestine. Since it was not a Jewish monopoly a careful distinction between them had to be made. How this was done is unclear. Personal acquaintance with a muries producer might be enough to allay any apprehension.[172] Another way, and one more important for our purposes, was declared by Rabbi Abbahu (fl. ca. late 3rd cent. A.D.) in Caesarea. He states that fish-entrails and fish-eggs could be purchased by anyone since one may assume that they came from Pelusium or Aspamia.[173] Although it appears from this statement that, at least in the period of Rabbi Abbahu, only kosher fish were being imported into Palestine, this is highly unlikely. There must have been other means, unspecified in the Talmud, to differentiate the products.[174] It would also be rash at this point, considering what has been said above, to assume that Pelusium and Apamaea exercised any sort of monopoly on the fish trade along the coast.[175] Not enough is known of Spanish, nor indeed of Pontic trade in the area.

---

[168] The "Gaza" jars mentioned in several papyri in Egypt may refer only to the type of vessel or its shape. See esp. Daniel Sperber, "Objects of Trade Between Palestine and Egypt in Roman Times," *JESHO* 19 (1976): 144–45. But cf. Zemer Forms 49–51 found at Kassarwit and a papyrus fragment (*P.Colt* 87) from Nessana which mentions garum that may have come from Gaza. See Carol A. M. Glucker, *The City of Gaza in the Roman and Byzantine Periods*. BAR International Series, 325 (Oxford 1987), p. 95.

[169] *BT. Terumoth* 11.1 (Epstein, p. 245), *BT. Abodah Zarah* 34b (Epstein, pp. 166–67), *BT. Abodah Zarah* 39a (Epstein, pp. 197–200), *BT. Mo'ed Katan* 11a (Epstein, pp. 58–61), and *BT. Makshirin* 6.3 (Epstein, p. 494). For ὀξύγαρον see Krauss, *Talmudische Archäologie*, 1: 112.

[170] Pliny *HN* 31.95. See esp. Thomas Corcoran, "Pliny's *Garum Castimoniarum*," *CB* 34 (1958): 69.

[171] Rome: *CIL* XV.4728(?); Pompeii: *CIL* IV.2569, 2609, 2611(?), 5660–62. See also Curtis, "Product Identification and Advertising ," pp. 223–24, and below pp. 165–66.

[172] *BT. Abodah Zarah* 34b (Epstein, pp. 166–67) and 40a–40b (Epstein, pp. 197–200). See also Sperber, "Social and Economic Conditions," pp. 11–12.

[173] *BT. Abodah Zarah* 39a (Epstein, pp. 197–200).

[174] See Sperber, "Fish and Fisheries," pp. 268–69; and *idem*, "Objects of Trade," pp. 119–23.

[175] Contra Sperber, "Fish and Fisheries," p. 265.

P.Rylands IV.627–39 provide perhaps the best examples of the availability of salted fish products in Syria and Palestine in the early fourth century A.D. These papyri form a collection of memoranda and daily accounts of Theophanes, an official of the Prefect of Egypt, who in ca. A.D. 317–23 made an extended journey from Antinoopolis in Upper Egypt to Antioch in Syria and returned. We are able to trace his route fairly accurately as he travelled to Alexandria and Pelusium in Egypt, thence to Gaza in Palestine, where he turned north toward Antioch, passing through Askalon, Caesarea, Tyre, Sidon, and Laodicea. Although several lacunae appear in these accounts as extant, we do have an almost complete record of his stay in Antioch for the month of Pauni (June). During this month Theophanes purchased τάριχος or γάρος an average of almost once every two days.[176] Although his purchases of salted fish products while travelling are less well-known, he did indicate that he bought γάρος at Askalon in Palestine and γάρος and τάριχος at Pelusium in Egypt.[177] There is every reason to believe that he had no trouble finding salt-fish merchants at the many other stops along his route, which was almost completely along the coast, and purchased whatever he needed for his entourage.

Salted fish products formed part of merchandise carried along the caravan routes moving inland into Arabia, Mesopotamia, and probably farther east. The Tariff of Palmyra, dating to A.D. 137 but with portions datable to the first century A.D., for example, places a tax of ten denarii on each camel-load of salted fish brought into or carried out of the city and three denarii for each donkey-load. Although the tax law concerns primarily the local economy of Palmyra and its territory, the salt-fish most likely formed part of caravan commodities coming from the coast bound for Palmyra or beyond.[178] Palmyra lay on the route between Damascus and cities lying on the Euphrates River, such as Dura Europus. Γαρέλεν, a mixture of garum and oil, whether of local production or imported is unknown, apparently formed part of a sacred meal for worshippers of Mithra in the third century A.D. mithraeum at Dura Europus.[179] At Nehardea near Babylon in the third century A.D. the Exilarch, the official head of the Babylonian Jewish com-

---

[176] *P.Ryl.* IV.629. He purchased τάριχος on days 1–8, 10–11, 16–17, 20–21, and τιμ(ῆς) βοριδίων εἰς τὸ γάρος on day 6. During his last two weeks in Antioch, roughly July 6–20, he purchased salted fish products even more frequently (*P.Ryl.* IV.630*).

[177] *P.Ryl.* IV.637$_{428}$ (Askalon), 637$_{495, 498}$ (Pelusium). Prices charged for these products cannot be computed since where we know the price paid we do not know how much was purchased. One hundred drachmae was the usual daily amount spent on τάριχος or γάρος. The size of Theophanes' party is unknown. For a list of foodstuffs, including garum, on an ostrakon of the Byzantine period found in Palestine see *SEG* 32 (1982): 418, no. 1511.

[178] *IGRR* III.1056, ii.35. See J. F. Matthews, "The Tax Law of Palmyra: Evidence for Economic History in a City of the Roman East," *JRS* 74 (1984): 157–80, esp. p. 176, lines 52–53.

[179] The fish sauce is listed along with other food items in a graffito scratched on the wall. For the graffito see M. I. Rostovtzeff, Frank E. Brown and C. B. Welles, *The Excavations at Dura-Europos: Preliminary Report of the Seventh and Eighth Seasons of Work* (New Haven 1939), p. 125, no. 862; and in M. J. Vermaseren, *Corpus Inscriptionum et Monumentorum Religionis Mithriacae* (The Hague 1956–60), p. 71, no. 65.

munity, served his high ranking guests salted fish.[180] Xenocrates claims that salted sea bream, although not very esteemed, were imported into the Mediterranean from India. The accuracy of this claim is questionable given the inexactness of the use of the adjective "Indian" by ancient authors. These products may have originated instead from Eastern North Africa, Egypt, or perhaps the Red Sea area.[181] If these fish products came from India, they may have used the east-west caravan routes or, more probably, carried in ships using the monsoon winds, arrived in the Red Sea ports where they were off-loaded and sent north into Syria and Asia, west to Egypt, and perhaps to Rome itself.

---

[180] *BT. Mo'ed Katan* 11a (Epstein, pp. 58–61). Fish salting seems to have been practiced in the Persian Gulf at Ras Abaruk. No vats were found, but discarded fish bones formed a large mound measuring fifteen meters across and 250 cm. deep. There also existed a complex of small, rustic structures, probably all relating to the salting activity. The area was apparently used as a temporary or seasonal site for curing fish, which were then transported elsewhere for consumption or sale. The dating of the site is uncertain, but seems to fall into the first few centuries A.D. See P. S. Garlake, "A Fish-curing Complex on Ras Abaruk, Site 6," in *Qatar Archaeological Report: Excavations 1973*. Beatrice de Cardi, ed. (Oxford 1978): 136–46.

[181] Xenocrates *ap*. Orib. 2.58.147: τρίγλαι γὰρ καὶ φάγροι σκληροὶ ἐκ τῆς Ἰνδικῆς κομιζόμενοί εἰσι μὲν κητώδεις, οὐκ ἐνάριθμοι δὲ τοῖς καθαριωτέροις θαλαττίοις. For the imprecise use of the adjective "Indian" in ancient authors, see Raschke, "New Studies," pp. 651–52. Spanish salt-fish products made their way to Arikamedu in India, probably by the Red Sea route. See Elizabeth Lyding Will, "The Roman Shipping Amphoras from Arikamedu," *AJA* 91 (1987): 293.

CHAPTER SIX

PRODUCERS AND MERCHANTS

Organization for Production and Commerce

Manilius, in *Astronomica* 5.656–81, describes individual fishermen processing their catch of tunny on the shore. This scale of operation was small and simple, necessitating little help beyond the fisherman's individual efforts. The facilities were modest, such as dolia or vats of a temporary nature, or at best a few permanent basins if the fishermen used the same area repeatedly. This was certainly the type of operation practiced at Tonnara del Cofano on Sicily, at several locations around the Bay of Douarnenez in Armorica, and many other places which had only two or three vats. One can also assume that much of the salting activity along the Nile River in Egypt likewise consisted of individual fishermen or small groups of fishermen, perhaps family operations. The survey of provinces has shown how frequently villas were closely connected with salting installations. Some were situated near large salteries, but others, such as many in Lusitania and Baetica, had only a few salting vats. Apparently it was not uncommon for owners of maritime villas to engage in small-scale economic activity, producing what they needed of fish products and perhaps selling a certain amount for an income.[1] In the latter cases, slaves living in the villa probably processed the fish, perhaps under the management of a *vilicus*. Fish could be caught by villa workers themselves or purchased from local fishermen.

Moderate to large scale operations naturally required a more or less formal organizational structure. How large an establishment had to be to demand a well-defined organization is difficult to say. Factories of the size of Lixus in Africa, Caetobriga and Baelo in Spain, or Tyritake and Chersonesos on the Black Sea definitely would need one. Those located around the Bay of Douarnenez which had as many as twenty basins probably did also. Fish salteries of significant size were usually located near an urban center and in all likelihood were operated by the owner, his family members, freedmen, and slaves, or even operated for the owner by slaves under a slave or freedman manager. An organization of this type seems to have existed at Pompeii, the only place for which evidence is plentiful. The or-

[1] For economic self-sufficiency of the villa described by Petronius, see Schmeling, "Trimalchio's Menu and Wine List," pp. 248–51. For the economic side of villas in the area of the Bay of Naples see D'Arms, *Commerce and Social Standing*, pp. 72–96. For the suggestion that this arrangement appertained to many places along the southern coast of Lusitania, see Edmondson, *Two Industries*, pp. 128–30.

ganization of workers at salteries in other places remains a matter of speculation.[2]

Since tunny are migratory fish, salting operations were no doubt seasonal in nature and the supply of particular species of other fish probably varied from year to year, sometimes sharply.[3] More workers would be needed in-season than off-season, and in bad years most workers could not depend on any work in the salteries. In lean years or when the tunny had passed, salting operations would be reduced, but probably not completely halted. Fishermen, who probably lived a permanent existence in nearby towns, would continue to fish for other species which could be salted or dried. Other types of meat, such as pork, might also be processed. Those workers no longer needed would have to take up another occupation until the next season or else attempt to follow the tunny in its migration to other places. A possible scenario might look something like this. The tunny migration from the Atlantic would provide work for many saltery workers during the late spring when they enter the Mediterranean and late summer when they migrate back to the Atlantic. In the meantime other types of fish could be caught and processed. Extracting purple dye from the murex could occupy the late winter and early spring months, while other meats, such as pork, could be salted year round if necessary.[4] Saltery managers presumably remained permanently at the saltery, perhaps living in the villa located nearby.[5]

The determination of ownership of salteries poses a more difficult problem, since literary and archaeological sources are completely silent on this point. Since fishermen could also prepare their catch on the shore as an integral part of their occupation, salting activity must have also come under the right of fishing (*ius piscandi*). This seems to be implied in the fact

---

[2] The owners of sizable installations may have derived most or all of their income from the industry and had little or no connection with agriculture. The workers were probably slaves and members of the local populace. This seems indicative of the large factories around Caetobriga in Lusitania. See Edmondson, *Two Industries*, pp. 130–34.

[3] Edmondson (*Two Industries*, pp. 110–15, and Table 5.3), for example, illustrates the varied tonnage of different species of fish caught off the Portuguese coast between 1971 and 1980. Tunny varied between a low of 21 tons in 1973 to a high of 4600 in 1980, mackerel from 21,988 tons in 1973 to only 4952 tons seven years later. The sardine catch was more consistent, ranging from a low of 75,489 tons in 1974 to a high of 106,324 tons in 1980. This somewhat sporadic supply of fish probably appertained in the Eastern Mediterranean as well. Nevertheless, as I have tried to show, fish salting was actively practiced throughout the Mediterranean, although most of the archaeological evidence so far discovered comes from the West where for various reasons archaeologists have been more active. The model proposed by T. W. Gallant (*A Fisherman's Tale* [Gent 1985], pp. 40–44) is far too pessimistic. The literary and archaeological evidence bespeaks a greater role for preserved fish products than merely "a short-term famine response"(p. 43).

[4] Tunny: Bourge, "Étude," pp. 85–97; purple: Pliny *HN* 9.133; pork: Columella *Rust.* 12.55.4. See also K. D. White, *Roman Farming* (Ithaca, N.Y. 1970), pp. 320–21.

[5] Ponsich believes that in Spain the managers, following the tunny, crossed back and forth between Spain and Mauretania Tingitana. See Ponsich, "Détroit de Gibraltar," pp. 675–77.

that in Latin *cetarius* refers not only to those who catch large fish but also to those who salt them. In addition, at least in Egypt, fishermen and fish salters seem indistinguishable.[6] Since the *ius piscandi* also included the right to dry, store and repair nets, and even to construct shelters on the shore, anyone with the inclination, manpower and resources could establish and operate a saltery on the seashore.[7] The size of the operation would depend upon the amount of capital available. Operation of a large saltery might frequently require two or more people to pool their resources to form a *societas*; that is, a private corporation whose purpose it was to acquire a profit from processing fish.

Although the sea and the fish in it were considered common to all people (*res nullius*), it seems apparent that the state did claim ownership of some fisheries and perhaps some salteries as well. The state derived considerable revenue by frequently leasing out the fishing rights to companies *(societates)* or imposing a tax on individuals wishing to fish in certain areas.[8] A dedicatory inscription found at Leeuwarden in the Netherlands, for example, names a Q. Valerius Secundus as *manceps* of a *societas* which apparently had purchased from the state the right to fish the Atlantic waters in that area.[9] There may be a similar state connection with C. Varenius Varus mentioned in a dedicatory inscription found on the beach at Ris, at Douarnenez, the location of the greatest concentration of Armorican salteries. Varus was a *curator* of a small conventus of Roman citizens residing in Armorica in Gaul probably for the purpose of trading in, if not producing and exporting, salted fish products manufactured in the area.[10] A first-century A.D. dossier on the fishing rights of Histria, a city lying on the Black Sea coast of Moesia Inferior near the mouth of the Danube River, shows that

[6] Nonius Marcellus *De compend. doct.* s.v. *cetari* (*genus est piscatorum quod maiores pisces capit*); and Columella *Rust.* 8.17.12: *salsamentorum omnium pergamenta, quae cetariorum officinis everruntur.* Cf. Terence *Eunuchus* 257. See also the sixth century A.D. glossator Luctatius Placidus *Glossae* s.v. *cetarii*: *cete dicitur genus marinae belvae. ab hoc vero genere abusive piscatores cetarii dicuntur et qui tractant ea, quae ex piscibus fiunt. ut sunt liquaminarii, qui ex corporibus piscium humorem liquant.* See also *CGL* IV.32, 23: *Cetari liquaminari*; and IV.318, 7: *cetari qui salsamenta vendunt.*

[7] Roman law viewed the sea and by extension the shore bordering on it as common to all people (*res nullius*). The right of fishing (*ius piscandi*) derived from the status of the sea. Thus no one could be forbidden to fish from the shore. In effect, the sea and the fish in it were not owned by the state. See Percy Fenn, Jr., *The Origin of the Right of Fishery in Territorial Waters* (Cambridge, Mass. 1926), esp. pp. 17–29.

[8] Bohlen, *Fischerei*, pp. 44–51. In the Greek East, Greek cities and sometimes temples for fiscal reasons taxed fishing privileges in waters claimed by them. Installations erected on the shore associated with fishing could be privately owned. The Romans seem to have patterned themselves, in some cases at least, on this arrangement, though unlike the Greeks the Romans viewed the sea as common. See Jacques Dumont. "Liberté des mers et territoire de pêche en droit grec," *RD* (1977): 53–57.

[9] *CIL* XIII.8830. See also Bohlen, *Fischerei*, p. 46.

[10] Sanquer restores the inscription as follows: N(umini) AUG(usti)/ NEPTUNO HIPPIO/ C(aius) VARENIUS VOLTIN(ia tribu)/ VARUS C(urator) C(ivium) R(omanorum) IIII/ POSUIT. See Sanquer, "L'inscription à Neptune," p. 225, and *idem*, "Les industriels des salaisons," pp. 148–56.

the Roman government taxed the fishing and fish salting revenues of the city.[11] This was not a tax directly on the salteries but on the municipal revenues derived from the salteries which may have been owned by the city or whose owners may have paid a tax or rent to the city. But even this level of state interference may not have existed elsewhere. The fishing and salting industries were quite active in Pompeii during the first century A.D., for example, yet no evidence exists to show that the state exercised any control. Apparently at Pompeii the fish sauce business was completely in the hands of private citizens, such as the Umbricii Scauri, who produced and sold salted fish products for their own profit. Villas located near salteries were also probably owned by private citizens who operated the salteries to their own advantage.

The fact that imperial salteries operated alongside large corporations, small *societates*, and even individuals in Spain has already been remarked upon. A few additional words on the *societas* of New Carthage, however, should be added. The exact nature of this organization remains unknown, but a connection with the Roman state cannot be ruled out. It has been suggested that such a long-lived organization must have been authorized by the state, and to be so, it could, like the mining companies, only lease the rights on public domain. Consequently, the *societas* was not formed to produce fish products, but instead to farm the salt works around the city of New Carthage. The salting of fish was a secondary activity prompted by the control of the salt necessary to process fish.[12] It is impossible to judge if this arrangement, even if correct for New Carthage, prevailed anywhere else. The salteries at Lixus, Baelo, and Caetobriga, for example, were quite large, yet we have no evidence that a similar organization operated those installations.

From available evidence, one must conclude that little can be said definitively concerning the ownership of Roman salteries. The large number of salting installations having only a few basins, however, speaks strongly for the conclusion, however tentative, that most salteries were small privately owned industries working independently of the state and in competition with each other. Many had so few vats that it is hard to imagine that the output satisfied anything more than personal requirements, with possibly

[11] See above, p. 128; Bohlen, *Fischerei*, pp. 47–48. Cyzicus and Byzantium in the first century B.C. received revenue from their fisheries and presumably paid a tax to the Roman government. See Strabo 7.6.2. The Roman state could derive an income from salted fish products passing through ports and down rivers since it retained ownership rights of harbors and inland waters, which were considered *res publicae*. See Fenn, *Right of Fishery*, p. 11. Fishery products passing through customs stations, such as Zarai in Africa (*CIL* VIII.4508), in the Fayum in Egypt (*P.Wisc.* II.80), and at Palmyra in Syria (*IGRR* III.1056) were also taxed, either by the Roman or local government. See Sijpesteijn, *Customs Duties in Graeco-Roman Egypt*, esp. pp. 1–7, 16–26, 40–50.

[12] Étienne, "Garum sociorum," pp. 297–313. For the analogy with mining companies see also André Piganiol, Preface to Ponsich and Tarradell, *Garum*, p. viii.

some for sale in the local area. Others, however, did produce for export as well. How long this situation continued is uncertain. Some level of state control, on commerce at least, is implied in the constitution of Valentinian, Valens, and Gratian in A.D. 368, which forbade the selling of liquamen, oil, and wine to people living outside the empire.[13] The fact that such a decree was necessary may imply that it was being done by merchants not under the control of the state. It is also a matter of speculation whether large corporations distributed as well as produced their products, although this does seem likely from the fact that salteries frequently have kilns located nearby for making commercial containers.

The wide variety of terms designating merchants in salted fish products seems to imply a high degree of specialization. This is probably misleading, however. Since all salted fish products were made at the same time in the salting process, a merchant may have dealt in the entire range of salted fish products but assumed a specific title to distinguish himself. The title would, therefore, by a kind of synecdoche, indicate that he traded in a number of related products of which his appellation indicated only one. P. Clodius Athenio, who belonged to a *societas* from Malaca stationed in Ostia, for example, called himself a *negotians salsarius*, while Tiberius Claudius Docimus, an imperial freedman from Africa who died in Rome, styled himself a *negotians salsamentarius et vinariarius*.[14] Both probably traded in salted meats of all kinds, including fish. Marcus Primus Secundianus was a *negotians muriarius* living in Lugdunum in Gaul, and there were several *negotiatores allecarii* operating in Germania Inferior.[15] It is hard to believe that fish sauce merchants traded in only one type of fish sauce. They probably traded in the other sauces as well. Whether a fish sauce merchant also traded in the more bulky salted or dried fish products is impossible to say, but it does seem likely.

Social and Economic Status

Macrobius (fl. ca. A.D. 400), in his discussion of jokes, says that it is a direct affront to ask someone "Have you forgotten because you used to sell salted

---

[13] *Cod. Iust.* 4.41.1: *Imppp. Valentinianus, Valens et Gratianus AA ad Theodorum, Magistrum militum. Ad barbaricum transferendi vini et olei et liquaminis nullam quisquam habeat facultatem, nec gustus quidem causa aut usus commerciorum.*

[14] P. Clodius Athenio: *CIL* VI.9677; Tiberius Claudius Docimus: *CIL* VI.9676. *CIL* VI.9873 may identify another *salsamentarius* (or *salsarius*), Lucius Poplicius Antiochis: L(ucii) POPLICI GN(aei) (?)/ ANTIOCHI SALS(amentarii?)/ IN FRONTE P(edes) XX/ IN AGRUM P(edes) XX. A fragmentary inscription from Vindonissa in Germania Superior (*CIL* XIII.5221) may identify a group of salt-fish and vegetable merchants: (ne)GOTIA(tores)/ (sal)SARI LEG(uminari?)/ (ci)VES RO(mani). . . . Merchants apparently traded in a variety of products related only in the broadest sense, such as liquids. The Auli Atinii, for example, traded in oil, fish sauce, and probably wine; the Quinti Caecilii, in Spanish fish sauce and oil. For a discussion of these two *societates* (?), see Desbat et al., "Inscriptions peintes sur amphores: Lyon," pp. 156–59, 164–66.

[15] M. Primus Secundianus: *CIL* XIII.1966. For the *negotiatores allecarii* see Curtis, "*Negotiatores Allecarii*," pp. 147–58. This is the only instance of the term *allecarius* known from antiquity. For a *salgamarius* see above, p. 113, note 6.

fish?", but a good-natured joke to say, "We remember when you used to wipe your nose with your arm."[16] This picturesque caricature of the salt-fish dealer is common to both Greek and Latin literature and may extend back at least to the third century B.C.[17] That it accurately reflects the social status of those engaged in the production and commerce of salt-fish products, however, may be doubted.[18]

Greek literature portrays the salt-fish dealer (ταριχοπώλης) as no better than the fishmonger (ἰχθυοπώλης), to whom he was closely related by occupation. He was seen as a rascal, cheater, deceiver, and liar. Theophrastus, for example, describes the "shameless man" (ἀπονενοημένος) as one who visits the fish sellers and fish salters and shares in their profits.[19] The sons of Chaerephilus, the salt-fish dealer, who were granted Athenian citizenship, were named by Antiphanes, the comic poet, as the lovers of a prostitute; while Plato places the sellers of salt-fish on a par with shoe makers and servers of stew.[20] Diogenes Laertius (fl. early 3rd cent. A.D.), in his "Life of Bion," has Bion (fl. 3rd cent. B.C.) state that

> "My father was a former slave, accustomed to wiping his nose on his elbow,"—he clearly meant a salt-fish dealer—"an inhabitant of Borsythenes, having no legal standing, but only a decree concerning legality, a token of the bitterness of his master. My mother was of the sort this kind of man would marry, from a brothel."

And finally, Libanius (A.D. 314 - ca. 393) describes a certain Heliodorus, a fish sauce dealer (γάρου κάπηλος), who exchanged this career for that of lawyer. His unscrupulous character, however, remained as he grew wealthy, and he ended his career as a magistrate and the owner of land located throughout Greece.[21]

---

[16] Macrobius *Sat.* 7.3.6: *est autem loedoria huius modi: oblitusne ea quia salsamenta vendebas? scomma autem, quod diximus saepe contumeliam esse celatam, tale est: meminimus quando brachio te emungebas. nam cum res eadem utrobique dicta sit, illud tamen loedoria est, quod aperte obiectum exprobratumque est, hoc scomma, quod figuate.*

[17] Cf. Plutarch *Mor.* 631D: ὁ γὰρ εἰπὼν ταριχοπώλην αὐτόθεν ἐλοιδόρησεν, ὁ δὲ φήσας, μεμνήμεθά σε τῷ βραχίονι ἀπομυττόμενον, ἔσκωψεν. Suetonius *Horatii Poetae Vita. Praefatio: Horatius Flaccus, Venusinus, patre, ut ipse tradit, libertino, et exactionum coactore; ut vero creditum est, salsamentario; cum illi quidam in altercatione exprobrasset, Quotiens ego vidi patrem tuum cubito se emungentem.* Cf. Horace *Od.* 2.20.5–6. Auctor *ad Herennium* 4.67: *Per consequentiam significatio fit cum res quae sequantur aliquam rem dicuntur, ex quibus tota res relinquitur in suspicione; ut si salsamentarii filio dicas: Quiesce tu, cuius pater cubito se emungere solebat;* Diogenes Laertius (below, note 21).

[18] I have discussed this question in greater detail in "The Man Who Wipes his Nose on his Shirt Sleeve," *Laverna* 1(1990): 1–12.

[19] Theophrastus *Char.* 6.9: οὐκ ἀποδοκιμάζειν δὲ ἀλλ' οὐδὲ πολλῶν ἀγοραίων στρατηγεῖν καὶ εὐθὺς τούτοις δανείζειν καὶ τῆς δραχμῆς τόκον τρία ἡμιωβόλια τῆς ἡμέρας πράττεσθαι, καὶ ἐφοδεύειν τὰ μαγειρεῖα, τὰ ἰχθυοπώλια, τὰ ταριχοπώλια, καὶ τοὺς τόκους ⟨τοὺς⟩ ἀπὸ τοῦ ἐμπολήματος εἰς τὴν γνάθον ἐκλέγειν. See also Athen. 6.224b–228c; Alciphron *Ep.* 21(i.18); and Ps-Manetho *Apotelesmata* 459 Koechly.

[20] Antiphanes *ap.* Athen. 8.338e–39e; Plato *Charm.* 163B.

[21] Diogenes Laertius 4.46: ἐμοὶ ὁ πατὴρ μὲν ἦν ἀπελεύθερος, τῷ ἀγκῶνι ἀπομυσσόμενος—διεδήλου δὲ τὸν ταριχέμπορον—γένος Βορυσθενίτης, ἔχων οὐ πρόσωπον, ἀλλὰ συγγραφὴν ἐπὶ τοῦ προσώπου, τῆς τοῦ δεσπότου πικρίας σύμβολον· μήτηρ δὲ οἵαν ὁ τοιοῦτος ἂν γήμαι, ἀπ'

Salt-fish dealers frequently appear as foreigners and non-citizens. The sons of Chaerephilus were apparently so, and Demosthenes, in his speech "Against Lacritus," describes merchants from Phaselis trading in salt-fish between Athens and the Black Sea region. In the Roman period, Lucian speaks disparagingly of Phoenician salt-fish dealers sailing the waters of the Bosphorus and Aegean Seas.[22] Salt-fish itself was seen as food for the common soldier, servants, and farm hands.[23]

Unfortunately, archaeological excavation in the Greek East has produced little information which can be used to confirm or refute this picture. An Attic manumission text of ca. 330–322 B.C. names a former slave who was a salt-fish dealer. Two epitaphs of the Roman period, one from Lebanon and the other from Caria in Southwestern Turkey, record salt-fish dealers as well, but tell us nothing of their wealth or social standing.[24] All one can conclude is that they were well-off enough to afford a tomb or sarcophagus with inscription.

The most potentially fruitful source of information is Corinth where in the 460s B.C. the owner of a house located in the southwest part of what later became the Roman forum dedicated a portion of it to the importation of wine and salt-fish.[25] After renovations, the entire house was given over to the business. The status of the owner is only implied by the size of the house and the quality of its table pottery found there. It seems likely that he was prosperous, if not rich, and his business expanded so much that (if the same person continued to own the establishment) he devoted the entire structure to business and moved himself to separate (more luxurious?) quarters elsewhere in the city. It is unknown, however, if his increased prosperity translated into enhanced social status.

In summary, then, for Greek society the salt-fish producer and dealer often seem to have been persons of low social standing, mean character, and little wealth; no better than fishermen and fishmongers. He was usually a slave or ex-slave, often a foreigner, that is, non-Athenian. Evidence from Corinth may indicate another, more prosperous side to life in the salt-fish business, but not enough is known of the owner of this house.

Evidence for the social standing of the Roman salt-fish producer and dealer is at once more plentiful and revealing. Latin literary allusions mirror the portrayal seen in Greek literature; that is, he is a man of mean char-

οἰκήματος; Libanius *Or.* 62.46–48. For κάπηλος see Moses I. Finkelstein, "Ἔμπορος, Ναύκληρος, and Κάπηλος: a Prolegomena to the Study of Athenian Trade," *CPh* 30 (1935): 320–36, and Jean Rougé, *Recherches sur l'Organization du Commerce Maritime en Méditerranée sous l'Empire Romaine* (Paris 1966), pp. 270–71.

[22] Demosthenes *In Lacritum* 933; Lucian *Toxaris* 4.

[23] Plato Comicus fr. 193 Edmonds; Demosthenes *In Lacritum* 933; Aristophanes *Acharn.* 967, 1097–1102.

[24] David M. Lewis, "Dedications of Phialai at Athens," *Hesperia* 37 (1968): 369–74; Rey-Coquais, *Inscriptions de la nécropole*, pp. 158–60, esp. p. 159, note 2; and Bean, "Epitaphs at Alabanda," p. 53.

[25] Above, p. 115.

acter and low social standing who cavorts with the dregs of society. A Pompeian graffito, for example, links the *salsamentarius* with other base occupations, such as pistor, the common huckster, and makers of furniture, small bottles, and bronze trifles.[26] Association with the product also evoked the image of base character and lowly station. Fish sauce, for example, is the food both of the farm-hand and soldier.[27] Persius speaks of a man so poor that only on his birthday does he eat muria on his cabbage; while Plautus has Antamonides refer to Hanno the Carthaginian as *hallex viri*, "the dregs of a man."[28] Martial in several epigrams associates the object of his ridicule with the strong odor of allec and garum, and Petronius describes Trimalchio's servile cook as a man who reeks of muria and other condiments.[29]

Although salt-fish products could have a strong odor, the derogatory remarks of Roman writers form only part of the picture.[30] Some of the same authors who disparage garum also express an equally enthusiastic fondness for the sauce. Pliny, for example, calls it "a kind of exquisite liquor," and two sentences after he calls it "the secretion of putrefying matter," he declares that garum could be diluted to the color of honey wine and drunk.[31] Martial speaks of "noble garum" and even devotes an entire epigram in praise of garum sociorum, labelling it "the proud sauce."[32] Appar-

---

[26] *CIL* IV.10150: [cum] *de*[d]*uxisti octies, tibi superat, ut* (h)*abeas sedecies. coponium fecisti; cretaria fecisti; salsamentaria fecisti; pistorium fecisti; agricola fuisti; aere minutaria fecisti; propola fuisti; laguncularia nunc facis. si cunnu*(m) *linx*⟨s⟩*e*⟨e⟩*ris, consummaris omnia.*

[27] Cato *Agr.* 58; *SHA. Aurel.* 9.6

[28] Persius *Sat.* 6.20; Plautus *Poen.* 1310. The meaning of "big toe," given for hallex in this passage by Lewis and Short (*A Latin Dictionary*, s.v. *allex*) is dubious. Antamonides calls Hanno many things which connote foul-smelling foods: *Ligula, i in malam crucem./ tune hic amator audes esse, hallex viri,/ aut contrectare quod mares homines amant?/ deglupta mena, sarrapis, sementium,/ manstruca, halagora, sampsa, tum autem plenior/ ali ulpicique quam Romani remiges.* In addition, Plautus' audience would have been aware that the Carthaginians were active in the salt-fish industry and would have recognized this connection. Cf. Gregor Maurach, *Der Poenulus des Plautus* (Heidelberg 1988), p. 172.

[29] Martial 3.77: Baeticus shows his mean character by eating such things as onions floating in allec, small useless fish (gerres), and salt-fish (melandrya); 6.93: Thais smells worse than an amphora of spoiled garum; 7.94: Papylus turns perfume into garum; 11.27: Flaccus is a man of steel who can love a mistress who eats garum and salt-fish (cybium) and whose maid carries allec for her to eat. See Petronius *Sat.* 70: *muria condimentisque fetentem.*

[30] For the strong odor of salted fish see Aristotle *Hist. Animal.* 534ᵃ21 and Pliny *HN* 9.92; for fish sauce, see Pliny *HN* 31.90, Horace *Sat.* 2.4.64–66, and Apicius *De re coq.* 1.7.

[31] Pliny *HN* 31.93: *liquoris exquisiti genus*. The word *liquor* can sometimes mean "putrefaction." See Vergil *Georgics* 3.484. For garum as a drink, see Pliny *HN* 31.95: *sicuti garum ad colorem mulsi veteris adeoque suavitatem dilutum, ut bibi possit.* But cf. Artemidorus *On.* 1.66 and Alciphron 3.4.

[32] Martial 13.82: *nobile garum*; 13.102: *fastosum garum*. Martial alludes more often to fish sauce than any other non-medical author, fourteen times in twelve epigrams. A brief survey shows that he employs fish sauce as he feels the need, relying on its negative qualities (usually strong odor) to criticize certain individuals (3.77; 6.93; 7.94; 11.27, twice), and its positive features to indicate a preference of one sauce over another or to emphasize the elegance which it can impart to certain culinary dishes (7.27; 13.40, 82, 102, 103). Twice he mentions fish sauce in describing an event in which the sauce has no real part other than, by implication, to fulfill a

ently, fish sauce had its good side. Archaeological and epigraphical evidence, discovered at numerous Roman salting installations and in towns and port facilities throughout the Roman world as well as among cargoes of many shipwrecks found in the Western Mediterranean, presents a picture of individuals occupied in fish preservation and its trade at once informative and not entirely at odds with this dichotomous view of the Roman sauces.

Many salting places are little more than temporary fixtures for fishermen-salters similar to those described by Manilius. Since at these locations and even at larger installations habitations for saltery workers have yet to be found and since fish salting was basically a seasonal occupation dependent upon the abundance of annually migrating fish, such as tunny, one can perhaps conclude that workers lived in temporary shelters which have failed to survive the centuries. If saltery managers remained permanently at the saltery, perhaps living in the villa commonly located nearby, even when a portion of it may have been given over to salting vats, their living conditions were much better than the poor workers who eked out a meager existence. In some places, such as in North Africa, burials of poor people found in the vicinity of salting installations have utilized terra-cotta tiles or, somewhat ironically, garum pots and transport vessels for salt-fish.[33] It remains possible that in some instances the overseer (*vilicus*) and perhaps some workers as well lived in the villa and operated it for an absentee owner who resided in or near an adjacent town. The house in Corinth may have functioned similarly in its second phase. In any case, the relative size of the salting installation, such as those at Baelo in Baetica, Troia in Lusitania, and Lixus in Mauretania Tingitana, implies extensive wealth for the owner. Unfortunately, we do not know the identities of any of the owners of these large salting factories.

Merchants in salt-fish products, who in most cases were probably distinct from those who produced them, were quite active and have left their records in stone and terra-cotta. Both Romans and non-Romans participated in this trade. The *negotiatores allecarii* of the late second or early third century A.D., operating between Britain and the Atlantic coasts of Gaul and Germania Superior, included a Roman citizen of Celtic origin (C. Gatullinus Seggo). Two others (L. Secundius Similis and T. Carinius Gratus), Roman citizens of uncertain origin, together dedicated an altar to Nehalennia

customary function, such as that of a condiment (3.50; 10.48). On only four occasions is fish sauce portrayed as expensive (7.27; 13.82, 102, 103), but there is no indication of it being particularly extravagant; this, even though two of the four instances (13.102, 103) involve garum sociorum, which is never referred to in a derogatory manner. On the other hand, Martial also speaks of an inexpensive fish sauce (muria) on three occasions (4.88; 10.48; 13.103), two of which refer specifically to the product from Antipolis in Southern Gaul, a product which Pliny (*HN* 31.94) notes as worthy of praise.

[33] Ponsich, *Tanger*, pp. 325, 332 (Tomb no. 9), 335 (Tomb no. 15).

and probably were partners in business.[34] Many, but by no means all, names which frequently appear written on Roman salt-fish containers are Greek, and these frequently of freedman status. The *titulus* on a Spanish amphora of Pelichet 46 found in Pompeii, for example, apparently contained garum sociorum. Included in the label were the initials *CCH*, probably standing for C. Cornelius Hermeros, a merchant or shipper known to have traded in wine and fish sauce.[35] Names recorded in *tituli picti* of vessels found near the Praetorian camp in Rome as well as funerary inscriptions in Italy and Gaul likewise indicate servile origin. The *negotians salsarius* from Spain residing in Ostia, P. Clodius Athenio, and the *negotians salsamentarius et vinariarius* from Africa, Tiberius Claudius Docimus, who died in Rome, were both ex-slaves. A *sevir augustalis*, living in Lugdunum and serving as *curator* of Rhodanian sailors operating on the Arar, M. Primus Secundianus, styled himself a *negotians muriarius*.[36] Servile names appear in *tituli picti* of Spanish salt-fish vessels; such as, Insequens, Artemidorus, and Iosippus. These, however, appear among names of those apparently free born; such as, L. Purellus Gemellus, A. Atilius Macer, Q. Granius Iunius, P. Cordus Gratus, the Quinti Caecilii and Aulii Atinii.[37] Beltrán Lloris presents strong circumstantial evidence that two members of a prominent family in New Carthage, M. Numisius Nicer and L. Numisius Silo, belonged to the famous *societas* of that city.[38]

Most instructive is the example of A. Umbricius Scaurus of Pompeii, the local producer and merchant in fish sauce who lived in a luxurious house complete with a fish pool and secondary atrium elaborately decorated with a mosaic design advertising his fish products.[39] His son, before he died, had been elected first aedile, then duovir of Pompeii and honored with an equestrian statue in the forum. The Umbricii Scaurii, therefore, apparently grown wealthy through the business ventures of the elder Scaurus, joined the local aristocracy through the political success of the younger. The latter, however, no doubt owed much to the former. Scaurus' garum shops employed both freedmen and freemen, possibly family members. Names of

---

[34] Bogaers, "Nehalennia en de epigrafische Gegevens," pp. 32–43; Hassall, "Britain and the Rhine Provinces," pp. 41–48; and Curtis, "*Negotiatores Allecarii*," pp. 147–58.

[35] *CIL* IV.5651. Cf. *CIL* IV.2588 (liquamen), 5638 (CoD), 5597 (wine).

[36] *CIL* VI.9677 (P. Clodius Athenio); *CIL* VI.9676 (Tiberius Claudius Docimus); *CIL* XIII.1966 (M. Primus Secundianus).

[37] Insequens (*CIL* XV.4706), Artemidorus (*CIL* XV.4729), Iosippus (*CIL* XV.4731), L. Purellus Gemellus (*CIL* XV.4719), A. Atilius Macer (*CIL* XV.4720), Q. Granius Iunius (*CIL* XV.4724), P. Cordus Gratus (*CIL* XV.4722, 4737, 4740), A. A. Atinii (*CIL* XV.4695–4700, 4739, 4744; cf. *CIL* XV.3639–41, 4701–02, 4742). For the Auli Atinii and Quinti Caecilii see Desbat et al., "Inscriptions peintes sur amphores: Lyon," pp. 156–59, 164–66. The determination of their proper role in the commerce of salt-fish products is difficult since the interpretation of names written on amphorae remains a matter of conjecture. See Appendix III.

[38] Beltrán Lloris, *Las ánforas romanas*, pp. 597–98; *CIL* XV.4708 (M. Numisius Nicer), 4709 (L. Numisius Silo).

[39] Below, pp. 167–69.

other people, both free and freed, appear among *tituli picti* on Pompeian vessels.[40] These individuals, apparently unassociated with Scaurus, operated businesses presumably in competition with Scaurus and perhaps with similar, but less dramatic success.

The picture of the salt-fish dealer in Roman society is in essence two pictures. First, workers were generally poor and of the lower classes, freedmen and slaves. Retailers probably ranked with those of other products, poor or marginal. The picture here is unclear, since the only garum shop thus far identified, at Pompeii, seems more a wholesale warehouse than a retail shop. Second, the owners of sizable factories and large-scale merchants were probably well-to-do, even rich in some instances. Although many of the latter were undoubtedly freedmen and frequently Greek, not all were. Scaurus, about whom the most is known, certainly was not. Locally they might become upstanding community leaders; their sons might even become members of the ordo, the municipal elite. The archaeological evidence, therefore, at least for Roman society, serves to refine and in some ways to correct the pejorative and stereotypical picture of the salt-fish producer and dealer found in literary sources.

---

[40] Curtis, "A. Umbricius Scaurus," pp. 31–33.

CHAPTER SEVEN

MERCHANDISING

Marketing

A successful businessman must attract potential customers to his product or service and must demonstrate that it surpasses that of his competitors. To these ends he must resort to advertisement. The Roman merchant, like his modern counterpart, was confronted with this necessity but lacked the highly sophisticated means of communication available today. Nevertheless, energetic entrepreneurs employed various, frequently innovative methods to present their products to a clientele which, as the Roman economy expanded with Roman power, was able to exercise more discrimination in what it bought and from whom it purchased them. These methods include shop signs, in the form of paintings on the outside or inside of shops or of mosaic designs in floors of shop entrances, stipulating the product or service offered. These devices might also include terra-cotta or stone plaques with relief sculpture depicting the product made in the shop. Graffiti, like billboards, could be scribbled by anyone, even by professional sign painters, on a vacant wall to describe the product sold or to give directions to the shop location. A well-to-do businessman might even pay to have his shop or product mentioned in a published literary work. All of these advertising schemes have been previously recognized and commented upon, but product advertising on transport containers has received little attention. [1]

Product identification has been the least studied part of the *titulus pictus*, probably because, although often in abbreviated form, it is the aspect of the label which presents the least difficulty in its interpretation. The consumer could readily recognize amphorae containing fish products, since vessel shape probably made general recognition easy, while the *titulus pictus* identified the specific contents. The large number of Spanish salt-fish amphorae bearing *tituli picti* and dating to the first two centuries A.D. and particularly the numerous container labels on vessels found in Pompeii and Herculaneum, datable also to the first century A.D., present a body of ma-

[1] G. Raskin, *Handelsreclame en soortgelijke praktijken bij Grieken en Romeinen* (Philologische Studiën, Teksten en Verhandelingen, 13–15) (Leuven 1936), passim; E. T. Sage, "Advertising among the Romans," *CW* 9 (1916): 202–08; W. Schlenker, "Geschäftsreklame in Pompeji," *F&F* 5 (1929): 193–95; A. P. Ball, "A Forerunner of the Advertising Agent," *CJ* 2 (1907): 165–70; and T. Frank, "A New Advertisement at Pompeii," *AJPh* 59 (1938): 224–25. This section on marketing appeared earlier in slightly altered form in "Product Identification and Advertising on Roman Commercial Amphorae," *Ancient Society* 15-17 (1984–86): 209–28. I wish to thank the editor for permission to incorporate this material here.

terial defined by fairly narrow geographical and chronological limits. Of 282 *tituli picti* consulted, 70 per cent came from Campania, while the majority of the others appear on Spanish amphorae found in Rome, in various shipwrecks in the Mediterranean Sea, and in the provinces of Gaul, Raetia, Noricum, Britain, and Germania Superior.[2]

Since one of the purposes of the product label was to identify the contents of the vessel, merely listing the name of the product with a single word, such as garum or liquamen, would suffice. This simple designation is indeed found on many vessels, but most *tituli picti* are more elaborate, including one or more adjectives or nouns which further define the product contained in the vessel. These words are sometimes substantive in nature, but frequently are almost worthless except for eye appeal and for advertisement. These expanded labels provide a "neon sign," as it were, to catch the eye of a potential customer, to show him that this product stands out above the rest and that only this one will satisfy his needs.[3] So widespread and common were these labels that they became, like inscriptions on stone, basically formulaic and so were frequently abbreviated. A sufficient number of unabbreviated ones exists, however, to allow us to understand the manner in which the product is being lauded or described. *Tituli picti* of this kind fall into three general categories: adjectives expressing the quality of the merchandise, modifiers identifying the point of origin of the product, and words relating something unusual or noteworthy about the ingredients or method of preparation of the commodity.

The most common mode of advertisement and the one which exhibited the greatest variety was that which designated quality. By far the most frequently used qualifier was the word *flos* (Pls. 7a-b).[4] This word is usually preceded on the same line by the single letter G or by three letters GAR neither of which allows one to know the grammatical form of the word

---

cluded from this study because of uncertainty in their interpretation. These include *CIL* IV.2611, 5651, 5728, 5841, 10320, 10335, 10749–50; XV.4514, 4570, 4737–38; and Egger and Görlich, "Der Lebensmittelimport," p. 412: [liqua]M(en) GARI . [r]ITE.

[3] It is unknown in each case who painted the *titulus pictus* on the vessel, or indeed if all parts of it were painted on by the same person. Since each label seems to be the work of one hand (except where the vessel has been reused and so a second or even a third *titulus pictus* has been applied, e.g. *CIL* IV.2574, 5705, 5711, 10280; XV.4718), the most likely candidate is the producer of the commodity. The producer could also be a merchant (*mercator*) in his own city, but for the export trade the vessel might change ownership. For the purpose of consistency I shall assume that the producer *qua* merchant is the advertiser. This does not, of course, exclude the possibility of a second or third party adding a new *titulus pictus*, or additional elements to a previously existing one (cf. CIL IV.9415, and Liou and Marichal, "Les inscriptions," p. 137), if ownership of the product has changed hands.

[4] Over 150 *tituli picti* recorded in *CIL* IV and XV alone use the word *flos* or its abbreviation F in referring to fish sauce. Early fascicles of *CIL* expanded the abbreviation F to F(actum), for example, *CIL* IV.2570–72, 2575–76. That it stands instead for F(los) can be seen from many examples where the full word *flos* is spelled out; for example, *CIL* IV.5706, 5714, 5734, 9388, 9414, 10737, 10743.

garum. On the analogy of *salis flos, olei flos*, and others, the genitive form GARI seems certain.[5] *Gari flos* is expressed in full on several vessels in Pompeii and in Noricum.[6] So common was the expression felt to be that frequently the *titulus pictus* consisted only of two letters G F, designating G(ari) F(los).[7] Interestingly, one does not find a two-letter abbreviation for *liquaminis flos*; and the word *flos* never appears with allec in any form.[8]

Some difficulty arises in understanding the meaning of *flos* with respect to the product sold. Two possibilities exist. First, *Gari flos*, "the flower of garum," may have referred to the first portion of liquid, and hence the best portion, drawn off during the production process. Pliny uses *flos* in this way when referring to oil drawn off after olives have been pressed for the first time. Perhaps more to the point is *nuoc-nhut*, the first liquid drawn off in the production of Vietnamese *nuoc-mam*.[9] The second possibility, and one closely related to the first, is that the word *flos* was used to emphasize, and hence to advertise, the quality of the sauce. Certainly this is the case where *flos* is repeated on a subsequent line of the label; for example, from Pompeii we find LIQ(uamen)/ FLOS/ FLOS and GAR(i) F(los)/ FLOS.[10] In a few instances the abbreviation G F F appears in product labels. If, as has been suggested, the initials stand for G(arum) F(los) F(loris), "garum, the flower of the flower," then the effort at advertisement becomes more apparent.[11] For if the best garum is that drawn off first in the preparation process, what in that process would make the best better? Obviously, the second *flos* is superfluous if not for the purpose of advertisement. I would suggest that the single use of flos carried the same message. *Flos* was an indication of quality used to advertise the product and hence to make the garum more

[5] Pliny *HN* 31.90 (*salis flos*); *Edict. Diocl.* III.1 (*olei flos*). See especially, J. Kapp, *Thesaurus Latinae Linguae*, s.v. *flos*, 6 (1912–26): 932–33.

[6] *CIL* IV.5663, and Egger and Görlich, "Der Lebensmittelimport," p. 412. This general rule would apply as well to abbreviations of liquamen, muria, and allec. When *flos* appears in a line different from that of the product (e.g. *CIL* IV.5714 and 9414), the latter term remains in the nominative case (cf. *CIL* IV.10743; XV.4715, 4723). The Romans were not entirely consistent, however. In Pompeii, for example, in contradiction to the usual rule one finds on one line GARU(m) FLOS (*CIL* IV.5666), and on separate lines GARI/ FLOS (*CIL* IV.10268). Apparently the Romans saw no difficulty with either method of expression. V. Väänänen (*Le latin vulgaire des inscriptions pompéiennes* [Berlin 1959], pp. 117–18, 129) attributes the use of a noun in apposition, in lieu of an epexigetic genitive, as characteristic of the syntax of vulgar Latin in Pompeian graffiti. For consistency, where the *titulus pictus* permits a choice, I shall use the genitive case in expanding abbreviations.

[7] Pompeii: *CIL* IV.2570, 5667, 5669–72, 9389–91, 9399: for M(uriae) F(los), see *CIL* IV.9430–34, 10291; Rome: *CIL* XV.4688–89, 4691–94, 4696, 4699, 4701, 4703–04, 4706–07, 4711.

[8] Most common is LIQ(uaminis) F(los). Cf. *CIL* IV.2588 (= 5716), 5706; XV.4715, 4719.

[9] André, *L'alimentation*², p. 196; Pliny *HN* 15.23: *quod vero post molam primum expressum est, flos*. For *nuoc-nhut*, see above p. 21. Cf. also Manilius *Astron.* 5.671, who in describing the process of garum production from tunny refers to the sauce as the "flower of the blood" (*floremque cruoris*).

[10] *CIL* IV.5673, 5706.

[11] August Mau, in his commentary to *CIL* IV.5668.

appealing to a potential customer. In this sense, *flos* signified the "best garum," and *flos floris*, "the flower of the flower," represents a sort of one-upmanship on the part of some merchants to assert a special case for their products.

After *flos* the most frequently used adjective is *optimum*, "the best."[12] But what could be better than *flos*? Does *optimum* refer to a sauce which has been drawn off after the *flos* has been extracted? If so, what can be made of the label LIQUAMEN/ FLOS/ OPTIMUM? Where does the sauce GAR(um) PRAE(cellens), found in Herculaneum, and LIQUAMEN/ PRIMUM, found in Pompeii, fit in?[13] One must conclude that these adjectives express the quality of the product and do not necessarily represent a specific sauce associated with a particular process or stage in a process. The adjectives are merely synonyms of high quality used by the producer or merchant to make the product more appealing. They were sometimes used in combination to emphasize further the high quality of the product. One merchant from Pompeii advertised his product as LIQ(uaminis) F(los)/ EXC(el)LENS, while another from Herculaneum declared his sauce to be LIQUAM(en)/ FLOS/ PRIMUM.[14] Labels denoting sauces of inferior quality are far less frequently found, but do exist. Sauces labelled SEC(undum) have been found in Rome and Noricum, and in Pompeii the adjective *penuarium*, perhaps indicating a "mere" food item, followed the word liquamen. Even if the liquamen was merely a food item, it nevertheless was an "excellent" one: LIQUAME(n)/ PENUA(rium)/ EXSELL(ens).[15] This distinction among qualities of fish sauce shows up in the fourth century A.D. in the Price Edict of Diocletian where top quality fish sauce (*liquamen primum*) has a higher price ceiling than that of lower quality sauce (*liquamen secundum*).[16] Of 282 examples of *tituli picti* consulted, only three denoted a sauce of inferior quality; if one includes those labels which have no qualifying adjective, the figure would rise only to 41. A grouping of the qualitative adjectives from Campania and elsewhere (in parenthesis), used alone or in combination with other modifiers, yields the following results:

---

[12] *CIL* IV.2589–92, 2593(?), 2594, 5689, 5707–14, 5717–19, 6924, 7110, 9397, 9407–11, 9415–19, 10278–81a, 10744–46.

[13] *Liquamen flos optimum*: *CIL* IV.5714; *Garum praecellens*: *CIL* IV.10735; *liquamen primum*: *CIL* IV.2593(?), 2595; *hallex optima*: *CIL* IV.5717–18, 5719(?), 9407–11. The spelling *hallex* is the only one found in *tituli picti* and is found but once in literature (Plautus *Poen*. 1310).

[14] Pompeii: *CIL* IV.2588, 5716, 9414; Herculaneum: *CIL* IV.10743. Cf. from Rome a Spanish vessel (*CIL* XV.4719) of LIQ(uaminis) FL(os)/ EXCEL(lens); and Pascual Guasch, "Dos ánforas, pp. 205–09. From Augusta Vindelicorum (Augsberg) in Raetia, see *CIL* III.12010.48.

[15] Pompeii: *CIL* IV.2596. Cf. from Rome, *CIL* XV.4741. Rome (*CIL* XV.4726): MUR(ia) SEC(unda); Magdalensberg (Egger and Görlich, "Der Lebensmittelimport," p. 412): GAR(um) SEC(undarium). Cf. Pliny *HN* 14.82 (*secundarium passum*). For *penuarium* cf. Liou, "Inscriptions peintes sur amphores: Fos (suite)," pp. 114–16 (Dressel Form 14 , lacking a product designation). Cf. also *P.Erl.* 16_{15} (5th–6th cent. A.D.): γάϱον χηδέον(= χυδαίον), "ordinary garum." The previous line had listed γάϱον.

[16] *Edict. Diocl.* III.6–7: *liquaminis primi/ liquaminis secundi*.

Modifier	Garum	Liquamen	Muria	Hallex
Flos	100(36)	5(5)	12(9)	0(0)
Optimum	4(0)	33(0)	0(0)	8(0)
Primum	2(0)	4(0)	0(0)	0(0)
Excellens	0(2)	2(5)	0(4)	0(0)
Praecellens	1(0)	0(0)	0(0)	0(0)
No qualifying adjective	5(1)	13(10)	5(3)	1(0)
Penuarium	0(0)	1(0)	0(0)	0(0)
Secundarium	0(1)	0(0)	0(1)	0(0)

From these figures one may draw three tentative conclusions. First, most *tituli picti* have an adjective expressing high quality, or else no adjective at all. Second, if *flos* represented the liquid first drawn off in the production process and hence the best fish sauce, one would reasonably expect it to cost far more than other products and to appear less frequently because fewer people could afford it. Yet, if these numbers can be taken to reflect the relative popularity of the different fish sauces, then *gari flos* was the preferred one, followed by *liquamen optimum* (at least in Pompeii). Since most *tituli picti* advertise *gari flos* and since vessels bearing this label are found throughout Pompeii in cauponae, thermopolia, villas, elegant and simple houses alike, one can reasonably conclude that this product must have been well within the budget of most Pompeians of all social strata.[17] Some kinds of garum must have been expensive, but apparently most were not, even that advertised as *gari flos*. And finally, comparative figures from scattered evidence outside Campania, primarily on Spanish vessels, show little difference proportionally from those collected in Pompeii and Herculaneum.

Although a customer might from the shape of a vessel recognize its point of origin, it was not uncommon for the label to designate the province or city from whence it came. A container of GAR(um) POMPEIAN(um) found in Rome, for example, informed the customer that he was purchasing the brand imported from Pompeii. This would have had special significance for the patron since, as Pliny verifies, Pompeii was especially noted for its garum.[18] The inscription on a vessel found in Herculaneum, labelled HAL(lex)/ HERC(u)LAN[e(n)sis] (or HERCLAN(io)), advised a potential customer that he would be buying a local product.[19] Unless the amphora was awaiting exportation, it is puzzling why the producer felt compelled to state the sauce's provenance. A buyer could probably assume that the sauce was a local product unless informed otherwise. Of nearly 200 inscribed fish sauce containers found in Pompeii, for example, not one claims

[17] Villa: *CIL* IV.5671–72, 9396, 9401–02; houses of modest character: *CIL* IV.9390, 9399, 9409; houses of luxurious character: *CIL* IV.9388, 9403–04, 9412. On the price of salt-fish products see below pp. 170–75; for commercial establishments see below note 63.

[18] *CIL* XV.4686; Pliny *HN* 31.94. But see below, note 33, p. 166.

[19] *CIL* IV.5720. Cf. *CIL* IV.4299, for the local ablative *Herclanio* used for *Herculanei*.

to be the Pompeian specialty. Yet the origin of most of the products is made obvious by the appearance of the name of a local dealer, such as Aulus Umbricius Scaurus. In one instance, the name of the *societas* which produced and exported the product was sufficient to identify the point of origin. Garum sociorum always identified the famous fish sauce from New Carthage in Spain.[20] Other extant *tituli picti* advertise products from Ostia and Antium in Italy, and perhaps Antipolis in Gaul.[21] Some labels name only the province from which the sauce came. Vessels containing G(arum) HISPA(num) and MUR(ia) HISP(ana), for example, have been found at Augst (Augusta Raurica) in Germania Superior and from Poetovio in Pannonia.[22]

The third mode of advertisement includes those words which reveal something about the ingredients or method of preparation. The most frequent ingredient designated is the type of fish used. Some labels include the name of a particular fish, in the genitive case; for example, G(ari) F(los) SCOMBR(i) or GAR(i) F(los)/ FLOS/ MUREN(ae). In these instances the producer wished to emphasize that the sauce was made entirely from one type of fish. By far the fish most frequently named is the *scomber*, or mackerel (Pls. 7a-b).[23] Although extant *tituli picti* attest only to the mackerel and eel (*murena*), literary sources indicate that fish sauce could be made from an infinite variety of fish, not only separately but also mixed together.[24] Some customers who preferred a pure sauce could buy G(ari) F(los) PER SE, "the flower of garum, by itself," that is, without additives. This would constitute

---

[20] *CIL* IV.5659. Cf. *CIL* IV.5651: (garum?) SOC(iorum).

[21] For Italy, see LIQ(uamen) ANTIA(tinum): *CIL* XV.4712; G(arum) OST(iense): Egger and Görlich, "Der Lebensmittelimport," p. 412. For Gaul, see G(arum) V(etus) Q(?)/ EXC(ellens)/ ANTIP(olitanum): Liou and Marichal, "Les inscriptions," p. 167. See also Martial 4.88.5–6 (Antipolis). For a probable reference to a site in Lusitania (possibly Esuris) associated with the goddess Luna, see G(ari) F(los) S(combri)/ LUNEN(se): Wright and Hassall, "Roman Britain in 1973," p. 467, no. 44 and note 41. This attribution to Lusitania is a tentative suggestion by the authors; for the association with Esuris specifically, see Alarcão, *Roman Portugal*, 1: 146, note 108. Cf. *CIL* XV.4570 (garum from Gades?), 4537 (muria from Malaca?).

[22] If not a designation of origin, it might indicate a sauce made according to the recipe of a certain Hispanus. Cf. below pp. 166–67. Bohn, "Pinselschriften," pp. 202–04 (Augst); Bezeczky, *Roman Amphorae from the Amber Route*, pp. 22–23 (Poetovio). Bohn's suggestion that the adjective possibly designates a Spanish recipe seems a less likely explanation.

[23] Murena: *CIL* IV.5673; mackerel: at least 73 examples published in *CIL* III, IV and XV or in scholarly journals.

[24] Sauces made from a single fish include the maena: Pliny *HN* 26.23, 27.127, 31.83, 32.88; Marcellus Sidetes *Medicina de piscibus* 101; Galen *De simplicium medicamentorum temperamentis ac facultatibus* 11.13 (12.377K); silurus: Galen *ibid.*; Rufus of Ephesus (Daremberg-Ruelle, p. 338); Oribasius *Ad Eunap.* 4.116.19; tunny: Martial 4.88.5, 13.103; Manilius *Astron.* 5.656–81; lupus: Pliny *HN* 31.95; mullet: *ibid.* 9.66. Pliny (*HN* 31.95) says that allex was made from an infinite variety of fish, while Isidore (*Orig.* 20.20.19–20) says the same thing of garum. The preparations described by Ps-Gargilius Martialis and the author of the *Geoponica* include many different kinds of small and large fish mixed together. That a sauce was made from two kinds of fish may be the message of *tituli picti* which record the contents as GEM(inus): *CIL* IV.5826–27, 9392–93, 10272–10273. The possibility that this term refers to the special recipe of Geminus is remote, since, unlike the *tituli picti* of Romulius and Lucretius (below, pp. 166–67), the name appears on the same line as the product identification and in the place where the species of fish (e.g. *scomber*) is usually found.

an important distinction because garum could be prepared with wine, oil, vinegar, or herbs and spices, such as argemonia.[25]

Some labels refer specifically to the production process itself. The vessel of LIQUAMEN/ OPTIMUM/ SACCATUM, "the best strained liquamen," no doubt contained a particularly clear liquid, free of any sediment.[26] Another amphora label advertises the contents as MUR(ia) VE(tus), "aged muria."[27] *Vetus* is an adjective common to wines, but its applicability to fish sauce is rarely attested for antiquity. Ancient recipes state that fish sauce production could take up to three months, but none says that a sauce was deliberately aged beyond the period necessary for its preparation. Since modern production processes, so similar to ancient methods, do frequently prescribe aging, the likelihood seems strong for antiquity as well. The letters AIIIIA found in Rome on a container of MUR(iae) F(los) has been interpreted to mean that the product was four years old.[28]

The best example of an adjective revealing either ingredients or method of production and one which shows astute commercial acumen is the use of the adjective *castum* or *castimoniale*. Pliny the Elder in his discussion of garum says (erroneously) that "In truth, another (garum) has been designed for the religious belief of abstinences and especially for Jewish rites, because it is made from fish without scales."[29] Abstinence was not practiced by Jews alone; devotees of Apis, Isis, and Magna Mater abstained from certain kinds of food as a purificatory rite. The Pythagoreans, who abstained from most kinds of fish, would avoid fish sauce altogether.[30] The

---

[25] *CIL* XV.4723: MUR(ia) ARG(uta)/ FLOS; and from Windisch, MUR(iae) ARG(utae)/ EX(cellentis)/ FLO[s] (=Bohn, "Pinselschriften," p. 206). See also Concepción Fernández-Chicarro, "Actividades arqueológicas en Andulacía," *AEA* 26 (1953): 440–41. The expression *per se* invariably appears on the same line of the label as the product identification. See *CIL* IV.2571–73, 5674–78, 9394, 10274, 10738. For wine and herbs and spices used in making garum, see *Geoponica* 20.46.3–4; Ps.-Gargilius Martialis 62; and Ps-Rufius Festus, *Breviarium*. For mixed garums see R. Zahn, "Garum," *RE* 7 (1912), cols. 844–47. No extant *titulus pictus* refers to a mixed garum, not even to oenogarum, but γαρέλεν (oil and garum) appears in a graffito found in the third century A.D. Mithraeum at Dura Europus. See above p. 146.

[26] *CIL* IV.7110. See also Apicius *De re coq*. 7.6.14 (*allecem colatum*). See also Ps-Gargilius Martialis 62 and *Geoponica* 20.46.2. A Dressel Form 6 amphora found in Northern Italy had a label identifying the contents as *garum geticum* (or *coktum*); the reading is apparently uncertain. See André Tchernia, *Le vin*, p. 132, note 23.

[27] *CIL* IV.5726. Cf. Bohn, "Pinselschriften," p. 203, and Liou and Marichal, "Les inscriptions," p. 167.

[28] *CIL* XV.4724. For a discussion of the use of the adjective *vetus*, see *CIL* XV, p. 682, and Liou and Marichal, "Les inscriptions," p. 135. For aging fermented fish products, see above p. 21.

[29] Pliny *HN* 31.95; but cf. *Deuteronomy* 14.10, and *Leviticus* 11.10–12. See also Corcoran, "Pliny's *Garum Castimoniarum*," p. 69. Cf. *BT. Hullin* 66a-b (Epstein, pp. 356–58).

[30] For groups practicing abstinence see Tertullian *De ieiun*. 2 and Plutarch *Mor*. 670D and 728D–730F. See also P. R. Arbesmann, *Das Fasten bei den Griechen und Römern* (Giessen 1929), pp. 50–53. Palladius (*Opus Agri*. 3.25.12) mentions a sauce made from pears (*liquamen de piris castimoniale*), but this is not a fish sauce. Cf. also the fishless sauces mentioned by Dioscorides *De mat. med*. 2.32 (meat) and Ps-Galen *De remediis parabilibus* 2 (14.546–48K) (unleaven bread and herbs and spices). Cf. Julius Africanus (Κεστοί 7.19) who describes a garum not destined for an abstemious group, but a kind of "ersatz" fish sauce for soldiers on campaign or short of the real item. It does contain, nevertheless, some fish material (ἀβδόμιοι = Lat. *abdomia*). See

Jews, however, would be faced with the problem of avoiding only certain kinds of fish sauce; that is, products made from scaleless fish, such as the murena, or from shellfish of all kinds. To be safe Jews would probably shun all sauces not specifically labelled with the name of the fish, since there would always remain doubt as to whether or not it was kosher.[31] Vessels labelled GAR(um) CAST(um)/ SCOMBRI are found alongside those advertising MUR(ia) CAST(a) and GAR(um) CAST(um), all apparently aimed at a clientele which practised abstention. It is unknown to whom they would appeal, but the Jewish customer would certainly be safe in purchasing the first example since the mackerel had scales.[32]

Some *tituli picti* have a name written in the neuter nominative case on the line following the product identification. Its precise meaning is unclear, but it has been plausibly suggested that it designates that the sauce was made according to the special recipe of the person named; for example, G(ari) F(los)/ ROMULIANUM, found in Pompeii. This technique might be useful for producers selling in local areas where he would be known to potential customers, but its practical advantage for a product exported to another city or province where the producer would be unknown is difficult to imagine. A label written on a Spanish vessel found in Rome, for example, mentions G(ari) F(los)/ LUCR(etianum).[33] Lucretius was perhaps not deterred by the lack of recognition his special brand might receive outside Spain; it was apparently enough for him that prospective customers knew that the rec-

---

Vieillefond, *Les 'Cestes' de Julius Africanus*, pp. 180, esp. note 126, p. 347 and note 149, p. 350.

[31] For allec from shellfish see Pliny *HN* 31.95; murena, *CIL* IV.5673. For allec, see also *BT. Abodah Zarah* 38b-39a (Epstein, pp. 190–91). Daniel Sperber, in his discussion of muria (or muries) mentioned in Rabbinic literature, says that muria "was made out of tunny or mackerel (both kosher fish) and no other fish." (Sperber, "Social and Economic Conditions," p. 11). This is incorrect. Although muria was frequently made from these species, it could be made from other kinds, including non-kosher ones, as well. Muria referred, in general, to any salt solution, such as that used to preserve turnips, olives, and other food items (Col. *Rust*. 12.56.2; Cato *Agr*. 88). More specifically, muria referred to the liquid used to preserve fish. This use in fish preservation can be seen in such references as *muria salsamentorum* (Pliny *HN* 31.83) and *duratos muria pisces* (Quint. *IO* 8.2.3), where no species are specified. Cf. also Cato *Agri*. 88, Pliny *HN* 9.92, and Col. *Rust*. 12.55. Sperber seems unaware of muria from the silurus (catfish), a fish lacking in scales and hence not kosher, mentioned in Galen *De simplicium medicamentorum temperamentis ac facultatibus* 11.13 (12.377K).

[32] *CIL* IV.2569, 2609, 2611(?), 5660–62; XV.4728(?). Examples of liquamen castum and allec casta have yet to be found, but production of garum castum would obviously yield the latter sauce as a by-product. See *BT. Abodah Zarah* 39a, where the *scomber* is specifically listed as a fish permitted to Jews to eat. Pompeii had a Jewish community, but of what size is uncertain. See A. Varone, *Presenze giudaiche e cristiane a Pompei* (Naples 1979), esp. pp. 11–25.

[33] ROMULIANUM: *CIL* IV.5681, 10270, 10276–77. See Heinrich Dressel's commentary on *CIL* XV.4691: LUCR(etianum). Cf. Desbat et al., "Inscriptions peintes sur amphores: Lyon," pp. 154–56: LIQ(uamen)/ APIC(ianum)/ G(ai) RUFI. The vessel, found in Lyon, was of local manufacture, the sauce probably imported and refined according to the prescriptions of a certain Apicius. The *titulus* GAR(um) POMPEIAN(um), written on a vessel of unknown form (*CIL* XV.4686) found on the Esquiline Hill in Rome, could conceivably designate a product made by a certain Pompeianus rather than indicate the sauce's origin. Unlike the labels of Romulius and Lucretius, however, the name is on the same line as the product designation.

ipe was his own, even if they did not know him or the details of his recipe.

The success of Aulus Umbricius Scaurus, Pompeii's leading producer and merchant of fish sauce, must have been in no small part due to his advertising practices. Most of his *tituli picti* had the usual product identification emphasized by one or more adjectives of quality and frequently indicated the fish used in its preparation.[34] Scaurus' advertising campaign went even farther. In his labels he often associated himself explicitly with his product; so much so that his name must have become inextricably linked with Pompeian fish sauce. He did this in three ways. Following the product identification he placed his name in the genitive case to designate that he was the owner of the product and its producer as well. Sometimes he used his full name, other times only the cognomen appears (Pls. 7a-b). This was particularly important when the sauce was produced at the shop of one of his freedmen.[35] Secondly, Scaurus' name or the name of one of his slaves, freedmen, or family members appears with the preposition *ab* to indicate the consignor of the container.[36] And finally, Scaurus indicated that the product came directly from his shop with the words *ex officina Scauri*.[37] One of his *tituli picti* in particular illustrates the advertising acumen of this highly competitive, shrewd businessman: G(ari) F(los) SCOMBR(i)/ SCAURI/ EX OFFICINA AGATHOPI, "the flower of garum, made from the mackerel, a product of Scaurus, from the shop of Agathopus."[38] The label has named the product, declared its high quality, disclosed its ingredients, identified the ultimate owner of the product, and given the name of the distributor, a sort of subsidiary of the owner. Modern labels hardly provide more information.

Scaurus has also provided us with a unique example of ancient advertising at its best. He lived in a palatial old house in the most ancient part of Pompeii, at Region VII, *Insula Occidentalis* 12–15 (Fig. 5). This elegant house of the second century B.C. was composed of many rooms, a peristyle with fish-pool, and a private bath. In an extension of the original house, probably of the reign of Tiberius, he installed a personalized floor mosaic in the atrium of entrance 15.[39] The black-and-white mosaic of *opus tessellatum* has as its primary decoration at each corner of the impluvium, outside the standard meander pattern circumscribing the pool, the design of an urceus of Pompeian Form VI, the one-handled vessel which at Pompeii normally

---

[34] In all extant cases, the fish so named was the mackerel.

[35] SCAURI: *CIL* IV.2575–76, 5682–83, 5686–88, 5690–94, 6921, 9400–06; A. UMBRICII SCAURI: *CIL* IV.2587, 5704–05, 5711, 9399. Sometimes both forms appear: *CIL* IV.2574. For shops of his freedmen, see Agathopus (*CIL* IV.2580[?], 5690, 7110, 9403–04, 9405[?]); Abascantus (*CIL* IV.5689).

[36] *CIL* IV.2576, 5661, 5670–71, 5674–76, 5684–85, 5688, 5710, 5723–24, 6921, 9410, 9418–19, 10262.

[37] *CIL* IV.2572(?), 2574, 2577, 5694, 9406.

[38] *CIL* IV.9403–04.

[39] Curtis, "Personalized Floor Mosaic," pp. 557–66.

contained fish sauce (Pl. 7a).[40] On each mosaic urceus the mosaicist has placed a different inscription:[41]

Urceus A:	G(ari) F(los) SCO[m](bri)/ SCAURI/ EX OFFI[ci]/NA SCAU/RI
Urceus B:	LIQUA(men)/ FLOS
Urceus C:	G(ari) F(los) SCOM(bri)/ SCAURI
Urceus D:	LIQUAMEN/ OPTIMUM/ EX OFFICI[n]/A SCAURI

The mosaic vessels are in silhouette, a white vessel set into a black field, and, averaging 0.645 m. in height, are greater in size than actual vessels of this form.

Since the bare shape of the vessel in outline would have been sufficient for any visitor to associate the urcei and the owner of the house with the fish sauce business, no further elaboration was needed. But Scaurus apparently wanted more, and the mosaicist obliged by placing an interior design within the silhouetted vessels. With a single row of black tesserae he delineated a *titulus pictus* for each mosaic vessel in imitation of labels painted on commercial urcei. The desire to include the inscriptions demanded that the vessels be moved outside the meander band; otherwise they would have been too small to be read easily, and it would have been more difficult to cut and lay stones small enough to be included within a silhouetted vessel much reduced in size. The placement of the mosaic designs outside the standard meander pattern common to atrium mosaics and into the field surrounding it is a significant break with tradition. The motivation for this move lies not with the mosaicist, but with Scaurus himself. The message of the mosaic determined the motif and its placement. The mosaic inscriptions were designed to function in the same way as *tituli picti* on actual urcei. The motivation was advertisement.[42]

Placing the mosaic vessels outside the meander was unusual and bound to attract attention. Placing a garum vessel on diagonally opposite corners and the same for liquamen vessels guaranteed that the spectator would see examples of both no matter on which side of the impluvium he stood. In

[40] A survey of 199 vessels listed in *CIL* IV as bearing a fish sauce *titulus pictus* and found in Pompeii and Herculaneum shows that 141 were on urcei of this form. Thirty-six were on amphorae and 22 on vessels other than amphorae and urcei or on containers unspecified in the commentary. Only one label on an urceus of Pompeian Form VI specified a different product. *CIL* IV.5738 mentions lomentum. Ten other urcei of Form VI lacked a *titulus pictus* identifying the product.

[41] Curtis, "Personalized Floor Mosaic," pp. 559–61, esp. Plate 74, Figs. 3–6.

[42] It is not impossible that Scaurus may have used this secondary atrium as a shop from which to conduct business; that is, selling urcei of fish sauce probably prepared elsewhere. The mosaic "shop signs" in the Piazzale delle Corporazioni in Ostia immediately come to mind, although these were not retail shops. Cf. below note 43. See also G. Becatti, "Alcune caratteristiche del mosaico bianco-nero in Italia," in *La mosaïque gréco-romaine* (Paris 1965), p. 22, who, after discussing motifs of marine life in baths, athletic games in palaestrae, craters in wine shops, and so on, observes that, "Questa armonica fusione di *utilitas* e di *decor* è uno degli aspetti più significativi ed originali dell'arte musiva romana."

this way the mosaicist has invited the visitor, indeed required him, to move around the impluvium to observe the figures from up to four different positions. By attracting the viewer's attention to the designs and inscriptions and engaging his interest by requiring him to move around to see all of them, the mosaicist has accomplished Scaurus' primary goal: to advertise his business, his wealth, and most of all Scaurus himself. This mosaic is the only one known from antiquity which uses a motif unequivocally referring to the owner's occupation, that of producer and merchant in fish sauce. He does this by employing the design of a specific type of utilitarian transport container undeniably associated with a particular product and includes, as on actual urcei, inscriptions designed to advertise the merchandise.[43]

In summary, although product labels display a limited vocabulary which was so commonly used throughout the Western Roman Empire that, in some cases, they became formulaic and could be highly abbreviated, enterprising businessmen showed ingenuity and sophistication in employing that vocabulary in a variety of combinations designed to attract potential customers and to promote recognition of their products and of themselves. Of the 282 *tituli picti* examined for this study, there were 60 variations in product identification alone (Appendix II). Some described their product simply as garum or muria; others proudly praised their product as *gari flos* or *hallex optima*. Still others, more enthusiastic, presented the "hard sell," frequently combining qualitative adjectives and employing words descriptive of the ingredients or method of production. The most indifferent person would surely have to look twice at a vessel labelled G(ari) SC(ombri) [F(los)] EX(cellens) V[etus], "the flower of garum, made from the mackerel, an excellent product, aged!"[44]

Why should there exist this vast array of varied *tituli picti*? Why was the need felt to attract the attention of a potential customer? Surely competition lay at the root of these efforts. Competition is more easily seen within individual cities, such as Pompeii, where the producer *qua* merchant would be daily vying with others to sell to the local population. His livelihood depended upon it. Competition among merchants on the provincial or interprovincial scale is less clear; the number of extant inscribed vessels is fewer and their chronological range far wider. Nevertheless, the general pattern of product designation within the *titulus pictus* of all extant vessels with labels show a remarkable similarity and consistency. Those found on Spanish vessels of the first and second centuries A.D. mirror those found

[43] The closest parallel would again be the mosaic floors in the Piazzale delle Corporazioni in Ostia. Most of these, however, display general emblems, such as a ship denoting *negotiatores*, or emblems signifying grain, such as the modius and the *mensor frumentarius*. Some have inscriptions indicating the origin of the product, but none mentions specific individuals unquestionably involved in the trade. See G. Becatti, *Scavi di Ostia* 4: *Mosaici e pavimenti marmorei* (Rome 1961), pp. 64–85, esp. Plates 83–138.

[44] Bohn, "Pinselschriften," p. 203.

on Pompeian containers. One can reasonably conclude, therefore, that this general standardization, not imposed to be sure but doubtless developed over a period of time by trial and error, insured that a common message would be recognized by Romans everywhere. How this competition worked when a merchant sold a product in a province (or city within a province) different from the one in which it was made is unclear, but must have been similar to its functioning locally. Although ownership of the amphora and its contents could change hands (for example, producer to merchant to retailer), the product message of the *titulus pictus* on the vessel was as valid where the contents were ultimately sold and consumed as where the label was first applied.

Price

The determination of prices of salt-fish products for any period is difficult because of scarce and fragmentary evidence. The example cited by Cato to illustrate the growth of luxury and extravagance among the youth of Rome in the early second century B.C., that is, that a single jar of Pontic salt-fish cost 300 drachmae, tells us little about the usual price for these products.[45] Cato's example may say something about the cost in Rome of salt-fish products imported from the Black Sea, but nothing of local products or of those available from western sources, such as Spain or Sicily. This price, probably exaggerated, is oft-repeated by later writers to illustrate the growth of luxury brought about by increasing exposure to things Greek and so probably adds to the notion that all imported salt-fish products were expensive.[46] A better, but still somewhat anomalous example comes from the late third century B.C. tariff at Akraiphia in Boeotia. It divides salted tunny (θουννόκειτος) into three categories. The most expensive is οὐπογάστρια (stomach portion) at two obols, two chalchoi per mina; some other tunny portions sold for perhaps one and one-half obols. Θουννίδια, or tunny cut into quarters, was the cheapest at one obol, two chalchoi. These prices also seem high and may derive from the cost of transporting large sea fish vis-à-vis the other species named into the interior of Greece. The elevated price may also result from an attempt by fishmongers to soak visitors to the nearby sanctuary. The need for such a tariff may indicate that even greater price gouging occurred beforehand. Prices elsewhere, not near religious sanctuaries, were probably less, but one can only guess.[47] The consistent reference to salt-fish as food for the poor, the soldier, or the disreputable, however, points strongly to the conclusion that preserved fish was not expensive, although at certain places at specific times the price charged might

[45] Polybius 31.25.5: ταρίχου Ποντικοῦ κεράμιον τριακοσίων δραχμῶν.
[46] Diodorus 37.3.6; Athenaeus 6.274f–275a; Plutarch *Mor.* 668c.
[47] See Salviat and Vatin, "Le Tarif," pp. 95–109.

be so beyond the norm as to call for special notice by a writer or for action by government officials.[48]

Customs duties of the Roman Period provide a little help in determining the general value, but again not the price, of salt-fish. In Egypt, for instance, in A.D. 114 the tax collected at the toll house at Bacchias on one chlibion (χλίβιον) of salt-fish carried on a donkey was seven drachmae, one obol (ca. 1.75 den.). The Tariff of Palmyra of A.D. 137 placed a ten denarii impost on a camel-load of salt-fish and three denarii for a donkey load. How these taxes compare with each other is uncertain, since in either case we do not know what was a normal donkey load and for the former instance the exact value of a chlibion, probably a basket of some sort, is unknown. It is interesting to note, however, that in the same papyrus from Bacchias a donkey load of fresh fish was taxed at two drachmae (ca. 0.5 den.). Why a tax on salt-fish should exceed by over three times that for fresh fish is puzzling. Perhaps a donkey could carry a much larger load of the former than of the latter.[49] On two different days in September of A.D. 199, salt-fish imported through the toll house at Arsinoë was taxed at 9 drs. (2.25 den.) and 67 drs. (16.75 den.), respectively. Again the unit of measure is unknown, since the means of transportation was listed only as "fishing boat" (ἁλιευτικὸν πλοῖον).[50]

Evidence of *tituli picti* as advertising vehicles on fish sauce containers found at Pompeii and Herculaneum, among cargoes of shipwrecks, and at other locations throughout the empire implies an attempt to sell to a market at once significantly large and financially able to purchase these products.[51] Modern scholars, nevertheless, persistently interpret the literary evidence regarding Roman fish sauces as proof of their great expense. This is somewhat misleading, since most of the evidence derives from writers, such as Martial, Horace, and Pliny, who were looking for a way to criticize someone in particular or society in general or to praise a certain popular

---

[48] It is difficult to compare these prices with that given by Cato, separated as they are in time and geography, but the figure quoted by Cato for Pontic salt-fish would purchase about 1333 kg. of the cheapest tunny passing through Akraiphia some half-century earlier. I have assumed a value of 8 *choes*, or about 24 liters, per κεράμιον and 800 grams per mina, given by Walbank, *Historical Commentary on Polybius.*, 3: 500–01. Since one amphora as a unit of measure was roughly 26 liters, the price of 300 drachmas per κεράμιον equates to a price of 325 drachmas (denarii?) per amphora. For salt-fish as a common food for the poor, the soldier, and the disreputable, see above p. 154, note 23.

[49] Toll house at Bacchias: *P.Wisc.* II.80$_{\text{v.169}}$. Tariff of Palmyra: IGRR III.1056, ii.35. For the chlibion see Clauson, "Customs House Registry," p. 268. For fresh fish see Sijpesteijn, *Customs Duties in Graeco-Roman Egypt*, p. 62. For customs duty rates see *ibid.*, pp. 75–82. In Egypt there were 6 obols per drachma; 4 drachmae per denarius.

[50] *P.Coll.Youtie* I.31. See Sijpesteijn, *Customs Duties in Graeco-Roman Egypt*, pp. 118–19.

[51] I remain skeptical of Whittaker's suggestion that market forces, such as competition, supply, and demand, played a far less significant role in bringing commodities to Rome and Italy than did the political status of wealthy Romans or of provincial aristocrats living in Rome both of whom owned provincial property and imported goods produced on their estates for distribution to clients. He does accept that some of these goods reached the marketplace but at

commodity by exaggerating its price in the capital. Garum was a product in widespread and frequent use throughout the Graeco-Roman world and, hence, was easily recognizable for its peculiar characteristics, especially the somewhat bizarre preparation process, the strong taste and odor of many types, and the expense of perhaps one in particular. Pliny says that two *congii* of garum sociorum sold for HS 1,000, or HS 4,000 per amphora, and adds that "scarcely any other liquid except perfumes has begun to be held in greater esteem, even to the families of the nobility." Both Seneca and Manilius call garum expensive (*pretiosum*), and Martial implies that garum made from the mackerel would only be sent as a gift to a rich man.[52] There is no doubt that garum was a common item on the table of the wealthy and even reached into the imperial household.[53] That the enjoyment of this food item was outside the means of the average Roman, however, is not borne out by archaeological evidence.

Tituli picti provide no help in determining the price of any processed fish product, since all items which might be associated with the value of the contents of the vessel, such as the export tax, are absent from extant fish sauce amphorae. The Tariff of Zarai, which dates to A.D. 202, however, lists the customs duty on one amphora of garum as one sestertius. If one assumes a tax of two and one-half per cent of the value of the merchandise, this impost yields a price of forty sesterces per amphora in Africa Proconsularis.[54] This price compares favorably with those of other food items mentioned in the same tariff, such as, for example, an equal quantity of wine which cost the same as garum. The Price Edict of Diocletian, promulgated in A.D. 301, provides a better example, since it separates fish sauce into two categories based on quality. The finest fish sauce (*liquamen primum*)

---

prices unreflective of the actual cost of production and transport. See C. R. Whittaker, "Trade and the Aristocracy in the Roman Empire," *Opus* 4 (1985): 49–75.

[52] Pliny *HN* 31.94; Seneca Ep. 95.25: Manilius *Astron*. 5.671; and Martial 13.103. Martial (13.102), also speaking of garum sociorum, calls it *munera cara*. The mackerel sauce referred to by Martial in 13.103 must be garum sociorum, which in 13.102 he called the "first blood of the mackerel" (*scombri de sanguine primo*). In 7.27, Martial mentions an *arcanum garum*, which Jardin ("Garum," p. 85) identifies with garum sociorum. Martial's partiality to the Spanish product is understandable, since he was born in Bilbilis and would know of it by reputation if not first hand. Most *tituli picti* which indicate the fish from which the sauce is made specify the *scomber*. The mackerel is plentiful throughout the Mediterranean, not just in Spanish waters. Consequently, garum sociorum may have been made exclusively from the mackerel, but not all mackerel sauce is garum sociorum. Pliny (*HN* 31.94) says that the mackerel is used for no other purpose than to make fish sauce. Cf. Martial 3.50, 4.86; and Catullus 95.8. For the migration of the mackerel see Thompson, *Greek Fishes*, pp. 243–45.

[53] Prefect of Egypt: *P.London* III.1159 (2nd cent. A.D.), *P.Ryl*. IV.627–39 (4th cent. A.D.); Caracalla for his visit to Egypt in A.D. 216: *P.Got*. 3. Cf. also *SHA. Elagab*. 29.5.

[54] Tariff of Zarai: CIL VIII.4508. See also Darmon, "Note sur le Tarif de Zaraï," pp. 6–23. Tenney Frank ("On the Export Tax of Spanish Harbors," *AJPh* 57 [1936]: 87–90) suggests that the letters (*áá* and *áás-*, for example) which sometimes appear in *tituli picti* on amphorae found on Monte Testaccio in Rome refer to the export tax on goods leaving Spain. Frank estimates this tax at 2.5 per cent of the price of the goods in the container. Though this thesis has been generally accepted, it has recently been seriously challenged. See Dali Colls et al., *L'épave Port-Vendres II*, esp. pp. 95–98.

had a price ceiling of sixteen denarii for one sextarius, while second quality sauce (*liquamen secundum*) could not exceed twelve denarii per sextarius.[55] These prices figure out to about HS 3,072 for one amphora of the best fish sauce, and HS 2,304 for a like quantity of second quality sauce. Both prices are considerably higher than the HS 40 per amphora of African fish sauce sold in A.D. 202. Increasing inflation rates combined with periodic currency devaluations experienced between the first and fourth centuries A.D. render difficult any comparison of prices.[56] The ceiling price of fish sauce in A.D. 301, however, does compare favorably with other food items listed in the same edict. Since garum sociorum was consistently described as an expensive brand of sauce by ancient authors, it would no doubt be priced at the ceiling for first quality sauce.[57] In the Edict, however, the best fish sauce was less expensive than a like quantity of both first and second quality honey. It costs the same as one sextarius of boiled down must, one pound of second quality fish, and a pound of the best salted pork. It exceeded in price one sextarius of ordinary oil, but was cheaper than the same amount of second quality oil.[58]

It seems apparent that in the third and fourth centuries A.D. the price of garum was not out of line with prices for other ordinary items. Garum sociorum was a sauce of the first quality and consequently cost more than other sauces. It did not, however, far exceed other food items in price, and in many instances was priced below them. The high price of garum sociorum quoted by Pliny might reflect food prices in Rome, which were generally higher than those in other areas of Italy and in other provinces. Even if Pliny is correct in his assertion, there is little reason to believe that this price prevailed elsewhere or, for that matter, in Rome in subsequent years. It was, after all, higher than that registered in Diocletian's Price Edict over two centuries later. In fact, the tenor of Pliny's statement implies that the price was unusually high, well beyond the norm.[59]

Ordinary, less expensive garum did exist. Diocletian's Price Edict states as much, and the garum mentioned in the Tariff of Zarai was probably of

---

[55] *Edict. Diocl.* III.6–7.

[56] Richard Duncan-Jones, *The Economy of the Roman Empire* (Cambridge 1974), p. 8, note 2. See now Michael H. Crawford and Joyce Reynolds, "The Publication of the Prices Edict: A New Inscription from Aezani," *JRS* 65 (1975): 160–63, and Mireille Corbier, "Dévaluations et évolution des prix (Ier–IIIe Siècles)," *RN* 28 (1985): 69–106.

[57] Ausonius (*Ep.* 25) provides evidence that garum sociorum was still being produced in the fourth century A.D.

[58] *Edict. Diocl.* III.10: *mel optimum* (40 den.); III.11: *mel secundum* (24 den.); II.15: (vinum) *decoctum* (16 den.); V.2: *piscis secundus* (16 den.); IV.7: *laridum optimum* (16 den.); III.3: *oleum cibarium* (12 den.); III.2: *oleum sequens* (24 den.) For limitations on the use of prices found in Diocletian's Price Edict, see Duncan Jones, *Economy*, pp. 366–67.

[59] For prices in Rome see Duncan-Jones, *Economy*, pp. 250, 345–47, 364–65. In one sixth century A.D. receipt from Egypt, a λαγήνιον, or about 5.7 liters (a little less than two congii, which equals ca. 6.5 liters), of γάρον αἱμάτιον cost five keratia of gold. At about the same time or a little earlier at Anazarbus in Cilicia an unknown amount of γάρον was taxed at a rate of one keration of gold. The rates for carob (1/2 k.) and garlic (1/3 k.), with wine and salt at even

this character. Evidence from excavations at Pompeii indicates that garum was inexpensive and readily available to the average Pompeian. Of 199 fish sauce vessels bearing labels and edited in *CIL* IV approximately 58% held garum, 26% liquamen, 10% muria, and 5% allec. If garum were the most expensive sauce one would expect that fewer people could afford it and that the frequency with which vessels of this sauce would be found would be small. This is obviously not the case. Since garum vessels are far more abundant at both Rome and Pompeii, these figures are unlikely to be the result of the accident of preservation.[60] Fish sauce was apparently well within the budget of most Pompeians who purchased garum and liquamen more often than either allec or muria. Garum sociorum was also available at Pompeii to those who could afford it; those who could not might easily purchase a variety of other brands.[61]

The accessibility of fish sauce to people of all classes can be seen as well at Pompeii and Herculaneum where sauces of every type, particularly the "flower of garum," reputed to be the best quality, have been found throughout the cities in houses both of the wealthy and of the poor or average citizen. Private homes have yielded the majority of fish sauce containers, with many being found in areas where cooking or eating normally took place, such as kitchens, dinning rooms, and gardens.[62] They have also been found in commercial establishments, such as inns, food shops, hot drink shops, and wine shops.[63] This picture is reflected as well in many references to salt-fish products in non-literary papyri from Graeco-Roman Egypt. In most cases, however, these are local products. The price ultimately paid by the consumer for an imported product would probably also

---

lower rates, show that garum was valued higher than ordinary food items, but it does not exceed that for fenugreek, taxed at the same rate. In comparison a slave was taxed at 9 keratia, saffron at 4 keratia. The fish sauce, therefore, may have been an imported product, whereas the wine, a Cilician specialty, and the other food items were probably of local origin. For the receipt from Egypt, see Worp, "Deux papyrus," pp. 132–34; and Shelton, "Garum rouge Sang," p. 156. For the Cilician customs document see Dagron and Feissel, *Inscriptions*, pp. 170–85.

[60] In Rome (*CIL* XV), the relative frequency of finds is similar to that in Pompeii. Of 46 vessels, 70% contained garum, 17% liquamen, 9% muria, and 4% allec.

[61] Only three vessels of garum sociorum have been found to date. See *CIL* IV.5651(?), 5659. Even the assumption that garum made from the mackerel was always the most expensive must be doubted. At Pompeii and Herculaneum 53, or approximately 25%, of the vessels contained sauce made from this fish. In Rome the figures are 8 of 46 containers, or 17%. One of these (*CIL* XV.4731) may have held allec made from the mackerel. *CIL* XV.4687, 4695, 4697, 4705, 4709–10. It is also of interest that Scaurus in the mosaic design of his atrium used only garum and liquamen vessels, even though labels on actual urcei indicate that he sold allec and muria as well (*CIL* IV.5723–24, 9410, 10262).

[62] Kitchens: *CIL* IV.5667, 5712, 9397, 9403–04, 9411, 9418; in or near dining rooms: *CIL* IV.6922, 10269, 10271, 10279–81, 10291; gardens: *CIL* IV.5675, 5684, 5700, 5709, 5722, 9394, 9417, 10274.

[63] Inns: *CIL* IV.9389, 9398, 9406, 10262; food shops: *CIL* IV.5667, 5714, 9395, 9405, 9433; hot drink shop: *CIL* IV.5679; wine shop: *CIL* IV.5664, 5684, 5707, 5709, 5718, 5721, 5667. See also Wilhelmina F. Jashemski, "A Pompeian Vinarius," *CJ* 62 (1967): 193–204.

be influenced by transportation costs, including payment of tariffs along the way. Since salted fish products are almost invariably part of mixed cargoes, it seems reasonable to conclude that in some cases transportation of other, high-value commodities, such as metals, may have served to subsidize the transport costs of salt-fish products and other export items and so to reduce their price to consumers.[64] Apparently, the majority of preserved fish products of all qualities were priced so as to be affordable by most of the people who consumed large quantities, particularly of the fish sauces, in their daily diet simply because they liked them.

---

[64] See D. J. Mattingly, "Oil for Export? A Comparison of Libyan, Spanish and Tunisian Olive Oil Production in the Roman Empire," *Journal of Roman Archaeology* 1 (1988): 52–53. But cf. Whittaker, "Trade and the Aristocracy," pp. 54–55.

CHAPTER EIGHT

SUMMARY AND CONCLUSIONS

Fermented fish products, especially the sauces, played an important role in Graeco-Roman society both as a food and as a medicine, often simultaneously. As a medicine they functioned to cure internal and external problems alike. Salt-fish, being bulkier, figures more prominently in ancient dietetic theory than does fish sauce; but the ancients gave to garum a greater therapeutic value. The latter often served as an additive to create an acceptable consistency for a complex medicinal recipe and at the same time as a condiment to render a concoction more palatable. Salt used in its preparation apparently lay at the heart of the ancient view that garum had the powers of heat and dryness, since as a drug, it was designed to combat afflictions characterized by the opposite properties. These supposed remedies, however, frequently were based on nothing more than superstition. Unbeknownst to the Greeks and Romans was the real dietary contribution of fish, both fresh and fermented, to the ancient diet.

Fish was, as it is today, an excellent source of protein and some important vitamins and minerals. Exactly what proportion of the ancient daily diet fish constituted is unknown, but in processed form it seems to have been significant. This must have been especially so in the case of the lower classes who probably could not afford much fresh fish. A recent study involving the chemical analysis of 97 of 139 skeletons found at Herculaneum, and so datable to A.D. 79, though preliminary in some respects, concludes that the Herculaneans derived most of their animal source protein from seafood.[1] Since Roman society lacked the necessary means of refrigeration and rapid transportation to market, preservation of fish by salting, smoking, and drying was essential. The ready availability of these food items could contribute to a healthful diet. If the lower classes in general consumed the lower-quality salt-fish products which were poorer in nitrogen content and so less nutritious than those of better quality, their diet may not have been as healthful as those higher up on the social ladder. The lower classes, however, would probably, as is the case in Vietnam today, have consumed greater quantities of it. Although this might have supplied the nutrition needed, it might also have brought with it serious health con-

[1] Sarah Bisel, "The Skeletons of Herculaneum, Italy," in *Wet Site Archaeology*. Barbara A. Purdy, ed. (Caldwell, N.J. 1988), pp. 213–15. In light of recent suggestions that the good dental health of modern Vietnamese may be attributable at least partially to their consumption of large amounts of fermented fish products in their daily diet (above, p. 34), it may be significant that Bisel's study concludes that the ancient Herculaneans had "slightly better teeth than the Hellenistic Greeks and much better teeth than modern Americans." *Ibid*., p. 212, and Table 1.

sequences. If preliminary conclusions resulting from modern studies on the effect of a diet high in salty foods applied as well to the ancient Roman population, the apparently high frequency of consumption of fermented fish products, in addition to pickled vegetables, may have resulted in a high incidence of stomach cancer in the lower socio-economic strata of Roman society.

Ancient methods used to produce fermented fish products mirror in nearly all details those practiced today, particularly in Southeast Asia. Using modern methods as a guide one can answer with a reasonable degree of confidence several hitherto perplexing questions about ancient products and production methods. First, the recognition by the Romans of the fact, if not the cause, of rapid deterioration of fish muscle following death helps to explain the location of ancient saltery installations on or near the shore. The best fish products are those processed as soon as possible. Unrefrigerated transportation, even for short distances, permits the growth of bacteria leading rapidly to spoilage. Second, the term liquamen, the exact meaning of which has long eluded definition, referred probably to a sauce prepared in one of two ways. It seems more likely to have been the liquid drawn off after a second or subsequent washing with a brine of the residue of garum production. This would account for the close association of liquamen with garum, the eventual correspondence in literature of the two sauces, and the more frequent use of the term liquamen over garum prevalent in Latin literature from the third century A.D. and after. Less likely, liquamen may have been a sauce prepared by brining, whereby the pickle over a long period of time becomes diluted unless more salt is added. In both cases, therefore, liquamen probably had a salt concentration and keeping ability less than that of garum. Third, Pliny's claim (*HN* 31.95) that allex could be made for itself is borne out by modern methods for production of fish pastes. Allex, like the Philippine *bagoong*, was the residue of fish sauce production, derived from the near total autolysis of fish material. But, if the fermentation process is curtailed well before autolysis has reached completion, the result is a paste. Allex, therefore, is the ancient fish paste.

A survey of the provinces indicates that production and commerce of garum and salsamenta extended throughout the regions bordering upon the Mediterranean and Black Seas and in many areas fronting upon the Atlantic ocean. Archaeological investigation, however, yields an unequal picture of this industry. Information is sporadic, based primarily upon partial excavations at various places and a still imperfect understanding of the relationship between amphorae and their contents and point of origin. Only in Spain (Baetica and Lusitania, primarily), North Africa, Northwestern Gaul, Sicily, and the Cimmerian Bosphorus can the archaeological evidence be called plentiful. In many places, where based on literary sources one would expect to find significant remains, such as in Sardinia, Southern Italy, and Egypt, the results have been disappointing. Frequently, one can only infer the presence of a saltery or commercial activity in salted fish products from scattered and disparate evidence; Cosa, for example. Nevertheless, archaeological excavation combines with literary, epigraphical, and papyrological sources to yield a reasonably clear picture of the production and commerce of salted fish products between the first century B.C. and the third century A.D.

Although there is a long tradition of fish preservation and trading in salted fish products in the Eastern Mediterranean dating back possibly to the seventh century B.C., the earliest remains so far discovered date only to the first century A.D. The technical knowledge of salting fish probably spread throughout the Western Mediterranean from the East by way of Greek and Phoenico-Punic colonists. Punic salting factories dating to the early fifth century B.C. have come to light in the area of Gades, and finds of Punic amphorae at several locations in Sicily and Africa attest to Punic salting activity there during the following century. There may have been some Italian commerce in salt-fish products from Cosa in the third century B.C., but the earliest Roman remains of salting installations date only to the first century B.C. The period of greatest Roman activity in the Eastern and Western Mediterranean seems to have been the first and second centuries A.D., with a perceptible disruption during the following century. Many factories continued to operate during the late third and fourth century; in some places, such as in Northern Spain at Rhode and in Western Gaul in Armorica, there was apparently a rejuvenation of activity. On the whole, it seems, however, that most installations functioned primarily on the local level and at a reduced rate of activity during the fifth century, with some possibly continuing into the sixth century A.D. Recent studies, however, suggest that there existed more sixth-century salting activity than once thought.

Roman salteries followed a general format in the arrangement of facilities. The size and number of buildings and vats varied depending upon the degree of salting activity associated with the particular site. Salteries were usually installed on sites which provided three necessary items: salt, fish, and fresh water. It was no accident that salteries appeared along the shore of the migration route of fish, particularly the tunny. This was especially true in the narrow strait of Gibraltar between North Africa and Southern Spain through which the tunny had to pass when entering and leaving the Mediterranean, and around the shore of the Black Sea, in particular the Cimmerian Bosphorus. Salteries invariably lay near the mouth of a river, bay, or estuary which could supply fresh water for cleaning fish, preparing the brine, or washing the facilities. Some factories, lacking sufficient water, employed cisterns or aqueducts. Processing centers obtained salt from nearby salt mines or marshes, or constructed apparatus to abstract it from salt water. Salteries usually were emplaced outside a city, but a few, such as at Baelo, Tyritake, and Pompeii (at least a wholesale building where some refining of the product may have occurred), were within the city walls. The

Byzantine zoning regulation from Palestine may imply that others were inside urban centers as well.

Roman salting facilities, called *cetariae* in the sense of a collection of individual basins (*cetaria*), varied little in their architectural features from one province to another.[2] Within the factory, basins were usually arranged in a square or semi-circular formation or in parallel series of two or three files. The salteries at Punta de l'Arenal and Chersonesos are exceptions in that basins were not grouped together but appeared randomly scattered throughout the area. Frequently, factories used rooms of buildings constructed to allow for good ventilation to locate the basins, while others had vats lying open to the sun, but probably covered by a roofed structure of wood and tiles to keep out the rain, insects, and sand.

Three basic types of vat, the most characteristic aspect of Roman salteries, differed little, except as necessitated by their physical location. Salteries built on or near a beach employed a vat constructed of broken tiles and bricks mixed with mortar. These might be sunk into the ground and exposed to the open air or roofed in some basic fashion. Other vats of a similar type might be installed inside a building of some sort. Those salteries, such as at Punta de l'Arenal in Jávea, erected on rocky areas utilized basins cut directly into the rock or were constructed identically to the first type but sat upon the ground like a tub. Left in rough state on the exterior, salting vats were coated on the interior with a smooth layer of finely crushed tiles mixed with mortar (*opus signinum*) to ensure a water-tight container. This mortar imparted a reddish tint to some vats in Gaul and the Cimmerian Bosphorus. The corners of the vats were rounded at the top, and the interior angles were reinforced with an ovolo. This served to strengthen the corners and to aid in cleaning the vat. Many basins had scooped out of the bottom a round hole of a few centimeters in width and depth which also aided in the cleaning process. At Rhode in Tarraconensis and Alcazarseghér in Mauretania Tingitana, some vats lacked this hole but had provision near the bottom for draining the liquid material into a sump located nearby. Salting basins took divers shapes—rectangular (most common), square, pear-shaped, or round—and varied in size. The larger ones held salsamenta, as finds of fish bones attest, while the smaller ones, usually round, were probably devoted to the preparation of fish sauce. Sometimes dolia, or pithoi, substituted for small vats. In Gaul and the Cimmerian Bosphorus roof tiles found in vats probably served to press down the materials during fermentation.

Roman salting installations had a variety of other structures, such as

---

[2] The Punic vats at Gades have not been fully published, but preliminary descriptions seem to show construction techniques similar to those used by the Romans; i.e. square or rectangular shape, interior coated with a mortar of lime and crushed ceramic to provide a water-proof container, and lack of drainage.

heated rooms or buildings set aside near the vats for speeding up processing time for at least some of the garum produced. Ancient literary sources, where mentioned at all, do not stress the heating of garum, except for immediate use. In modern methods in use in Southeast Asia likewise curing periods, sometimes lengthy, at ambient temperatures predominate. Heating at temperatures in excess of 45° C actually produces a product of lower quality. It seems likely, therefore, that only small amounts of the product were actually heated. This would explain the appearance of small cooking pots at some installations and their apparent absence at others. Installations often had kilns to produce these cooking pots and commercial containers used to transport the finished products. A few salteries, such as the one at Barbate in Spain, Antipolis in Gaul, and perhaps at Cosa in Italy, possessed holding tanks, or *piscinae,* to keep fish alive or fresh until processed. And finally, villas seem to be an omnipresent structure at Roman salteries. Villas, not always directly physically connected with the factory, were perhaps also used as a residence by the owner or manager. The workers probably lived in temporary shelters which have unfortunately left no remains.

Spain, especially Baetica, exceeded all other provincial areas in the production and commerce of salted fish products up to the late second or early third century A.D. No less than ninety salting establishments dot the Atlantic and Mediterranean coasts from Lisbon to Rhode. Spanish salt-fish amphorae appear in great numbers along the *limes* in many northern provinces, in numerous shipwrecks in the Mediterranean basin, in Italy, and in many places in the Greek East. A caveat may be appropriate here. The archaeological evidence paints a picture of a market saturated with salted fish products from Spain. This almost complete control of the market by Spanish merchants may be more apparent than real. This impression arises from the finds of numerous salting installations in Spain and the many amphorae identified by their shape or clay content as Spanish vessels containing preserved fish products. Little is known of amphorae from other provinces where archaeological excavation also proves the existence of fish salting establishments. Further refining of our knowledge of amphorae from these provinces should allow future scholars to draw a more balanced picture of trade in these products. Even so, there is no doubt that up until the early third century A.D. Spain did capture the lion's share of the market, although it did not maintain a complete monopoly. After the early or mid-third century A.D., Africa seems to have garnered a larger share of at least the Italian market. How much and for how long is unknown. In the East, the Black Sea salteries seem to have dominated the markets, although Spanish products did enter eastern ports, for example, in Egypt and Palestine. How much of the eastern market they serviced is unknown. Eastern provinces sent some salt-fish products to Rome, but the bulk of it, at least that produced in the Black Sea area, probably went to supply surrounding provinces. Egyptian salteries served primarily the needs of its own population, but did export some to Africa and to Syria and Palestine, where locally produced salt-fish apparently did not satisfy demand.

Little is known about the organization for production or commerce in salted fish products. Fishermen could process their own catch, producing both salsamenta and fish sauce. Larger operations required permanent facilities which might need more capital than one man could supply. A *societas* could be formed between two or more individuals to meet this requirement. Certain ones, such as the company from New Carthage which operated over a long period of time, no doubt contained many partners. It seems that most salteries were privately owned by individuals or corporations and were operated on a day-to-day basis by slaves and freedmen under a manager, also probably a freedman. This seems to have been the arrangement at Pompeii, the only place for which clear evidence exists. The state claimed control neither of the salting industry nor of the commerce in salted fish products, although imperial producers did exist, at least in Spain. Although the evidence is far from definitive, it seems that the state may have assumed a position toward salteries similar to the one it took with respect to fisheries; that is, it claimed the revenue of certain fisheries only and farmed out the fishing, and perhaps the salting and distribution rights, to corporations and individuals. Apparently much of the distribution was in private hands and reached a rather high level of organization. Some *societates*, such as the one from Malaca, established permanent representatives in other provinces (in this case, Italy) to facilitate trade. The state derived some profit from this trade through customs duties collected in ports and customs stations. The army probably received the bulk of its supplies through merchants who contracted with the state to deliver the products required.

Literary sources for the most part accurately reflect the archaeological evidence. Methods and ingredients for producing garum, not the facilities or production methods for manufacturing salsamenta, attracted the attention of ancient writers. For this reason we can judge the evidence for fish sauce more accurately than that for salt-fish. With respect to garum, references to fish used, to small containers and production facilities, and to storage vessels can be corroborated by finds at many sites. Literary sources speak frequently of Spanish activity in preserved fish commerce; archaeological excavation in the Western Mediterranean points to a near monopoly of the market in these products by Spanish producers and merchants, at least up to the mid-third century A.D. And finally, salted fish products, including fish sauce, were not rare items in Roman commerce. Salted fish and most fish sauces were well within the budget of most Romans everywhere and served as a staple food in the diet of Romans of all social classes. Garum was not a luxury product, although one, garum sociorum, enjoyed a high reputation and demanded a higher price.

In the promotion of commerce ancient entrepreneurs often used *tituli picti* on transport containers to advertise their products. These labels represent a keen sense of what might attract the attention of a potential customer. Sixty documented variations illustrate that labels taut the products for their high quality, origin, and special preparation process. One producer, A. Umbricius Scaurus of Pompeii, even displayed a unique mosaic design in a secondary atrium of his luxurious home to advertise his products. The advertising efforts were aimed at meeting the demands of competition, but the available evidence does not allow a full understanding of this activity, except at Pompeii where archaeological and epigraphical evidence implies that competition was quite strong in Campania during the first century A.D.

Individuals from all levels of society participated in one aspect or another of production and commerce. Workers at installations were poor, generally slaves and freedmen. For most of them fish processing was probably a second occupation. In the off-season they returned to work on farms or in nearby towns. Many salteries may have continued to process year-round, but at a reduced level of activity, since annex industries, such as the manufacture of purple dye and the salting of meats other than fish, such as pork, beef, and sheep, would have utilized the same facilities. For some workers, therefore, salting would have been their sole occupation. Factories were operated by the owner or by slave or freedmen overseers who probably resided permanently at the factory where a villa was closely associated with it. Owners of large factories were apparently well-off, if not wealthy. Their social standing is difficult to gauge since only a few can be definitely identified as producers. At least one, A. Umbricius Scaurus, a man of freeborn status, grew quite wealthy from his business concerns. His son no doubt used this wealth to finance his political career in Pompeii, becoming first aedile, then duovir, thereby enrolling his family among the local aristocracy. Many merchants in salt-fish products, were freedmen, but free men also participated. Most usually traded in other products, such as wine, in addition to salt-fish, but some, such as the *negotiatores allecarii*, concentrated their efforts in preserved fish.

In sum, literary, archaeological, epigraphical, and papyrological evidence allows one to trace the path of preserved fish products from the point of production through intermediaries who transport the items to local merchants who sell the products to the ultimate consumer. Preserved fish prepared by local fishermen in small or temporary facilities probably landed up on the fishermen's table or in nearby markets. Large installations produced for local consumption and for export. The producer would bottle the salt-fish or fish sauce in amphorae of specific shapes produced by his own kilns or for him by owners of independent kilns. Some vessels he marked with a *titulus pictus* identifying the contents and perhaps the name of the merchant or shipper who would transport them. The filled amphorae might be delivered to market by the producer or sold to a merchant. Some amphorae might even be delivered to a local wholesale merchant who further processed the product to his own specification before sale or exportation.

The merchant or producer would deliver the amphorae to the harbor where they would be stored until ready for shipment. They would be consigned to a shipper (*negotiator*) who would add them to his mixed cargo of perhaps wine, lead ingots, and so forth. The shipper might be an individual or a *societas* working privately or on contract to the Roman government. The *negotiator* then transported the products to their foreign destination, paying any taxes or tolls on them and delivering them to a specified person, perhaps a merchant or a representative of the company, who might further transship the amphorae by river or land transportation to inland markets, such as those along the *limes* in Germany or across the Channel in Britain. Some would go to government contractors supplying army units, others to local merchants. This latter individual (*salsamentarius*, γαροπώλης, or various other appellations) would then sell the product wholesale or retail in competition with local products and with those imported from other provinces. The consumer, perhaps enticed by some snappy advertisement written on the vessel or persuaded by an energetic entrepreneur, would purchase the product in an amphora or, more likely, in a smaller container for home use, as a food, or a medicine as the need arose. The salt-fish dealer or consumer could smash the empty amphora or else re-use it for a like product or for various other purposes.

The importance of fish in the Graeco-Roman diet has been recognized for decades, but when commerce in drugs and foodstuffs is discussed processed fish products, if mentioned at all, are only commented upon in passing, being overshadowed by commerce in wine, oil, and grain. This study has tried to show that, even if they did not surpass the big three in volume, processed fish products formed a significant part of ancient commerce and should be given their proper place in any discussion of the Roman economy, especially in the realm of food, medicine, and trade.

CHAPTER NINE

EPILOGUE

Production and commerce of salted fish products did not cease in the fifth or sixth century A.D., but the level of activity, at least until the eleventh century and then primarily in Northern Europe, never approached what it had been in the first two centuries A.D. The available sources for the post-classical period are mostly literary in nature, are scattered geographically and chronologically, and are difficult to interpret. This latter problem is further compounded by the lack of any identifiable archaeological evidence relating to production and commerce of these products. What seems certain is that the dietetic and therapeutic uses of these items of materia medica continued in both the Eastern and Western Mediterranean areas and that there was some level of trade in them as well. One cannot, however, cleary determine the degree to which they continued to play a practical role in medicine nor can one judge the level of production and commerce before the Early Modern Period. By that time salt-fish, particularly herring and sardines, were quite popular, but the fish sauces were little used and played no significant role in Mediterranean and Atlantic trade.

For the Western empire the evidence comes primarily from Italy and Gaul. Anthimus, a Greek physician and emissary of the Ostrogothic king Theoderic the Great to the Franks in the late fifth century A.D., in his dietetic handbook *De observatione ciborum*, written in Latin in the early sixth century, refers ambiguously to liquamen. In his discussion of domestic pork, he states that if pork loins are rather hard to chew, they should be dipped in pure salt: "For we prohibit liquamen from every part." Whether he implies some measures taken to prevent its importation into Ostrogothic Italy is unknown. Cassiodorus (ca. 490–ca. 583), on the other hand, writing a little later in the same century, mentions salting factories (*garismatia*) operating in Histria in Northern Italy at the upper reaches of the Adriatic Sea.[1] The best source, however, is Gregory, Bishop of Tours (A.D. 538–94) in Merovingian France. In Book IV of his *Historiae* he describes a controversy precipitated by the theft of seventy vessels (*orcae*) of oil and liquamen from a *negotiator* who had brought the goods into port at Massi-

[1] Anthimus *De observatione ciborum ad Theodoricum regem Francorum epistula* 9 (= *Corpus Medicorum Latinorum*. Edward Liechtenhan, ed. [Leipzig 1928], p. 7): *De porco domestico et elixae et assatae; quantum tamen recentiores sunt tantum leviores sunt et aptae ad digestionem; praeterea de lumbis porcellinis expedit assas manducare, quia aptae sunt et bene conficiuntur, ita, ut sale in aqua soluto cum pinnis, quando assantur, tangantur; et si duriores fuerint quando manducantur, melius est, sic tamen, ut in sale puro intingantur. nam liquamen ex omni parte prohibemus*; and Cassiodorus *Variae* 12.22.4.

lia. Unfortunately, he does not specify the origin of the products, although a western source may be implied since the cargo, apparently a mixed one, included oil, a product which, for example, could have come from Africa.[2]

The Frankish monk Marculf (fl. ca. mid-7th cent. A.D.) records among his collection of *formulae* (or *cartae regales*) a letter (*tractoria*) of an unnamed king to his functionaries (*agentes*) advising them to provide certain provisions for persons travelling on official business. Included among the food items was garum.[3] The items appear consciously, but loosely grouped into categories, such as meats, fowl, condiments, food for animals, and so on. The fish sauce appears within the group of liquids used for cooking and seasoning food: oil, garum, honey, and vinegar. Following this group are the spices: cumin, pepper, costum, cinnamon, and so forth. That the fish sauce does not appear directly among the list of spices may be significant in that it seems to imply that garum was not included among costly spices probably imported from the East. And finally, a diploma of Chilperic II, dated to April of A.D. 716, granted permission to the Abbot of Corbie to draw provisions, including garum, from the *cellarium fisci* at Fos. This diploma merely confirmed a similar grant to the abbey made by Clotair III (A.D. 657–73) and Childeric II (A.D. 673–75) in the seventh century.[4]

Apparently Massilia in the sixth and Fos in the seventh and eighth centuries A.D. continued to serve as a port for the receipt of goods bound for the interior of Gaul, much as they had done in the first century. Although these sources do not preclude the possibility that some fish sauce was imported, perhaps even from the East, two ninth century sources confirm that fish preservation was at that period still an important feature of the local economy. The Carolingian capitulary *De villis* lists garum as one of several items produced on Gallic villas, and a medical treatise, extant in a manuscript perhaps of the same period from the Abbey of Echternach, gives detailed instructions on how to prepare garum.[5] Fish sauce, either

---

[2] Gregory of Tours *Historia Francorum* 4.43 (=*MGH. Scriptores Rerum Merovingicarum*. Vol. 1, p. 177): *In regno autem Sigiberti regis, remoto ab honore Iovino rectore Provinciae, Albinus in loco eius subrogatur. Magnam enim inter eos inimicitiam haec causa congessit. Igitur advenientibus ad cataplum Massiliensim navibus transmarinis, Vigilii archidiaconi homines septuaginta vasa quas vulgo orcas vocant olei liquaminisque furati sunt, nesciente domino. Negotiator autem cum cognovisset, sibi rem furto ablatam fuisse, inquirere diligenter coepit, quo furtum in loco fuisset reconditum.* For the probable exportation of African olive oil in the Late Roman Empire, see Keay, *Late Roman Amphorae*, esp. pp. 303–50, 432–35; and Michel Bonifay, Gaëtan Conges, and Martine Leguilloux, "Amphores tardives (V^e–VIIe siècle) à Arles et à Marseille," in *Amphores Romaines et Histoire Économique. Dix Ans de Recherche.* Coll. de l'École Française de Rome, 114 (Rome 1989), pp. 660–63.

[3] Marculf *Formula* 1.11 (= *MGH. Legum Sectio V*, p. 49): *garo liberas tantas.*

[4] *MGH. Diplomata Regum Francorum* I, no. 86, p. 76: *garo modios* 30, and again *garo lib.* 1.

[5] *De villis* 34 (*MGH. Legum Sectio* II, p. 86): *omnino praevidendum est cum omni diligentia, ut quicquid manibus laboraverint aut fecerint, id ist lardum, siccamen, sulcia, niusaltus, vinum, acetum, moratum, vinum coctum, garum, sinape, formaticum, butirum, bracios, cervisas, medum, mel, ceram, farinum, omnia cum summo nitore sint facta vel parata.* For the medical treatise see Paris Bibliothèque Nationale Ms. Lat. 11219 (Appendix I-7). The Latin of the medical text leaves much to be desired and is probably corrupt in places. Its dating remains unknown, since the anony-

locally produced or imported, as mentioned in Merovingian and Carolingian sources, apparently served as an item both of medicine and of food.[6]

Inhabitants of the Mediterranean and North Seas continued to process fish. The Chronicles of the Monastery of Evesham for the year A.D. 709 mentions the herring fishery at Yarmouth in England and the same fish was being caught across the Channel at Fécamp, Calais, and Dieppe in 1031.[7] Herring fisheries, called *domus alleciariae*, operated in late thirteenth-century England, while the herring merchant in Northern France of the fourteenth century was called an *alleciarius*, both terms deriving from the Latin word allec, referring to the North Atlantic herring and to the Mediterranean anchovy and other related fish from which the Romans frequently made fish sauce of the same name. The terms recall also the Roman salt-fish merchant operating in Northern Europe in the third century A.D., the *negotiator allecarius*.[8] Between the fifteenth and eighteenth centuries the North Sea and Atlantic fisheries were critical to the economies of several European countries, such as Holland, while Mediterranean fisheries were less active.[9]

If Rabelais (ca. 1483–1553), a physician and former Franciscan and Benedictine initiate, can be taken as a guide, fish sauce, although continuing to be produced, but probably not imported, in the sixteenth century played a small role in the diet of most Europeans, and apparently was not a medicine in widespread usage either. Étienne Dolet (1509–46) dedicated a poem (*carmen*), entitled *De Garo Salsamento*, to Rabelais[10]:

---

mous Carolingian manuscript collects several medical texts, including an excerpt dealing with fish sauce from the *Origines* (20.3.19–20) of Isidore, the seventh-century A.D. Bishop of Seville. Isidore's discussion of garum is apparently derivative (cf. Pliny *HN* 31.93–95) and so says little of the role of salt-fish and fish sauce in seventh century A.D. Spain (Appendix I-6).

[6] Jean Lestocquoy, "Épices, médecine et abbayes," *Études mérovingiennes. Actes des journées de Poitiers, 1–3 Mai 1952* (Paris 1953): 179–86. For long-distance trade in the Carolingian period see Richard Hodges and David Whitehouse, *Mohammed, Charlemagne and the Origins of Europe. Archaeology and the Pirenne Thesis* (Ithaca, N.Y. 1983), passim.

[7] For the Chronicles of Evesham see Arthur M. Samuel, *The Herring* (London 1918), p. 58; for herring on the French coast, Charles L. Cutting, *Fish Saving. A History of Fish Processing from Ancient to Modern Times* (London 1955), pp. 54–56.

[8] For the herring fisheries of England see *Extract from the Account Rolls of the Abbey of Durham*. Publications of the Surtees Society 100 (1899): 500 (*domus allec. de Jaru*, in 1299); *ibid.*, 99 (1898): 66 (*magne domus alleciarie*, in Hartlepool in 1438–1439); and *Foedarium Prioratus Dunelmensis*. Publications of the Surtees Society 58 (1871): 24 (*magnam domum alleciariam*, in Hartlepool in 1420). For French herring merchants see *Ordonnances des roys de France de la troisiéme race*. Denis F. Secousse and E. J. De Lauriére, eds. (Paris 1723–1844), Vol. 6, pp. 404–14. See also Curtis, "*Negotiatores Allecarii*," pp. 147–58.

[9] For seafood in Europe from the fifteenth to the eighteenth century see Fernand Braudel, *The Structures of Everyday Life*. Vol. 1 of *Civilization and Capitalism, 15th–18th Century*. Siân Reynolds, transl. (New York 1981), pp. 214–20; and *ibid.*, *The Perspective of the World*. Vol. 3 of *Civilization and Capitalism, 15th–18th Century*. Siân Reynolds, transl. (New York 1984), pp. 188–90. See also Samuel, *The Herring*, passim; and Cutting, *Fish Saving*, passim.

[10] *Stephani Doleti Ad Franciscum Rabelaesum De Garo Salsamento Carmen*:

Tuo ingenio, Rabelaese, Garum Salsamentum
Aetate ab antiqua reductum est. Iam nostris,

> Rabelais, salted garum has been restored from the ancient age by your genius. Now, Marot, let it be eagerly celebrated by our verses, since it stimulates so delightfully the palate of each of us and restores the appetite with such a sweet-smelling odor. A thing so pleasing must not be concealed.

For his part Rabelais penned the following response, also entitled *De Garo Salsamento*[11]:

> Behold, I am sending to you garum, which once so many doctors of old valued but is unknown to ours. Add sour wine and oil, however much you wish. There are those to whom savory butter is better than oil. When you are busily devoted to your books, no medicine better restores to you a lost appetite. No medicine or liquids better clean out phlegm; no medicine will be able more conveniently to loosen the bowels. Rather more, after you have eaten garum, you will be astonished that no other sauce however much pleasant will please you.

Both Dolet and Rabelais imply that knowledge of garum was not widespread, even among physicians. Their discussion of it, as their phraseology suggests, derives not so much from practical knowledge as from their acquaintance with the ancient authors. Rabelais' experience with it, however, was probably not all theoretical. Guillaume Rondelet (1507–66), a contemporary of Rabelais, in his treatise on fish says that he personally observed the preparation of the "best and most agreeable garum" at the home of the Bishop of Montpellier in the south of France near the Mediterranean coast. Rabelais himself for a time between 1537 and 1539 lectured on medicine in Montpellier.[12]

It seems then that in the West preserved fish continued to be processed in areas where the Romans earlier had been active, but the North Sea fish-

---

Marote, versibus celebretur animosè.
Quando palatum utrique nostrum tam bellè
Irritat, et stomachum recreat tam odorato
Sapore. Res tam grata non est reticenda.

Les Oeuvres de Maistre François Rabelais. Ch. Marty-Laveaux, ed. (Paris 1873), p. 376.

[11] *F. Rabelaesi ad Doletum De Garo Salsamento*:

Quod medici quondam tanti fecere priores
Ignotum nostris, en! tibi mitto Garum.
Vini addes acidi quantum vis, quantum olei vis;
Sunt quibus est oleo plus sapidum butyrum.
Dejectam, assiduus libris dum incumbis, orexim
Nulla tibi melius pharmaca restituent.
Nulla et aqualiculi mage detergent pituitam:
Nulla alvum poterunt solvere commodius.
Mirere id potius, quantum vis dulcia sumpto
Salsamenta Garo nulla placere tibi.

The Works of Francis Rabelais. Albert Jay Nock and Catherine Rose Wilson, eds. 2 vols. (New York 1931), 1: 930.

[12] Guillaume Rondelet, *Libri De Piscibus Marinis* (Lugdunum 1554–55), p. 141: *alii antiquorum more in muria sinunt tabescere, ut garum faciant. Ex qua optimum et suavissimum garum paratum vidi, apud Gulielmum Pelicerium episcopum Monspelienem, virum summa laude dignissimum.* Dolet resided in Lyon (Lugdunum) for most of the final twelve years of his life.

eries outdistanced those of the Mediterranean. Fish sauce is rarely mentioned and its production may have essentially become concentrated in the Mediterranean areas of Southern France. The decline in popularity of fish sauce perhaps has its origin in the alimentary prohibitions of the early Christians. The example of St. Pachomius' proscriptions immediately comes to mind, as does the letter to Eustochium of St. Jerome.[13] Interdictions became even stronger in Catholic Europe of the Middle Ages and Renaissance. Salted, smoked, and fresh fish formed the main course during lent, but Rabelais indicates that the consumption of garum was forbidden.[14] A recent study argues that fish was a primary food for Lent since, appearing to be a cold, bloodless meat, it embodied the idea of penitence and mortification essential to the observance of abstinence. Additionally, fresh-water fish became, at least in France and England, more popular in the sixteenth and seventeenth centuries and remained so until the beginning of this century.[15] How this relates to the decline in popularity of garum can only be speculated. Perhaps fish sauce, made from small, whole fish and the intestines and blood of larger ones, was seen as too rich, too appetite-provoking to qualify as a food during periods of fasting. Though still being produced in a few places, it apparently served a local need which continuously declined as the number of days devoted to abstinence increased. Its medicinal usages were apparently minimal as well, the knowledge of them seemingly residing only with those acquainted with the ancient sources.[16]

Salted fish products continued to be produced and sold in the East. Several papyri attest to fish sauce production in Egypt between the fifth and eighth centuries A.D. A salt-fish dealer (σαλγαμάριος) was apparently operating in Corinth in the sixth century; and at about the same time garum, making its way into the interior of Cilicia, was taxed at the customs station at Anazarbus.[17] Whether it came from a coastal area of Cilicia or from some foreign source is unknown. A zoning regulation of unknown date, but of the Byzantine period and perhaps referring to the area of Phoenicia or Palestine, includes a provision restricting the erection of a fish sauce factory less than three stades from a town or village. Interestingly, the edict lumps

---

[13] St. Pachomius *Regula Sancti Pachomii* 46 (above, note 29, p. 35); St. Jerome *Ep.* 108.17 (above, note 120, p. 136).

[14] Rabelais, *Des faicts et Dicts Héroïques du Bon Pantagruel* 5.29. Rabelais in this instance uses the transliterated Greek form *garon*.

[15] Laurence Bérard, "La consommation du poisson en France: des prescriptions alimentaires à la prépondérance de la carpe," in *Anthropozoologica*, pp. 171–80.

[16] Besides Rabelais and Rondelet, see, for example, Carl Wittesteyn, *Vera Totius Medicinae Forma* (Antwerp 1588), esp. pp. 139–40, and Ludovicus Nonnus, a seventeenth century physician in Antwerp. *Ludovici Nonni Diaeteticon sive De Re Cibaria Libri IV* (Antwerp 1627), esp. Book III, chapters 44–45.

[17] For example, *P.Oxy.* XIV.1656, XVI.1924, XXXIV.2732; *P.Apollo* 85, 93, 96; *P.Amst.* I.44, II.156; *P.Oslo* III.147; *BGU* II.377; *P.Erl.* 16; *P.Got.* 17; *SB* I.1960; *Stud.Pal.* XX.151; *P.Lond.* I.113. For σαλγαμάριος see Robert, "Épitaphs," pp. 39–46; for Cilicia see Dagron and Feissel, *Inscriptions de Cilicie*, pp. 170–85.

fish sauce producers (γαρεψοί) with cheese makers (τυροποιοί). It prohibits the erection of new installations because of the offensive odor, but allows those already operating or granted an easement to remain.[18] Liutprand, Bishop of Cremona, visiting Constantinople in June of 968 as representative of Otto I, the Holy Roman Emperor, describes a luxurious evening meal sent to him by the Byzantine emperor Nicephorus II Phocas to appease him for an insult suffered earlier. The main dish consisted of roasted goat covered with onions, leeks, and garum.[19] These few literary and epigraphical sources, however, do not allow one even to trace the outlines of what trade existed in these products in the Byzantine period; archaeological evidence is non-existent.

Knowledge of the therapeutic and dietetic properties of preserved fish products continued as it had done in the West. Rhazes, the Persian physician who practiced in Baghdad in the early tenth century A.D., recommends the fish sauce of Nabataea for the treatment of small pox. Symeon Seth (fl. 11th cent. A.D.), who apparently borrowed from Arabic sources and knew and sometimes disagreed with Galen, in his work "On The Properties of Foods" refers occasionally to γάρος.[20] Other Byzantine medical texts, including collections of recipes and dietetic handbooks, such as the tenth or eleventh-century medical calendar extant under the name of Hierophilus the Sophist, likewise include references to salt-fish products. This work, among other things, prescribes certain alimentary regimens according to the particular month of the year.[21] But again, as for the West, it

---

[18] Constantine Harmenopulus 2.4.22 (= *Constantini Harmenopuli Manuale Legum sive Hexabiblos*. Gustav Ernest Heimbach, ed. (Leipzig 1851), pp. 248–50): Ἐπαρχικὸν ΠΕΡΙ ΓΑΡΕΨΩΝ. Ἡ τέχνη τῶν γαρεψῶν καὶ ἡ τῶν τυροποιῶν οὐ τὴν τυχοῦσαν ποιεῖ τοῖς παρακειμένοις βλαβήν· πολλὴ γὰρ ἡ ἀπ' αὐτῆς ἀτμὶς δυσώδης τε ἀμέτρως ἐστὶ καὶ ἐπιβλαβὴς ἐπὶ πολὺ διάστημα. Ὅθεν χρὴ τοὺς τοιούτους παντάπασι μὲν πόλιν μὴ οἰκεῖν μηδὲ κώμην. Εἰ δὲ χρεία τούτων εἴη πρὸς τὰς χρήσεις τῶν πόλεων καὶ τῶν κωμῶν, ἀφεστᾶναι στάδια τούτους δεῖ τρία. Εἰδέναι δὲ χρὴ ὡς ταῦτα πάντα τὰ προειρημένα ἐπὶ τῶν ἐκ νέου κατασκευαζόντων εἴρηται· εἰ δὲ χάρται εἰσὶ παλαιοὶ ἢ καὶ δουλεία τις προλαβοῦσα, κεχρῆσθαι δεῖ τοῖς ἐξ ἀρχῆς περὶ αὐτῶν συμπεφωνημένοις. See also John Pairman Brown, *The Lebanon and Phoenicia* (Beirut 1969), Vol. 1, pp. 51–52.

[19] Liutprand *Relatio de legatione Constantinopolitana* 20 (*Script. Rerum Germ.*, Vol. 41 [Hanover 1915], p. 186): *sed lenivit dolorem meum imperator sanctus munere magno, mittens mihi ex delicatissimis cibis suis haedum pinguem, ex quo ipse comederat, allio, cepe, porris laute suffarcinatum, garo delibutum, quem vestrae tunc mensae inesse optavi, ut, qui delicias sancti imperatoris faustas esse non creditis, saltem his perspectis crederetis.*

[20] Rhazes, cited in Jardin, "Garum," p. 94; Symeon Seth *De alim. fac.* (= *Simeonis Sethi Syntagma De alimentorum facultatibus*. Bernhard Langkavel, ed. [Leipzig 1868], pp. 24–25, 49, 65, 87–88, 90, and passim). Cf. also the tenth century Byzantine physician Theophanes Nonnos *De omnium particularium morborum curatione* (Hieremia Martius, ed. Strasburg 1568) chapt. 156, pp. 177–79: *De stomachi, ventriculi et praecordiorum affectibus, et cibi fastidio, quod Graeci* ἀνορεξίαν *appellant* ; chapt. 158, pp. 180–81: *De canino appetitu*; and chapt. 162, pp. 183–84: *De cruditate ventriculi*. In each case ὑδρόγαρον is among medicinal foods recommended. See also Herbert Hunger, *Die hochsprachliche profane Literatur der Byzantiner*. Handbuch der Altertumswissenschaft, XII.5. 2 vols. (Munich 1978), 1: 308–09.

21. *Anecdota Atheniensia et Alia*. A. Delatte, ed. 2 vols. (Paris 1939), 2: 455–66, esp. for the months of January, April, June, and July. Delatte collects also several anonymous Byzantine texts attributable to Hippocrates and Galen which include references to preserved fish prod-

is impossible to gauge the practical use of fish sauce as part of everyday Byzantine materia medica.

The preservation of fish, therefore, was never completely forgotten in the East or West, although fish sauce as a condiment may have maintained a greater popularity in the former area, particularly in Turkey.[22] One hundred years after the fall of Constantinople to the Arabs and at about the same time that Rondelet was publishing his treatise on fish, a French traveler, Pierre Belon, visited the city and reported that fish sellers, called *cetarii,* also made garum. He observed further that in Italy the *cetarii* were called *piscigaroli,* a word formed by the combination of *piscis* and garum.[23] The link between ancient processed fish products and those of today, however, is nowhere more obvious than in India, Japan, and many countries of Southeast Asia, particularly Vietnam, Cambodia, and the Philippines, where the production process for fish sauce parallels almost exactly that used by the ancient Romans two thousand years ago.[24]

---

ucts. See, for example, *ibid.*, pp. 485–87 (Περὶ ἰχθύων), 488–89 (Περὶ τῶν ταριχευομένων ἁπάντων τῶν ζῴων τε καὶ πετεινῶν καὶ ἐνύδρων), and 489 (Περὶ γάρου). I wish to thank Prof. John Scarborough for bringing these citations to my attention. See also Hunger, *Die hochsprachliche profane Literatur*, esp. pp. 309–10.

[22] Bérard ("La consommation du poisson," p. 172) says that the western and eastern churches agreed on the role of fish in the observance of fasting. For this reason, the same causes of decline in the popularity of garum postulated for the Western Mediterranean may apply as well for the eastern part.

[23] Pierre Belon, *Les observations de plusiers singularitez et choses memorables, trouvées en Grece, Asie, Iudée, Egypte, Arabie, et autres pays estranges* (Antwerp 1555), Chapt. 25, p. 72: *Il y eu une liqueur nommée Garum, qui estoit anciennement en aussi grand usage à Rome, comme nous est le vinaigre pour l'heure presente. Nous l'avons trouvée en Turquie en aussi grand cours qu'elle fut iamais. Il n'y a boutique de poissonnier qui n'en ait à vendre en Constantinople. Tels vendeurs estoyent nommez Cetarii, qui n'ont encor gaigné aucun nom François, qui ne les voudroit nommer Harenniers, et toutesfois ont bien trouvé appelation vulgaire en Italie. Car les Romains les nomment Piscigaroli: qui est diction procedente de l'appellation du poisson et du garum. Les Piscigaroles de Constantinople sont pour la plus part en Pere, qui apprestent iournellement des poissons fraiz, et les exposent en vente desia frits: desquels ostants les tripes et ouyes, et les mettants tremper en la saulmure, la font convertir en Garum.*

[24] The question of the origin of the knowledge of fish preservation in Southeast Asia and other Far Eastern countries is one that must be left for others to pursue.

APPENDIX I

ANCIENT RECIPES

1. Columella *Rust.* 12.55.4 (1st cent. A.D.):

est et alia salsura, quae etiam locis calidis omni tempore anni potest usurpari. cum ab aqua pridie sues prohibitae sunt, postero die mactantur, et vel aqua candente, vel ex tenuibus lignis flammula facta glabrantur, nam utroque modo pili detrahuntur caro in libraria frusta conciditur: deinde in seria substernitur sal coctus, sed modice ut supra diximus infractus: deinde offulae carnis spisse componuntur, et alternis sal ingeritur. sed cum ad fauces seriae perventum est, sale reliqua pars repletur, et impositis ponderibus in vas comprimitur: eaque caro semper conservatur, et tanquam salsamentum in muria sua permanet.

2. Pliny *HN* 31.93–95 (1st cent. A.D.):

(93) *Aliud etiamnum liquoris exquisiti genus, quod garum vocavere, intestinis piscium ceterisque, quae abicienda essent, sale maceratis, ut sit illa putrescentium sanies. hoc olim conficiebatur ex pisce, quem Graeci garon vocabant, capite eius usto suffitu extrahi secundas monstrantes,* (94) *nunc e scombro pisce laudatissimum in Carthaginis spartariae cetariis—sociorum id appellatur—, singulis milibus nummum permutantibus congios fere binos. nec liquor ullus paene praeter unguenta maiore in pretio esse coepit, nobilitatis etiam gentibus. scombros et Mauretania Baeticaeque etiam Carteia ex oceano intrantes capiunt, ad nihil aliud utiles. laudantur et Clazomenae garo Pompeique et Leptis, sicut muria Antipolis ac Thurii, iam vero et Delmatia.* (95) *vitium huius est allex atque inperfecta nec colata faex. coepit tamen et privatim ex inutili pisciculo minimoque confici. apuam nostri, aphyen Graeci vocant, quoniam is pisciculus e pluvia nascatur. Foroiulienses piscem, ex quo faciunt, lupum appellant. transiit deinde in luxuriam, creveruntque genera ad infinitum, sicuti garum ad colorem mulsi veteris adeoque suavitatem dilutum, ut bibi possit. aliud vero est castimoniarum superstitioni etiam sacrisque Iudaeis dicatum, quod fit e piscibus squama carentibus. sic allex pervenit ad ostreas, echinos, urticas maris, mullorum iocinera, innumerisque generibus ad sapores gulae coepit sal tabescere.*

3. Manilius *Astronomica* 5.656–81 (1st cent. A.D.):

Laeva sub extremis consurgunt sidera Ceti
Piscibus Andromedan ponto caeloque sequentis.
hoc trahit in pelagi caedes ut vulnera natos
squamigeri gregis, extentis laqueare profundum

retibus et pontum vinclis artare furentis;
et velut in laxo securas aequore phocas
carceribus claudent raris et compede nectent
incautosque trahent macularum nemine thynnos.
nec cepisse sat est: luctantur corpora nodis
exspectantque novas acies ferroque necantur,
inficiturque suo permixtus sanguine pontus.
tum quoque, cum toto iacuerunt litore praedae,
altera fit caedis caedes: scinduntur in artus,
corpore et ex uno varius discribitur usus.
illa datis melior, sucis pars illa retentis.
hinc sanies pretiosa fluit floremque cruoris
evomit et mixto gustum sale temperat oris;
illa putris turbae strages confunditur omnis
permiscetque suas alterna in damna figuras
communemque cibis usum sucumque ministrat.
aut, cum caeruleo stetit ipsa simillima ponto
squamigerum nubes turbaque immobilis haeret,
excipitur vasta circum vallata sagena
ingentisque lacus et Bacchi dolia complet
umorisque vomit socias per mutua dotes
et fluit in liquidam tabem resoluta medulas.

4. Ps-Rufius Festus *Brev.* (Förster, p. 23) (3rd cent. A.D.?):

Confectio gari

sume pisces minores salsos aut si salsi non fuerint, saliantur pauco sale. et mitte ex illis sextarium unum et de bono vino sextarios tres et coque in aereo vase usque dum duae partes consumantur et tertia remaneat. tum cola per saccum usque ad claritatem et refrigera. tum mitte in vitream ampullam et utere.

5. Ps-Gargilius Martialis 62 (=Rose, "Aringus, der Hering," pp. 226–27) (3rd cent. A.D.?):

Confectio liquaminis quod oenogarum vocant

capiuntur pisces natura pingues, ut sunt salmones et anguillae et alausae et sardinae vel aringi, et fit ex eis atque ex herbis odoratis aridis cum sale compositio talis. praeparatur vas bene solidum ac bene picatum capax trium vel quattuor modiorum, sumunturque herbae aridae bene olentes tam de horto quam de agro, utputa anetum coliandrum feniculum apium satureia sclareia ruta menta sisymbrium ligusticum puleium serpullum origanum vettonica argemonia, et ex his in fundo vasis primus ordo consternitur. tum ex piscibus si minores fuerint integris, si maiores in frusta concisis alter ordo componitur. super hunc tertius ordo salis binos digitos altus adicitur. atque in hunc modum his tribus herbarum et piscium salisque ordinibus supra in vicem alternantibus vas est usque ad summitatem implendum, tum addito operculo claudendum atque ita per dies septem dimittendum. quibus transactis per continuous viginti dies cottidie bis vel ter palo ligneo in modum remi formato compositio ista usque ad fundum est commovenda. quibus expletis liquor qui de hac compositione defluxit colligitur. atque in hunc modum ex eo liquamen vel oenogarum conficitur. sumuntur huius liquoris sestarii duo et cum dimidio boni vini sestario commiscentur, tum quattuor herbarum aridarum singuli manipuli in hanc mixturam coiciuntur, aneti videlicet et coliandri et satureiae atque sclareiae. feni graeci quoque seminis pugillus unus adicitur, et de aromatibus piperis grana triginta vel quadraginta, costi pondo denarii tres, cinnami similiter, caryophylli similiter. haec minute contrita eidem liquori permiscentur. tum vel in ferreo vel in aereo vase compositio haec tam diu coquenda est quousque ad unius sestarii mensuram perveniat. prius tamen quam percoquatur mellis despumati selibram in eam adici oportet. quae cum percocta fuerit more potionum per saccum colari debet usque ad claritatem, fervens tamen sacco infundenda est. eliquata vero et refrigerata in vase bene picato servatur ad obsonia condienda.

6. Isidore *Origines* (or *Etymologiae*) 20.3.19–20 (7th cent. A.D.):

(19) *Garum est liquor piscium salsus, qui olim conficiebatur ex pisce quem Graeci γάϱον vocabant; et quamvis nunc ex infinito genere piscium fiat, nomen tamen pristinum retinet a quo initium sumpsit.* (20) *Liquamen dictum eo quod soluti in salsamento pisciculi eundem humorem liquant. Cuius liquor appellatur salsugo vel muria.*

7. Paris Bibliothèque Nationale Ms. Lat. 11219 (=Jean Lestocquoy, "Épices, médicine et abbayes," *Études mérovingiennes. Actes des journées de Poitiers, 1–3 Mai 1952* (Paris 1952): 185–86 (8th-9th cent. A.D.):

Confectio ad garum faciendum

pisces mundos partes duos, sal partem unam, anetum partem unam; et agitas eum bene de die in diem: et de herbas quas ibidem mittere debes siccis, ad coquendum haec sunt: anetum manipulos duos, menta manipulos quattuor; nepita sclareia, origano, satureia, ambrosia, serpullo, fenogreco, de uniquaque manipulos II; et de herbis virides: cassia, salvia, savina, iva, ruta, abrotano, costo ortense radices, livestici radices, fenuculi radices, lauri folia, geniperi grana, de uniquique fasciculos duos; citonia sextarios II, poma similiter; nuces gallicas similiter, panes asatos IIII, cipiro radices pulvera sextarios II, ad unoquoque modio de pisces, mustodilce modios II, ad conjectandum postea III, et mel sextarios II; et coquis usque ad medium, ex tollis de foco, et mittis in saco, et clarare facias, et postea mittis in vaso bene picatum, ut nullum suspirium habeat.

8. *Geoponica* 20.46.1–6 (10th cent. A.D.):

Γάρων ποίησις

1) Τὸ καλούμενον λικουάμεν οὕτω γίνεται. τὰ ἔγκατα τῶν ἰχθύων βάλλεται εἰς σκεῦος, καὶ ἁλίζεται· καὶ λεπτὰ ὀψαρίδια, μάλιστα δὲ ἀθερίναι, ἢ λεπτὰ τριγλία, ἢ μαινίδια, ἢ λυκόστομοι, ἢ ὃ ἂν δόξῃ λεπτὸν εἶναι, πάντα ὁμοίως ἁλίζεται, καὶ ἐν ἡλίῳ ταριχεύεται πυκνῶς δονούμενα. 2) ὅταν δὲ ταριχευθῇ τῇ θερέᾳ, ἐξ αὐτῶν γάρος οὕτως αἴρεται. κόφινος μακρὸς πυκνὸς ἐντίθεται εἰς τὸ μεστὸν ἀγγεῖον τῶν προειρημένων ὀψαρίων, καὶ εἰσρεῖ τὸ γάρος εἰς τόν κόφινον, καὶ οὕτω διὰ τοῦ κοφίνου διηθηθὲν τὸ καλούμενον λικουάμεν ἀναιροῦντα· τὸ δὲ λοιπὸν πάτημα γίνεται ἄλιξ. 3) Βιθυνοὶ δὲ κατασκευάζουσιν οὕτως· λαμβάνεις κάλλιον μὲν εἰ μαινίδας μικρὰς ἢ μεγάλας, εἰ δὲ μή, λυκοστόμους, ἢ σαύρους, ἢ σκόμβρους, ἢ καὶ ἄλικα, καὶ πάντων μίγμα, καὶ βαλεῖς αὐτὰ εἰς μαγίδα ἀρτοκοπικήν, ἐν ᾗ εἰώθασι φυρᾶν τὸ ἄλευρον, καὶ εἰς τὸν μόδιον τῶν ἰχθύων ἁλὸς ξέστας β΄ Ἰταλικοὺς βαλὼν ἀναφύρασον, ὡς συγκραθῆναι τοῖς ἁλσί· καὶ ἐάσας ἐπὶ νύκτα μίαν βάλε ἐπὶ κεράμιον, ἀπώμαστόν τε τίθει ἐν ἡλίῳ ἐπὶ μῆνας β΄ ἢ γ΄, δονῶν αὐτὸ ῥάβδῳ ἐκ διαστημάτων, εἶτα λαβὼν καὶ πωμάσας ἀποτίθεσο. 4) τινὲς δὲ καὶ οἴνου ἐμβάλλουσι παλαιοῦ εἰς τὸν ξέστην τῶν ἰχθύων ξέστας Β΄. 5) Εἶτα εἰ βούλει εὐθέως χρήσασθαι τῷ γάρῳ, τουτέστι [τοῦ] μὴ ἡλιάσαι αὐτό, ἀλλ᾽ ἑψῆσαι, ποιήσεις οὕτως. ἅλμης στακτῆς δεδοκιμασμένης, οὕτως ὡς ᾠὸν ἐμβληθὲν ἐπιπλεῖν (ἐὰν δὲ βυθίζηται, οὔπω ἔχει ἅλας τὸ ἀρκοῦν), εἶτα βαλὼν εἰς τὴν ἅλμην τὸν ἰχθὺν ἐν κύθρᾳ καινῇ, καὶ ἐμβαλὼν ὀριγάνου, ἐπιτίθει πυρὶ αὐτάρκει, ἕως ἂν ἑψηθῇ, τουτέστιν ἕως ἂν ἄρξηται κἂν ὀλίγον ἀποποιεῖν· τινὲς καὶ ἕψημα προσβάλλουσιν· εἶτα ψυχθὲν βαλών εἰς ὑλιστῆρα δεύτερον καὶ τρίτον ἐπίῤῥιπτε τὸ αὐτὸ τῷ ὑλισττῆρι, ἕως ἂν καθαρὸν ἐκβῇ. καὶ πωμάσας ἀποτίθεσο. 6) Τὸ δὲ κάλλιον γάρος, τὸ καλούμενον αἱμάτιον, οὕτω γίνεται. λαμβάνεται τὰ ἔγκατα τοῦ θύννου μετὰ τῶν ἐμβραγχίων καὶ τοῦ ἰχῶρος καὶ τοῦ αἵματος, καὶ πάσσεται τὸ ἀρκοῦν ἅλας· καὶ ἐάσας ἐν τῷ ἀγγείῳ, [καὶ] μετὰ μῆνας β΄ τὸ πολύ, τρυπᾶς τό ἀγγεῖον, καὶ ἐξέρχεται γάρος τὸ καλούμενον αἱμάτιον.

APPENDIX II

PRODUCT DESIGNATION IN *TITULI PICTI*[1]

GARUM

Garum Flos (52)
Garum Flos Scombri (44)
Garum Flos Per Se (10)
Garum Flos Geminum (9)
Garum Scombri Flos (8)
Garum (6)
Garum Scombri (6)
Garum Flos Scombri Optimum (4)
Garum Castum (4)
Garum Flos Scombri Romulianum (3)
Garum Scombri Primum (2)
Garum Sociorum (3)
Garum Flos Flos (or Floris) (1)
Garum Flos Scombri Excellens Vetus (1)
Garum Flos Flos Murenae (1)
Garum Castum Scombri (1)
Garum Praecellens (1)
Garum Hispanum (1)
G(arum?) Histricum (1)
Garum Ostiense (1)
Garum Pompeianum (1)
Garum Vetus Excellens Antipolitanum (1)
Garum Flos Scombri Lunense (1)
Garum Secundarium (1)
Liquidum Gari (1)[2]
Garum Flos Romulianum (1)
Garum Flos Lucretianum (1)
Garum Apicianum (1)
Garum Ren(nianum) (1)[3]

---

[1] The variations are listed in an unabbreviated form without regard to individual abbreviations which may vary from one container to another. The possibilities in abbreviation have been discussed in the text. In parenthesis are found the total number of instances in which this particular form has been documented. The sources for these forms have been indicated in the text or footnotes, except where noted.

[2] Egger and Görlich, "Lebensmittelimport," p. 412.

[3] *Ibid*. This may refer to a sauce made according to the recipe of a certain Rennus or Rennius.

Garum Geticum (or coktum) (1)[4]

LIQUAMEN

Liquamen Optimum (30)
Liquamen (22)
Liquamen Flos (2)
Liquamen Flos Excellens (2)
Liquamen Flos Primum (2)
Liquamen Primum (2)
Liquamen Flos Flos (or Floris) (1)
Liquamen Flos Excellens Scombri (1)
Liquamen Flos Scombri Excellens (1)
Liquamen Optimum Scombri (1)
Liquamen Flos Optimum (1)
Liquamen Optimum Saccatum (1)
Liquamen Penuarium Excellens (1)
Liquamen Excellens (1)
Liquamen Antiatinum Excellens (1)

MURIA

Muria Flos (22)
Muria (8)
Muria Arguta Excellens Flos (2)
Muria Flos Arguta (1)
Muria Excellens (1)
Muria Casta (1)
Muria Vetus (1)
Muria Secunda (1)
Muria Flos Excellens (1)
Muria Flos Flos (or Floris) (1)
Muria Hispana (1)

HALLEX

Hallex Optima (8)
Hallex (1)[5]
Hallex Scombri (1)
Hallex Herculanensis (1)

---

[4] André, *Le vin*, p. 132, note 23. Cf. Lang, *Graffiti and Dipinti*, p. 74, no. Hd 3.

[5] A lead tessera, similar to those usually attached to amphorae (but in this case of unknown form) and found at Iulia Concordia in Histria, bore the inscription *allicium*. Though technically not a *titulus pictus*, lead tesserae did repeat some of the same elements. See Solin, "Tabelle plumbee," p. 157.

APPENDIX III

NAMES IN *TITULI PICTI*

The expectation that Romans everywhere over a period of two or three centuries (that is, the 1st to 3rd century A.D., the period which provides the bulk of our archaeological evidence) generally maintained consistency in the format of *tituli picti* may ultimately prove correct, but the state of research to date has not progressed thus far to prove it. Conclusions based on a study concentrating on a large body of material limited and well-defined in geographical area and time period would provide for greater confidence in the interpretation of names appearing in *tituli picti*. The evidence from Pompeii, Herculaneum, and neighboring villas destroyed by the eruption of Mt. Vesuvius in A.D. 79 supplies just such a source collection. It must be emphasized, however, that a rigorous proof of interpretations presented would necessitate a detailed investigation of all Pompeian *tituli picti* of all products and would require more space than is available for the present study.

As with a study showing the remarkable variety of expression in product advertisement in the fish sauce business,[1] a study of names appearing in fish sauce *tituli picti* in Campania may provide valuable clues for understanding those found in container labels for different products from other parts of the Roman Empire. This hope stems from the fact that Pompeian fish sauce labels, although they show a wide variety of forms, to a large extent belong to one man and his business organization. The name of A. Umbricius Scaurus or of someone connected with the *gens Umbricia* appears in more than fifty Campanian fish sauce *tituli picti*, over 28 percent of the total. With few exceptions these appear on urcei of Pompeian Form VI, a locally produced terracotta commercial container.[2] We know that Scaurus himself produced fish sauce in his own workshop, since some labels explicitly state as much: EX OFFICINA SCAURI. From similar labels we learn that he had freedmen who operated separate workshops.[3] Using this information

[1] Curtis, "Product Advertising," pp. 209–28. Fish sauce *tituli picti* on transport containers, primarily Italian and Spanish vessels datable to the first and second centuries A.D. and found throughout the Western Roman Empire, exhibit a remarkable variety of advertising expressions and show a high level of consistency in both format and abbreviation. This appendix appeared earlier in "A. Umbricius Scaurus of Pompeii," in *Studia Pompeiana et Classica in Honor of Wilhelmina F. Jashemski*. Robert I. Curtis, ed. 2 vols. (New Rochelle, New York 1988–89), 1: 19–49. I wish to thank the publisher for permission to reprint it here.

[2] The clay content is similar to that of amphorae produced by the Pompeian *gens Eumachia*. Liou and Marichal, "Les inscriptions," p. 165.

[3] See above p. 95.

as a kind of control data, we can, I believe, by comparison and judicious extrapolation create a reasonable list of criteria useful in interpreting other names appearing on Pompeian urcei. Names of known Pompeians (primarily members of the *gens Umbricia*) appearing on amphorae of foreign or indeterminable origin, but which were found in Campania, can also be classified according to their function *vis-à-vis* the container and its contents. Whether these criteria can be rigorously applied as well to names of non-Pompeians or of individuals of unknown origin, whose role in the fish sauce business is not precisely known from other sources and which appear on non-Pompeian amphorae, is uncertain and falls beyond the scope of this work. For the present study, therefore, I have adopted the following criteria in interpreting names appearing in *tituli picti* primarily on Campanian fish sauce vessels:

1. GENITIVE CASE

A. A name appearing in the genitive case following the phrase EX OFFICINA identifies a producer.

B. A name in the genitive case following the product identification designates either a producer or the owner of the vessel who at the same time is ultimately in charge of the production.[4] Confirmation of this latter case must come from other information identifying the person as a producer. If this information is lacking, then the person named may be a producer or someone who has purchased the vessel, for example, a retail customer, *negotiator*, or *navicularius*.[5]

C. A second name also in the genitive case probably identifies a second, or perhaps ultimate, owner of the vessel, unless information exists to indicate that the two persons mentioned are associated with each other, such as in a *societas*, and so function together as producer or merchant or shipowner.[6]

---

[4] Scaurus, a known producer, frequently placed his name in the genitive case following the product identification and preceding the indication of the workshop which produced the product; e.g. CIL IV.5690: G(ari) F(los) SCOMBR(i)/ SCAURI/ EX OFFICINA AGATHOPI. He sometimes even did this for products made in his own workshop; e.g. *CIL* IV.2574, 5694, 9406, and in mosaic urceus A of his home (Curtis, "Personalized Floor Mosaic," p. 559, and Fig. 3). There has been no example found to date, however, of one of Scaurus' freedmen who also operated a shop placing his name in the genitive case following the product identification.

[5] Andreau, *Jucundus*, p. 236; Panella, "Studio," p. 156, n. 32; Liou and Marichal, "Les inscriptions," p. 165 (Scaurus).

[6] Liou and Marichal ("Les inscriptions," p. 141) record the following label on a Dressel Form 14 amphora from Spain found at Fos-sur-mer: LIQ(uamen)/ EXC(ellens)/ SABINI ET AVITI. The names, written on the same line and joined together by the conjunction, apparently represent a *societas*, whether of producers or of merchants is indeterminable, but probably the latter. The possibility remains, however, though it seems less certain, that two names in the genitive case not joined by a conjunction and written in consecutive lines of the *titulus pictus* following the product identification might be associated together in a *societas* as well. Cf. the label GARUM SCOMBRI/ PRIMUM/ M. ACCEI TELEMACHI/ CAESIAE HELPIDIS, found in the House of the Ship Europa (Reg. I.xv.3). There is no evidence that Caesia Helpis, who was involved in the wine trade, had any connection with the *gens Accea*. Telemachus, who is otherwise unknown in Pompeii, may have been a fish sauce producer or, perhaps, a merchant who was an intermediary owner of the vessel. For the *gens Caesia*, see Della Corte, *Case*[3], p. 64, n. 2 and p. 164. I owe the reference to this label, recorded in the Daybook of Excavations at Pompeii for July,

D. A name in the genitive case following a name in the ablative case preceded by *ab* or following numbers or any other information probably designates the owner of the vessel; that is, a *negotiator* or *navicularius*.[7]

2. DATIVE CASE

A. A name appearing alone in the dative case identifies the recipient of the vessel or the intermediary owner, not a producer.[8]

B. A name in the dative case written in a color different from another *titulus pictus* on the container designates the recipient of the vessel; that is, the consumer or possibly a shopkeeper.[9]

C. A name in the dative case appearing before or after a name in the ablative case preceded by *ab* identifies the recipient of the vessel; that is, the consumer or the shopkeeper.[10]

3. FEMININE NAME IN -AE

The function of a person whose name appears as the feminine form in *-ae* without a cognomen is indeterminable, since one cannot distinguish the genitive from the dative case.[11]

4. ABLATIVE CASE

A name appearing in the ablative case preceded by *ab* identifies the consignor of the vessel. This person could be the producer himself or an employee in the workshop.[12]

1957, to the kindness of Prof. Wilhelmina Jashemski. For a vinarius who probably also sold fish sauce in his wine shop, see Wilhelmina Jashemski, "A Pompeian Vinarius," *CJ* 62 (1967): 193–204.

[7] Liou and Marichal, "Les inscriptions," pp. 131–35, no. 27; 165, no. 69; and *CIL* IV.5675.

[8] Scaurus' name never appears in the dative case. The only example I have found of a known producer whose name appears in the dative case alone is in *CIL* IV.5926: A. UMBRICIO/ ABASCANTO. Abascantus' name appears written in red paint on an amphora of undesignated form. The label lacks a product identification. This vessel, containing an unknown product, must have been sent to Abascantus. Cf. Liou and Marichal, "Les inscriptions," pp. 112–13. Other examples of names in the dative case alone on vessels found in Campania include CIL IV.5664 (Sextillus), 5722 (Junius Ampliatus), 9398 (A. Trebius Synhodus), 9429 (Pompeius Onesimus and Petutius Quintio), and most recently discovered among many Dressel Form 2–4 vessels in Villa B (Villa of L. Crassius Tertius) at Oplontis, Sextus Aconius Dorotheus (Adele Lagi De Caro, "Torre Annunziata-Oplontis-Villa B," *Bollettino dell'Associazione Internazionale Amici di Pompei* 1 [1983]: 371–72). A more doubtful example may be seen in CIL IV.10273, where the product identification appears on the shoulder of the vessel while two names in the dative case (one illegible, the other that of Pedius Leontius) were written on the handle.

[9] Andreau, *Jucundus*, p. 243; Panella, "Studio," p. 156, n. 32.

[10] Andreau, *Jucundus*, p. 243; CIL IV.5712, 6921 (Claudius Eulogus, after indication of consignor), 9394, 9418 (Claudius Eulogus, before indication of consignor), 9419. *CIL* IV.6921 presents the only example of the name appearing after that of the consignor.

[11] Andreau, *Jucundus*, p. 241; Panella, "Studio," p. 156, n. 32.

[12] Mau, *Pompei*², p. 507; *CIL* IV.2576, 5661, 5670–71, 5674–76, 5684–85, 5688, 5710, 5712–13(?), 5723–24, 5905, 6921, 9389, 9394, 9406, 9410, 9418–19, 10262, 10271. Both Umbricius Agathopus (*CIL* IV.5690, 5691 [=2580], 7110, 9403–04, 9405[?]) and Umbricius Abascantus (*CIL* IV.5689) operated their own workshops, but their names also appear in some *tituli picti* as consignors (Agathopus: *CIL* IV.5712, 6921, 9394, 9418–19; Abascantus: *CIL* IV.5671, 5685, 5724).

5. NOMINATIVE CASE

A. A name appearing in the neuter, nominative case following the product identification designates the producer or, more likely, a wholeseller who has further refined the product to his own specification.[13]

B. A name in the masculine or feminine, nominative case following or preceding the product identification probably designates the recipient or owner of the vessel, most likely the consumer as well.[14]

6. INITIALS

A name appearing as initials, almost always representing the *tria nomina*, has from the modern point of view an indeterminable function, since one cannot distinguish its grammatical case. Andreau plausibly speculates that it may represent the recipient of the vessel when the initials have been added, usually in a different color, to another *titulus pictus* and have been written in larger letters with less care. He adds that the recipient is probably an innkeeper or the like who sells the product; that is, he is a merchant himself.[15]

The criteria presented above are merely working hypotheses adopted for an attempt to describe the organization and operation of the fish sauce business in Campania. Deduced from the evidence available, they seem reasonable assumptions, but ones which have yet to be confirmed. No doubt new evidence will necessitate changes, additions, and further refinements.

---

[13] H. Dressel in his commentary to *CIL* XV.4691: G(ari) F(los)/ LUCR(etianum) / C. C(orneli) H(ermerotis). For *garum Romulianum* in Pompeii see *CIL* IV.5681, 10270, 10276–277. The garum shop at Reg. I.xii.8 may have functioned as a place where garum, prepared elsewhere, was further refined (above, pp. 92–94).

[14] *CIL* IV.5666, 9393(?).

[15] Andreau, *Jucundus*, pp. 241–42. Cf. Panella, "Studio," p. 156, n. 32. The initials C.S.D. (*CIL* IV.9402) and A.U.C. (*CIL* IV.5705) appear after Scaurus' name in the genitive case following the product identification. The initials A.U.C. could refer to an unknown freedman of Scaurus or to a family relation, but no name with these initials appears elsewhere in Pompeii. A.U.S. (*CIL* IV.5700), written in red paint on an amphora of Pompeian Form X, probably refers to Scaurus himself or perhaps to another freedman, such as A. Umbricius Successus of Puteoli (A. Maiuri in *NSc* [1927]: 333). Cf. *CIL* IV.5650, a *titulus* on an amphora of Pompeian Form VII with an illegible product designation, probably a Spanish fish sauce vessel. Below the major *titulus*, written in white on the neck of the amphora, are in red paint the initials D.C.F. and below them the name D. Caprasius Felix, written in the dative case. Here the initials and name appearing together confirm that initials should be interpreted as being in the dative case and so probably designating the recipient of the vessel.

BIBLIOGRAPHY

Alarcão, Jorge de. *Roman Portugal*. 2 vols. Warminster, England 1988.

Amano, K. "The Influence of Fermentation on the Nutritive Value of Fish with Special Reference to Fermented Fish Products of Southeast Asia," in *Fish in Nutrition*. Eirik Heen and Rudolf Kreuzer, eds. London 1962, pp. 180–200.

Aminullah Bhuiyan, A. K. M., W. M. N. Ratnayake, and R. G. Ackman. "Effect of Smoking on the Proximate Composition of Atlantic Mackerel (Scomber scombrus)." *Journal of Food Science* 51,2 (March–April 1986): 327–29.

———. R. G. Ackman, and S. P. Lall. "Effects of Smoking on Protein Quality of Atlantic Mackerel (Scomber scombrus)." *Journal of Food Processing and Preservation* 10,2 (1986): 115–26.

Amores, Fernando. "Una nueva factoría romana de salazones en Trafalgar (Cádiz)." *Habis* 9 (1978): 441–53.

Amphores Romaines et Histoire Économique. Dix Ans de Recherche. Collection de l'École Française de Rome, 114. Rome 1989.

André, Jacques, *L'Alimentation et la cuisine à Rome*. 2d ed. Paris 1981.

André, Patrick. "Les pêcheries romaines du Blavet." *Archéologie en Bretagne* 32 (1981): 43–45.

Andreau, Jean. *Les affaires de monsieur Jucundus*. Collection de l'École Française de Rome, no. 19. Rome 1974.

Andrews, Alfred C. "The 'Sardinian Fish' of the Greek and Romans." *American Journal of Philology* 70 (1949): 171–85.

Anselmino, L., et al. *Ostia IV*. Studi Miscellanei, 23. Rome 1977.

Applebaum, Shimon. "Economic Life in Palestine." in Vol. II, Chapter 14 of *The Jewish People in the First Century*. Section One of *Compendia Rerum Iudaicarum ad Novum Testamentum*. Philadelphia 1976, pp. 631–700.

Arteaga, Oswaldo. "Vorbericht über die Grabungskampagne 1976 auf dem Cerro del Mar." *Mitteilungen des Deutschen Archäologischen Instituts (Abt. Madrid)* 18 (1977): 101–15.

Arthur, Paul. "Roman Amphorae from Canterbury." *Britannia* 17 (1986): 239–58.

Athanassakis, Apostolos N., transl. and ed. *The Life of Pachomius* [*Vita Prima Graeca*]. Missoula, Montana 1975.

Bacci, G. M. "Antico stabilimento per la pesca e la lavorazione del tonno presso Portopalo." *Kokalos* 28–29 (1982–83): 345–47.

Baldacci, Paolo. "Alcuni aspetti dei commerci nei territori Cisalpini." *Atti del Centro Studi e Documentazione sull'Italia Romana* 1 (1967–68): 7–50.

Balil Illana, A. "Economía de la Hispania romana." *Estudios de economía antigua de la península ibérica*. Barcelona 1968, pp. 289–370.

———. "Un estudio sobre el 'garum'." *Archivo español de arqueología* 26 (1953): 183–85.

———. "Garum, salazones y pesquerías en el Mediterráneo hispánico." *Archivo español de arquelogía* 38 (1965): 188–89.

Baltar Veloso, R. "Una nueva interpretación de Edict. Diocl. 5, 12." *Hispania antiqua* 2 (1972): 61–68.

Baradez, Jean Lucien. "Nouvelles fouilles à Tipasa." *Libyca* 9 (1961): 7–199.

———. "Quatorze années de recherches archéologiques à Tipasa (1948–1961)." *Revue africaine* 105 (1961): 215–50.

———. *Tipasa. Ville antique de Maurètanie*. Alger 1952.

Bateman, Nic and Alison Locker. "The Sauce of the Thames." *The London Archaeologist* 4 (1982): 204–07.

Bates, Oric. "Ancient Egyptian Fishing." *Harvard African Studies* 1 (1917): 199–271.

Bean, George F. "Epitaphs at Alabanda." *Anadolu Araştirmalari* 1 (1955): 52–55.

Bebko, W. *Les épaves antiques du sud de la Corse*. Bastia 1971.

Beddows, C. G. "Fermented Fish and Fish Products." in *Microbiology of Fermented Foods*. Brian J. B. Wood ed. 2 vols. London 1985, pp. 1–39.

Belov, G. D. "Raskopki v Xersonese v 1961 g." *Soobščenija Gosudarstvennogo Ordena Lenina Érmitaža* 25 (1964): 62–65.
———. "Raskopki v Xersonese." *Soobščenija Gosudarstvennogo Ordena Lenina Érmitaža* 27 (1966): 81–83.
———. "Raskopki Xersonesa v 1961 g." *Soobščenija Xersonesskogo Muzeya* 3 (1963): 55–60.
Beltrán Lloris, Miguel. *Las ánforas romanas en España*. Monografías arqueológicas (Anejos de "Caesaraugusta") no. 8. Zaragosa 1970.
———. *Ceramica romana: tipología y clasificacion*. Zaragosa 1978.
———. "Problemas de la morfología y del concepto histórico-geográfico que recubre la noción tipo. Aportaciones a la tipología de las ánforas beticas." in *Méthodes classiques et méthodes formelles dans l'étude des amphores*. Actes du Colloque de Rome, 27–29 Mai 1974. Collection de l'École Française de Rome, no. 32. Rome 1977, pp. 97–131.
Benoit, Fernand. "Les abbayes du sel: L'héritage antique du delta au moyen-âge." *Delta* (*Revue économique et littéraire du delta du Rhône*) 3 (1961): 17–32.
———. "L'archéologie sous-marine en Provence." *Rivista di studi liguri* 18 (1952): 237–307.
———. "L'économie du littoral de la Narbonnaise à l'époque antique: le commerce du sel et les pêcheries." *Rivista di studi liguri* 15 (1959): 87–110.
———. "Épaves de la côte de Provence: Typologie des amphores." *Gallia* 14 (1956): 23–34.
———. "Nouvelles épaves de Provence." *Gallia* 16 (1958): 5–39.
———. "Nouvelles épaves de Provence (II)." *Gallia* 18 (1960): 41–56.
———. "Nouvelles épaves de Provence (III)." *Gallia* 20 (1962): 147–76.
———. *Recherches sur l'Hellénisation du Midi de la Gaule*. Aix-en-Provence 1965.
Bergonzoni, Franco. "Una industria romana nelle isole Egadi." *Antiqua* 7 (1977): 26–31.
Berti, Fede et al. *Le Terme del Nuotatore: Ostia II*. Studi Miscellanei 16. Rome 1968–1969.
Besta, Maria Carlotta. "Pesca e pescatori nell'Egitto greco-romano." *Aegyptus* 2 (1921): 67–74.
Bezeczky, Tamás. *Roman Amphorae from the Amber Route in Western Pannonia*. BAR International Series, 386. Oxford 1987.
Bisel, Sara. "The Skeletons of Herculaneum, Italy." in *Wet Site Archaeology*. Barbara A. Purdy, ed. Caldwell, N.J. 1988, pp. 207–18.
Bjelke, Erik. "Epidemiologic Studies of Cancer of the Stomach, Colon, and Rectum; With Special Emphasis on the Role of Diet." *Scandinavian Journal of Gastroenterology* 9, Suppl. 31 (1974): 1–235.
Blázquez, José Maria. *Economía de la Hispania romana*. Bilbao 1978. (Basically an updated collection of several articles on the economy of Roman Spain written since 1957).
Bodson, Liliane, ed. *Anthropozoologica*. 2d Special Number: *L'animal dans l'alimentation humaine. Les critères de choix*. Paris 1988.
Bogaers, J. E. "Nehalennia en de epigrafische Gegevens." in *Deae Nehalenniae*. Leiden 1971, pp. 32–43.
Bohlen, Diedrich. *Die Bedeutung der Fischerei für die antike Wirtschaft*. Hamburg 1937.
Bohn, Oskar. "Pinselschriften auf Amphoren aus Augst und Windisch." *Anzeiger für schweizerische Altertumskunde* (*Indicateur d'antiquités suisses*) 28 (1926): 197–212.
Bolkestein, H. *Economic Life in Greece's Golden Age*. 2nd ed. rev. by E. J. Jonkers. Leiden 1958.
Bonifay, Michel, Gaëtan Conges, and Martine Leguilloux. "Amphores tardives (V[e] - VIIe siècle) à Arles et à Marseille." in *Amphores Romaines et Histoire Économique. Dix Ans de Recherche*. Collection de l'École Française de Rome, 114. Rome 1989, pp. 660–63.
Bonneville, Jean-Noël, François Didierjean, Nicole Dupre, Pierre Jacob, Janine Lancha, Myriam Fincker, Claude Ney, and Jean-Louis Paillet. "La dix-huitième campagne de fouilles de la Casa de Velazquez à Belo en 1983 (Bolonia, province de Cadix)." *Mélanges de la Casa de Velazquez* 20 (1984): 439–86.
Bowman, Alan K. "Roman Military Records from Vindolanda." *Britannia* 5 (1974): 360–73.
Braekkan, Olaf R. "B-Vitamins in Some Fish Products." in *Fish in Nutrition*. Eirik Heen and Rudolf Kreuzer, eds. London 1962, pp. 141–45.
Brašinskij, I. B. "Recherches soviétiques sur les monuments antiques des régions de la Mer Noire." *Eirene* 7 (1968): 81–118.
Breasted, J. H. *Ancient Records of Egypt*. 5 vols. Chicago 1906.
Brisay, K. W. De and K. A. Evans (eds.). *Salt. The Study of an Ancient Industry*. Colchester 1975.
Brooks, Roger I. and G. A. Reineccius. "Identification of Neutral and Basic Flavor Compounds in Fermented Fish Sauce." Abstract, *Papers of the American Chemical Society* 172 (1976): AGFD 158.

Broughton, T. Robert S. "Some Notes on Trade and Traders in Roman Spain." in *Studies in Honor of Edward Togo Salmon*. Toronto 1974, pp. 11–30.

Brown, John Pairman. *The Lebanon and Phoenicia*. Vol. 1. Beirut 1969.

Buchi, Ezio. "Banchi di anfore romane a Verona. Note sui commerci Cisalpina." in *Il territorio veronese in età romana*. Atti del convegno del 22–23–24 Ottobre 1971. Verona 1972, pp. 531–650.

Callender, M. H. *Roman Amphorae*. London 1965.

Caprotti, Erminio. "Molluschi e Medicina nel I° Secolo d.C." *Conchiglie* 13 (1977): 137–44.

Carandini, Andrea and Clementina Panella et al. *Le Terme del Nuotatore: Ostia III*. (parte seconda). Studi Miscellanei 21. Rome 1972.

———. and Clementina Panella. "The Trading Connections of Rome and Central Italy in the Late Second and Third Centuries: the Evidence of the Terme del Nuotatore Excavations, Ostia." in *The Roman West in the Third Century*. Anthony King and Martin Henig, eds. 2 Vols. BAR International Series, 109. Oxford 1981, Part ii: pp. 487–503.

Cardoso, Guilherme. "Ânforas romanas no Museu do Mar (Cascais)." *Conimbriga* 17 (1978): 63–78.

Carignani, Andrea and Francesco Pacetti. "Anfore tardo-antiche dagli scavi del Palatino." in *Amphores Romaines et Histoire Économique. Dix Ans de Recherche*. Collection de l'École Française de Rome, 114. Rome 1989, pp. 610–15.

Cheftel, Henri. "The Processing of the Anchovy: Engraulis encrasilicholus Linnaeus." in *Fish as Food*. Georg Borgström, ed. 4 vols. New York 1965, 3: 219–25.

Cisneros, Maria Josefa Jiménez. "Beobachtungen in einen römischen Töpferbezirk bei Puerto Real, Prov. Cadiz." *Germania* 36 (1958): 469–75.

Clauson, N. Y. "A Customs House Registry from Roman Egypt (P. Wisconsin 16)." *Aegyptus* 9 (1928): 240–80.

Cleere, Henry. "Roman Harbours in Britain South of Hadrian's Wall." in *Roman Shipping and Trade: Britain and the Rhine Provinces*. Joan du Plat Taylor and Henry Cleere, eds. Research Report No. 24. London 1978, pp. 36–40.

Clergues, J. H. "Fichier d'archéologie sous-marine du secteur d'Antibes." *Cahiers d'archéologique subaquatique* 1 (1972): 53–62.

———. "Les fouilles de la plaine d'Antibes: Vaugrenier. Note préliminaire." *Rivista di studi liguri* 35 (1969): 171–88.

Colls, Dali et al. *L'épave Port-Vendres II et le commerce de la Bétique à l'époque de Claude. Archaeonautica* 1 (1977).

———. Claude Domergue and Victor Guerrero Ayuso. "Les lingots de plomb de l'épave romaine *Cabrera 5* (île de Cabrera, Baléares)." *Archaeonautica* 6 (1986): 31–80.

Corcoran, Thomas H. "Pliny's *Garum Castimoniarum*." *Classical Bulletin* 34 (1958): 69.

———. "Roman Fish Sauces." *Classical Journal* 58 (1963): 204–10.

———. "The Roman Fishing Industry of the Late Republic and Early Empire." Ph.D. dissertation, Northwestern University, 1957.

Cotte, J. *Poissons et animaux aquatiques au temps de Pline*. Paris 1944.

Creac'h, Paul. "Un actuel 'Garum' français: le Pissala. La pêche du Nonnat et de la Poutine." *Pêches Maritimes* (Institut Scientifique et Technique des Pêches Maritimes, Paris) 17 (1952): 57–60.

Crisan, Eli V. and Anne Sands. "Microflora of Four Fermented Fish Sauces." *Applied Microbiology* 29,1 (Jan. 1975): 106–08.

Curtis, Robert I. "A. Umbricius Scaurus of Pompeii." in *Studia Pompeiana et Classica in Honor of Wilhelmina F. Jashemski*. 2 vols. New Rochelle, N.Y. 1988–89, 1: 19–49.

———. "The Garum Shop of Pompeii (I. 12. 8)." *Cronache Pompeiane* 5 (1979): 5–23.

———. "In Defense of Garum." *Classical Journal* 78, 3 (Feb.-Mar. 1983): 232–40.

———. "*Negotiatores Allecarii* and the Herring." *Phoenix* 38 (1984): 147–58.

———. "A Personalized Floor Mosaic from Pompeii." *American Journal of Archaeology* 88 (1984): 557–66.

———. "Product Identification and Advertising on Roman Commercial Amphorae." *Ancient Society* 15–17 (1984–1986): 209–28.

———. "The Salted Fish Industry of Pompeii." *Archaeology* 37,6 (Nov.-Dec. 1984): 58–59, 74–75.

———. "Salted Fish Products in Ancient Medicine." *Journal of the History of Medicine and Allied Sciences* 39,4 (Oct. 1984): 430–45.

———. "A Slur on Lucius Asicius, the Pompeian Gladiator." *Transactions of the American Philological Association* 110 (1980): 51–61.

———. "Spanish Trade in Salted Fish Products in the 1st and 2nd Centuries A.D." *International Journal of Nautical Archaeology and Underwater Exploration* 17,3 (1988): 205–10.

Cutting, Charles L. *Fish Saving. A History of Fish Processing from Ancient to Modern Times.* London 1955.

———. "The Influence of Drying, Salting and Smoking on the Nutritive Value of Fish." in *Fish in Nutrition.* Eirik Heen and Rudolf Kreuzer, eds. London 1962, pp. 161–79.

———. "Smoking." in *Fish as Food.* Georg Borgström, ed. 4 vols. New York 1965, 3: 55–105.

Cuvier, Baron and M. Valenciennes. "Account of the Common Mackerel, (Scomber scombrus, Lin.) and the Garum of the Ancients." *Edinburgh Journal of Science* n. s. 6 (1832): 286–94.

Dagron, Gilbert and Denis Feissel. *Inscriptions de Cilicie.* Travaux et Mémoires du Centre de Recherche d'Histoire et Civilisation de Byzance. Monographies 4. Paris 1987.

Daniel, Robert W. and Rosario Pintaudi, "PSI XII 1263 recto: Conti amministrativi." *Aegyptus* 64 (1984): 61–67.

Dardaine, Sylvie and Jean-Noël Bonneville, "La campagne de fouilles d'Octobre 1979 à Belo." *Mélanges de la Casa de Velazquez* 16 (1980): 375–419.

Darmon, Jean-Pierre. "Néapolis." *Africa* 2 (1968): 271–83.

———. "Note sur le Tarif de Zaraï." *Les cahiers de Tunisie* 48 (1964): 6–23.

Degrassi, Attilio. "Aquileia e l'Istria in età romana." *Studi Aquileiesi offerti il 7 Ottobre 1953 a Giovanni Brusin nel suo 70. compleanno.* Aquileia 1953, pp. 51–65.

Desbat, Armand, Robert Lequément, and Bernard Liou. "Inscriptions peintes sur amphores: Lyon et Saint-Romain-en-Gal." *Archaeonautica* 7 (1987): 141–66.

——— and Stéfanie Martin-Kilcher, "Les amphores sur l'axe Rhône-Rhin à l'époque d'Auguste." in *Amphores Romaines et Histoire Économique. Dix Ans de Recherche.* Collection de l'École Française de Rome, 114. Rome 1989, pp. 339–65.

Desse, Georges. "Sur un condiment marin." in *Archéologie et Médecine. VIIèmes Recontres Internationales d'Archéologie et d'Histoire, Antibes, Octobre 1986.* Juan-les-Pins 1987, pp. 479–88.

Dias Diogo, A. M. "Fornos de ânforas do Monte da Enchurrasqueira e do Vale da Cepa. Notícia preliminar." *Conimbriga* 22 (1983): 209–15.

Donnadieu, A. "Les fouilles des ruines gallo-romaines de Villepey (Villa Podii) près Fréjus (Forum Julii)." *Mémoires de l'institute des fouilles de Provence et des Préalpes* 1 (1926–1929): 129–49.

Dressel, Heinrich. "Aus dem Bonner Provinzialmuseum." *Jahrbücher des Vereins von Alterthumsfreunden im Rheinlande* 95 (1894): 61–87.

———. "Di un grande deposito di anfore rinvenuto nel nuovo quartiere del Castro Pretorio." *Bullettino della commissione archeologica comunale di Roma* 7 (1879): 36–112, 143–95.

Driesch, Angela von den. "Osteoarchäologische Auswertung von Garum-resten des Cerro del Mar." *Mitteilungen des Deutschen Archäologischen Instituts (Abt. Madrid)* 21 (1980): 151–54.

Dumont, Jacques. "Liberté des mers et territoire de pêche en droit grec." *Revue historique du droit française et étranger* (1977): 53–57.

———. "La pêche dans le Fayoum hellénistique: traditions et nouveautés d'après le Papyrus Tebtynis 701." *Chronique d'Égypte* 52 (1977): 125–42.

———. "La pêche du thon à Byzance à l'époque hellénistique." *Revue des études anciennes* 78–79 (1976–1977): 96–117.

Eberl, Georg. *Die Fischkonserven der Alten.* Stadtamhof 1892.

Edelstein, Ludwig. "The Dietetics of Antiquity." in *Ancient Medicine. Selected Papers of Ludwig Edelstein.* Oswei Temkin and C. Lilian Temkin, eds. Baltimore 1967, pp. 303–16.

Edmondson, J. C. *Two Industries in Roman Lusitania: Mining and Garum Production.* BAR International Series, 362. Oxford 1987.

Egger, Rudolf and Walter Görlich. "Der Lebensmittelimport aus Italien auf den Magdalensberg." *Carinthia* 1 (1969): 410–16.

Estácio Da Veiga Affonso Dos Santos, Maria Luísa. *Arqueologia romana do Algarve.* 2 vols. Lisbon 1971.

Esteve Guerrero, Manuel. "Sanlúcar de Barrameda (Cadiz): Fábrica de salazón romana en La Algaida." *Noticiario arqueológico hispánico* 1–3 (1952): 126–33.

Étienne, Robert. "A propos du 'garum sociorum'." *Latomus* 29 (1970): 297–313.

———. *La Vie quotidienne à Pompéi.* 2d ed. Paris 1974.

Ettlinger, Elisabeth. "Aspects of Amphora-typology,—Seen from the North." in *Méthodes clas-*

siques et méthodes formelles dans l'étude des amphores. Actes du Colloque de Rome, 27–29 Mai 1974. Collection de l'École Française de Rome. Rome 1977, pp. 9–16.

———. and Christoph Simonett. *Römische Keramik aus dem Schutthügel von Vindonissa*. Veröffentlichungen der Gesellschaft pro Vindonissa. Bd. 3. Basel 1952.

Evans, A. K. B. "Pottery and History." in *Roman Pottery Research in Britain and North-West Europe. Papers Presented to Graham Webster*, Part ii. A. C. Anderson and A. S. Anderson, eds. BAR International Series, 123. Oxford 1981, pp. 517–35.

Fernández-Chicarro, Concepción. "Actividades arqueológicas en Andalucía." *Archivo español de arqueología* 26 (1953): 435–43.

Ferri, Silvio. "La pesca del tonno nell'Adriatico in una stele garganica." *Magna Graecia* 5, no. 11–12 (Nov.–Dec. 1970): 1–3.

Février, Paul-Albert. "Les récents travaux archéologiques effectués à Fréjus (Var)." *Bulletin de la société nationale des antiquaires de France* (1976): 25–30.

Filsinger, Beatriz E. "Effect of Pressure on the Salting and Ripening Process of Anchovies (engraulis anchoita)." *Journal of Food Science* 52,4 (July–Aug. 1987): 919–27.

———. C. A. Barassi, H. M. Lupin, and R. E. Trucco. "An Objective Index for the Evaluation of the Ripening of Salted Anchovy." *Journal of Food Technology* 17,2 (1982): 193–200.

Flower, Barbara and Elisabeth Rosenbaum. *Apicius: The Roman Cookery Book*. London 1958.

Foerster, Federico. "Spain: Riells-La Clota." *International Journal of Nautical Archaeology and Underwater Exploration* 7 (1978): 163.

Forbes, R. J. *Studies in Ancient Technology*. Vol. III. Leiden 1955.

Formazov, A. A. et al. "The Most Important Recent Archaeological Discoveries made in European Russia." in *Recent Archaeological Excavations in Europe*. Rupert Bruce-Mitford, ed. London 1975, pp. 188–226, esp. Section III by D. B. Shelov, "Scythians, Sarmatians and Greeks: Recent Works." pp. 208–20.

Formigé, Jules. "La station antique de Lero à l'île Sainte-Marguerite (Alpes-Maritimes)." *Gallia* 5 (1947): 146–55.

Foucher, Louis. "Note sur l'industrie et le commerce des salsamenta et du garum." in *Actes du 93e Congrès National des Sociétés Savantes, Tours, 1968. Section d'archéologie*. Paris 1970, pp. 17–21.

Frutos, G. de, G. Chic, and N. Berriatua. "Las anforas de la factoría preromana de salazones de 'Las Redes' (Puerto de Santa Maria, Cadiz)." in *Actas Ier Congreso Peninsular de Historia Antigua*. G. Pereira Menaut, ed. Santiago de Compostela 1988, 1: 295–306.

Gajdukevič, Viktor F. "Bosporskie goroda v svete arxeologičeskix issledovanij poslednix dvux desjatiletij." in *Arxeologija i Istorija Bospora*. Simferopol 1952, pp. 19–42.

———. *Das Bosporanische Reich*. Berlin 1971.

———. *Mirmekij*. Warsaw 1959.

———. "Raskopki Mirmekija v 1935–1938 gg." *Materialy i Issledovanija po Arxeologii SSSR*. No. 25. Moscow 1952, pp. 135–220.

———. "Raskopki Mirmekija i Tiritaki, arxeologičeskie razvedki na Kerčeskom poluostrove v 1937–1939 gg." *Vestnik Drevnej Istorii* 3–4 (1940): 300–17.

———. "Raskopki Tiritaki v 1935–1940 gg." *Materialy i Issledovanija po Arxeologii SSSR*. No. 25. Moscow 1952, pp. 15–134.

———. "Raskopki Tiritaki i Mirmekija v 1946–1952 gg." *Materialy i Issledovanija po Arxeologii SSSR*. No. 85. Moscow 1958, pp. 149–85.

Gallant, T. W. *A Fisherman's Tale*. Miscellanea Graeca, Fasc. 7. Gent 1985.

Galliou, Patrick. *L'Armorique romaine*. Braspars 1984.

———. "Celtic Permanence or Roman Change? Roman Brittany Revisited." *Oxford Journal of Archaeology* 5,1 (1986): 67–76.

———. "Les industries de salaisons en Armorique romaine." *Caesarodunum* 10 (1975): 141–47.

———. "Western Gaul in the Third Century." in *The Roman West in the Third Century*. Anthony King and Martin Henig, eds. BAR International Series, 109. Oxford 1981, pp. 259–86.

———. and René Sanquer. "L'industrie du garum et des salaisons en Armorique romaine." *Caesarodunum* 10 (1975): 157–58.

Gamer, Gustav. "Antike Anlagen zur Fischverarbeitung in Hispanien und Mauretanien." *Antike Welt* 18,2 (1987): 19–28.

García y Bellido, Antonio. "La industria pesquera y conserva española en la Antiqüedad." *Investigación y Progreso* 13 (1942): 1–8.

Garcia del Toro, Javier. R. "*Garum sociorum*. La industria de salazones de pescado en la Edad

Antigua en Cartagena." *Anales de la Universidad de Murcia* 36 (1979): 27–57.

Garlake, P. S. "A Fish-curing Complex on Ras Abaruk, Site 6." in *Qatar Archaeological Report: Excavations 1973*. Beatrice De Cardi, ed. Oxford 1978, pp. 136–46.

Gemmill, Chalmers L. "Silphium." *Bulletin of the History of Medicine* 40,4 (July–Aug. 1966): 295–313.

Georgacas, Demetrius J. *Ichthyological Terms for the Sturgeon, and Etymology of the International Terms Botargo, Caviar and Congeners*. Athens 1978.

Giacobbi-Lequément, Marie-France. "La céramique de l'épave *Fos 1*." *Archaeonautica* 7 (1987): 167–91.

Gibbins, D. J. L and A. J. Parker. "The Roman Wreck of c. AD 200 at Plemmirio, near Siracusa (Sicily): Interim Report." *International Journal of Nautical Archaeology and Underwater Exploration* 15,4 (1986): 267–304.

Gignac, Francis T. *A Grammar of the Greek Papyri of the Roman and Byzantine Periods*. Vol. II: *Morphology*. Milan 1981.

Glucker, Carol A. M. *The City of Gaza in the Roman and Byzantine Periods*. BAR International Series, 325. Oxford 1987.

Gorges, Jean-Gérard. *Les villas hispano-romaines. Inventaire et problématiques archéologiques*. Paris 1979.

Gren, Erik. *Kleinasien und der Ostbalkan in der wirtschaftlichen Entwicklung der römischen Kaiserzeit*. Uppsala Universitets Årsskrift, No. 9. Uppsala 1949.

Grenier, Albert. "Le garum de Fréjus." *Revue des études anciennes* 34 (1932): 291–92.

———. "Le matériel de la navigation les amphores." in Vol. 2 of *Manuel d'archéologie gallo-romaine*. Paris 1934, pp. 601–42.

———. and Thomas Monod. "Sur la véritable nature du 'garum'." *Revue des études anciennes* 54 (1952): 27–38.

Guha, B. C. "The Role of Fish in Human Nutrition." in *Fish in Nutrition*. Eirik Heen and Rudolf Kreuzer, eds. London 1962, pp. 39–42.

Haenszel, William, Minoru Kurihara, Mitsuo Segi, and Richard K. C. Lee. "Stomach Cancer Among Japanese in Hawaii." *Journal of the National Cancer Institute* 49 (1972): 969–88.

———. Minoru Kurihara, Frances B. Locke, Kiyoshi Shimuzu, and Mitsuo Segi. "Stomach Cancer in Japan." *Journal of the National Cancer Institute* 56 (1976): 265–74.

Hamm, William S. and John A. Clague. *Temperature and Salt Purity Effects on the Manufacture of Fish Paste and Sauce*. Fish and Wildlife Service Research Report, 24. Washington, D.C. 1950.

Hassall, Mark. "Britain and the Rhine Provinces: Epigraphic Evidence for Roman Trade." in *Roman Shipping and Trade: Britain and the Rhine Provinces*. Joan du Plat Taylor and Henry Cleere, eds. Research Report No. 24. London 1978, pp. 41–48.

———. and R. S. O. Tomlin, "Roman Britain in 1981. II. Inscriptions." *Britannia* 13 (1982): 417, nos. 60–62.

———. and R. S. O. Tomlin, "Roman Britain in 1983. II. Inscriptions." *Britannia* 15 (1984): 344, no. 37.

Hayes, J. W. "The Villa Dionysos Excavations, Knossos: the Pottery." *Annual of the British School at Athens* 78 (1983): 97–169.

Hennig, Dieter. "Die 'heiligen Häuser' von Delos." *Chiron* 13 (1983): 411–95.

Hesnard, A. "Un dépôt augustéen d'amphores à la Longarina, Ostie." in *The Seaborne Commerce of Ancient Rome: Studies in Archaeology and History*. MAAR, vol. 36. Rome 1980, pp. 141–56.

Hess, E. "Fishery Products of Indochina." in *The Technology of Herring Utilization*. M. Jul and M. Kondrup, eds. Bergen 1953, pp. 131–44.

Höppener, Henk. *Halieutica: Bijdrage tot de Kennis der oud-grieksche Visscherij*. Amsterdam 1931.

Hughes, John P. and R. Gordon Wasson. "The Etymology of 'Botargo'." *American Journal of Philology* 68 (1947): 414–18.

Iria, Alberto. "As pescarias no Algarve." *Conservas de Peixe* 8, no. 90 (September 1953): 13–15; 8, no. 91 (October 1953): 15–16; 8, no. 92 (November 1953): 15–16; 8, no. 93 (December 1953): 15–16.

———. "As ruínas de tanques de salga de peixe encontradas recentemente em Olhão." *Industria Portuguesa* 273 (1950): 727–32.

Ishidate, Morizo, Akio Tanimura, Yoshio Ito, Ayako Sakai, Hiroko Sakuta, Taro Kawamura,

Keiichi Sakai, Fumio Miyazawa, and Hiroshi Wada. "Secondary Amines, Nitrites and Nitrosamines in Japanese Foods." in *Topics in Chemical Carcinogenesis*. Proceedings of the 2nd International Symposium of the Princess Takamatsu Cancer Research Fund. Waro Nakahara, Shozo Takayama, Takashi Sugimura, and Shigeyoshi Odashima, eds. Baltimore 1972, pp. 313–21.

Jardin, Claude. "Garum et sauces de poisson de l'antiquité." *Rivista di studi liguri* 27 (1961): 70–96.

Jashemski, Wilhelmina. "A Pompeian *Vinarius*." *Classical Journal* 62,5 (1967): 193–204.

Jehasse, Jean. "Les fouilles d'Aléria (Corse): l'acropole et ses problèmes (1962)." *Gallia* 21 (1963): 77–109.

Jodin, André. *Les établissements du roi Juba II aux îles Purpuraires (Mogador)*. Tanger 1967.

Joncheray, Jean-Pierre. *Essai de classification des amphores découvertes lors de fouilles sous-marines*. Fréjus 1970.

Jones, W. H. S. "Ancient Roman Folk Medicine." *Journal of the History of Medicine and Allied Sciences* 12 (1957): 459–72.

Kadeev, Vladimir I. *Očerki Istorii Èkonomiki Xersonesa Tavričeskogo v I-IV vekax n.è.* Xar'kov 1970.

———. and S. G. Rižov. "Nova ribozasoljuval'na cisterna u Xersonesi." *Arxeologia* 12 (1973): 76–80.

Keay, Simon J. "The Conventus Tarraconensis in the Third Century A.D.: Crisis or Change?" in *The Roman West in the Third Century*. Anthony King and Martin Henig, eds. BAR International Series, 109. Oxford 1981, pp. 451–86.

———. *Late Roman Amphorae in the Western Mediterranean. A Typology and Economic Study: the Catalan Evidence*. 2 Vols. BAR International Series, 196. Oxford 1984.

Keen, Richard. "Great Britain: Guernsey, Channel Islands: Little Russel Amphora Site A." *International Journal of Nautical Archaeology and Underwater Exploration* 8,1 (1979): 87.

Keimer, L. "La boutargue dans l'Égypte ancienne." *Bulletin de l'institut d'Égypte*. Ser. 6, 21 (1938–39): 215–43.

Keller, Otto. *Die antike Tierwelt*. 2 vols. Leipzig 1909, 1913.

Köhler, [?]. "Τάριχος ou recherches sur l'histoire et les antiquités des pêcheries de la Russie méridionale." *Mémoires de l'Académie Impériale de Sciences de St. Petersburg*. Sixième série, tome 1, 1832.

Kolendo, Jerzy. "Parcs à huîtres et viviers sur un flacons en verre du Musée National de Varsovie." *Travaux du Centre d'Archéologie Méditerranéenne de l'Académie Polonaise des Sciences*. Tome 18. Études de Travaux IX. Warsaw 1976, pp. 143–58.

Koller, R. "Die Pökelung im Altertum." *Schlachthofwesen Lebensmittelüberwachung (Beilage zur Deutschen Tierärztlichen Wochenschrift)* 17 (1939): 549–51.

Kolonel, Laurence N., Abraham M. Y. Nomura, Tomio Hirohata, Jean H. Hankin, and M. Ward Hinds. "Association of Diet and Place of Birth with Stomach Cancer Incidence in Hawaii Japanese and Caucasians." *The American Journal of Clinical Nutrition* 34 (1981): 2478–85.

Krauss, Samuel. *Talmudische Archäologie*. 3 vols. Leipzig 1910.

Labrousse, Michel. "Recherches sur l'alimentation des populations gallo-romaines: escargots, huîtres et fruits de mer à Montmaurin." *Pallas* 8 (1959): 57–84.

Lang, Mabel. *Graffiti and Dipinti*. Vol. 21 of *The Athenian Agora*. Princeton, N.J. 1976.

Lassus, Jean. "Chronique l'archéologie algerienne en 1956." *Libyca* 5 (1957): 123–52.

Laubenheimer, Fanette. "Les amphores Gauloises sous l'Empire: recherches nouvelles sur leur production et leur chronologie." in *Amphores Romaines et Histoire Économique. Dix Ans de Recherche*. Collection de l'École Française de Rome, 114. Rome 1989, pp. 105–38.

Lauffer, Siegfried. *Diokletians Preisedikt*. Berlin 1971.

Lebedev, V. D. and Ju. E. Lapin. "K voprosu o rybolovstve v Bosporskom carstve." *Materialy i Issledovanija po Arxeologii SSSR*. No. 33. Moscow 1954, pp. 197–214.

Leglay, Marcel. "Cartennae, Ténès, région (Mauretania Caesariensis, Algeria: Alger). 5239: Fouilles et découvertes." *Fasti Archaeologici* 9 (1956): 377.

Lequément, Robert. "Une épave du Bas-Empire dans la baie de Pampelonne (presqu'île de Saint Tropez)." *Revue archéologique de Narbonnaise* 9 (1976): 177–88.

———. "Etiquettes de plomb sur des amphores d'Afrique." *Mélanges d'archéologie et d'histoire de l'École Française de Rome* 85 (1975): 667–80.

Lewis, David M. "Attic Manumissions." *Hesperia* 28 (1959): 208–38.

———. "Dedications of Phialai at Athens." *Hesperia* 37 (1968): 368–80.
Lijinsky, William and Samuel S. Epstein. "Nitrosamines as Environmental Carcinogens." *Nature* 225 (Jan. 3, 1970): 21–23.
Liou, Bernard. "France: Port-Vendres (Pyrénées-Orientales)." *International Journal of Nautical Archaeology and Underwater Exploration* 4 (1975): 373–74.
———. "Informations archéologiques. Corse du Sud." *Gallia* 40 (1982): 439–54.
———. "Inscriptions peintes sur amphores: Fos (suite), Marseille, Toulon, Port-la-Nautique, Arles, Saint-Blaise, Saint-Martin-de-Crau, Mâcon, Calvi." *Archaeonautica* 7 (1987): 55–139.
———. and P. Pomey. "Informations archéologiques. Pyrénées-orientales: Port-Vendres." *Gallia* 43 (1985): 547–51.
———. and Robert Marichal. "Les inscriptions peintes sur amphores de l'Anse Saint-Gervais à Fos-sur-mer." *Archaeonautica* 2 (1978): 109–81.
MacKendrick, Paul. *The Iberian Stones Speak*. New York 1969.
Mackie, I. M., R. Hardy and G. Hobbs. *Fermented Fish Products*. FAO Fisheries Reports, No. 100. Rome 1971.
MacKinney, Loren C. "Animal Substances in Materia Medica: A Study in the Persistence of the Primitive." *Journal of the History of Medicine and Allied Sciences* 1 (1946): 149–70.
Maia, Manuel. "Contribuição para o estudo das ânforas romanas de Tróia—ânforas do tipo 'Africano Grande'." *Setúbal Arqueológica* 1 (1975): 155–58.
Maiuri, Amedeo. "Dalle anfore esce l'odore della salsa di 2000 anni fa." *Corriere della Sera* (Milan). 26 January 1961, p. 3 (= "La Bottega del Salsamentario." in *Amedeo Maiuri Mestiere d'Archelologo* [Naples 1978], pp. 635–36).
Manacorda, Daniele. "Anfore spagnole a Pompei." in *L'instrumentum domesticum di Ercolano e Pompei nella prima età imperiale*. Quaderni di cultura materiale, 1. Rome 1977, pp. 121–33.
Maniatis, Y., R. E. Jones, I. K. Whitbread, A. Kostikas, A. Simopoulos, Ch. Karakalos, and C. K. Williams, II. "Punic Amphoras Found at Corinth, Greece: an Investigation of their Origin and Technology." *Journal of Field Archaeology* 11 (1984): 205–22.
Marquardt, Joachim. *Das Privatleben der Römer*. Leipzig 1882.
Martin, Gabriela. "Las pesquerías romanas de la costa de Alicante." in *Trabajos de arqueología dedicados a D. Pío Beltrán*. Papeles del laboratorio de arquelogía de Valencia, no. 10. Valencia 1970, pp. 139–53.
———. and Maria Dolores Serres. *La factoría pesquera de Punta de l'Arenal y otros restos romanos de Jávea (Alicante)*. Serie de trabajos varios, no. 38. Valencia 1970.
Martin-Bueno, Manuel, Jesús Liz Guiral, and María Luisa Cancela Ramirez de Arellano. "Baelo Claudia: Sector sur 1981–1983 (Avance)." *Mélanges de la Casa de Velazquez* 20 (1984): 487–96.
Martin-Kilcher, Stéfanie. "Fischsaucen und Fischkonserven aus dem römischen Gallien." *Archäologie der Schweiz* 13 (1990): 37–44.
Marty-Laveaux, Ch. *Les oeuvrés de Maistre François Rabelais*. Vol. 3. Paris 1873.
Masterman, E. W. G. "The Fisheries of Galilee." *Palestine Exploration Fund* (1908): 40–51.
Matthews, J. F. "The Tax Law of Palmyra: Evidence for Economic History in a City of the Roman East." *Journal of Roman Studies* 74 (1984): 157–80.
Mau, August. *Pompeii, Its Life and Art*. Francis W. Kelsey, transl. 2nd ed. New York 1902.
McCann, Anna Marguerite, Joanne Bourgeois, Elaine K. Gazda, John Peter Oleson, and Elizabeth Lyding Will. *The Roman Port and Fishery of Cosa*. Princeton, N.J. 1987.
Mesquita de Figueiredo, Antonio. "Ruines d'antiques établissements à salaisons sur le littoral sud du Portugal." *Bulletin hispanique* 8 (1906): 109–21.
Miller, S. A., H. A. Dymsza, and S. A. Goldblith. "The nutritive Value of Sardines." in *Fish in Nutrition*. Eirik Heen and Rudolf Kreuzer, eds. London 1962, pp. 295–97.
Milne, Gustav. *The Port of Roman London*. London 1985.
Minns, Ellis H. *Scythians and Greeks*. 2 vols. Cambridge 1913.
Mirčev, Milko. "Novi epigrafski pametnici ot Černomorieto." *Arxeologičesko Druženstvo (Varna), Izvestija* 12 (1961): 7–21.
Mongait, Alexander. *Archaeology in the USSR*. David Skvirsky, transl. Moscow 1959.
Monguilan, L. "Geographie commerciale de la Gaule. Un port romain dans le Golfe de Fos." *Caesarodunum* 12 (1977): 359–70.
Moreno Páramo, A. and L. Abad Casal. "Aportaciones al estudio de la pesca en la antiqüedad." *Habis* 2 (1971): 209–21.

Moulé, Léon. "La Zootherapie au temps de Dioscorde et de Pline." in *1er Congrès de l'Histoire de l'Art de Guérir (Anvers, 7–12 août 1920).* Anvers 1921, pp. 451–61.
Muñoz Vincent, Ángel, Gregorio de Frutos Reyes, and Nerea Berriatua Hernández. "Contribución a los orígenes y difusión comercial de la industria pesquera y conservera Gaditana a Través de las recientes aportaciones de las factorías de salazones de la Bahía de Cadiz." in *Congreso Internacional el Estrecho de Gibraltar Ceuta, Noviembre 1987* (Distancia 1989[?]), pp. 487–508.
Nicolini, Gérard. "Informations archéologiques: Charente-Maritime." *Gallia* 35 (1977): 376–77.
Nolla, J. M. and F. J. Nieto. "Una factoria de salaó de peix a Roses." *Fonaments* 3 (1981): 187–200.
Nolla-Brufau, J. M. "Excavaciones recientes en la ciudadela de Roses. El edificio Bajo-imperial." in *Papers in Iberian Archaeology*. T. F.C. Blagg, R. F. J. Jones, and S.J. Keay, eds. BAR International Series, 193 (ii). Oxford 1984, pp. 430–59.
Nutton, Vivian. "The Drug Trade in Antiquity." *Journal of the Royal Society of Medicine* 78,2 (1985): 138–45.
Oliver, James H. "Texts A and B of the Horothesia Dossier at Istros." *Greek, Roman, Byzantine Studies* 6 (1975): 143–56.
Orejana, Florian M. and John Liston. "Agents of Proteolysis and Its Inhibition in Patis (Fish Sauce) Fermentation." *Journal of Food Science* 47,1 (Jan.-Feb. 1982): 198–209.
Owens, J. D. and L. S. Mendoza. "Enzymically Hydrolysed and Bacterially Fermented Fishery Products." *Journal of Food Technology* 20,3 (June 1985): 273–93.
Pace, Biagio. *Arte e civiltà della Sicilia antica.* 2 vols. Milan 1935.
Padilla Monge, Aurelio. *La provincia romana de la Betica (253–422).* Écija 1989.
Pais, Ettore. *Storia della Sardegna e della Corsica durante il dominio romano.* 2 vols. Rome 1923.
Panella, Clementina. "Annotazioni in margine alle stratigrafie delle Terme ostiensi del Nuotatore." in *Recherches sur les amphores romaines.* Collection de l'École Française de Rome, no. 10. Rome 1972, pp. 69-106.
———. "Per uno studio delle anfore di Pompei." in *In Memoria di Giovanni Becatti.* Studi Miscellanei 22. Rome 1977, pp. 151–65.
Parássoglou, G. M. "A Lease of Fishing Rights." *Aegyptus* 67 (1987): 89–93.
Pareja, Félix. "Marques sur une amphore de l'île de Fraile (Aguilas)." *Cahiers d'Archéologie Subaquatique* 1 (1972): 107–08.
Parker, Anthony J. "Amphores Almagro 50 de l'épave de Randello (Sicile)." in *Amphores Romaines et Histoire Économique. Dix Ans de Recherche.* Collection de l'École Française de Rome, 114. Rome 1989, pp. 650–53.
———. "The Evidence Provided by Underwater Archaeology for Roman Trade in the Western Mediterranean." in *Marine Archaeology.* D. J. Blackman, ed. London 1973, pp. 361–79.
———. "Lead Ingots from a Roman Ship at Ses Salines, Majorca." *International Journal of Nautical Archaeology and Underwater Exploration* 3,1 (1974): 148.
———. "Lusitanian Amphoras." in *Méthodes classiques et méthodes formelles dans l'étude des amphores. Actes du Colloque de Rome, 27–29 Mai 1974.* Collection de l'École Française de Rome, no. 32, Rome 1977, pp. 35–46.
———. "Roman Amphoras: A Review Article." *International Journal of Nautical Archaeology and Underwater Exploration* 1 (1972): 225–29.
———. "Shipwrecks and Ancient Trade in the Mediterranean." *Archaeological Review from Cambridge* 3 (1984): 99–113.
———. "Sicilia e Malta nel commercio marittimo dell'antichità." *Kokalos* 22–23 (1976–77): 622–31.
———. and Jennifer Price. "Spanish Exports of the Claudian Period: the Significance of the Port Vendres II Wreck Reconsidered." *International Journal of Nautical Archaeology and Underwater Exploration* 10,3 (1981): 221–28.
Pârvan, Vasile. "La pénétration hellénique et hellénistique dans la vallée du Danube." *Académie Roumaine. Bulletin de la Section Historique, vol. 10.* Bucarest 1923, pp. 23–47.
Pascual Guasch, Ricardo. "Algunos aspectos del comercio antiguo según las ánforas." in *Comunicaciónes a la I reunion de historia de la economía antigua de la península ibérica.* Papeles del laboratorio de arqueología de Valencia, no. 5. Valencia 1968, pp. 67–79.
———. "Ánforas de garum en Culip." *Rivista de la Mar* (Centro de Recuperaciones e Investigaciones Submarinas) 6 (1959): 10–11.
———. "Dos ánforas del Pecio Gandolfo (Almería)." *Zephyrus* 11 (1960): 205–09.

———. "La evolución de las exportaciones béticas durante el Imperio." in *Produccion y comercio del aceite en la antigüedad. Primer Congreso Internacional*. María Blázquez Martínez, ed. Madrid 1980, pp. 233–42.
———. "El Pecio Gandolfo (Almería)." *Pyrenae* 4 (1968): 141–55.
———. "Sobre una estampilla anfórica de Ampurias." *Miscelánea Arqueológica*. Vol. 2. Barcelona 1974, pp. 139–44.
———. "Underwater Archaeology in Andalusia (Almeria and Granada)." *International Journal of Nautical Archaeology and Underwater Exploration* 2,1 (1973): 107–19.
Paunier, Daniel. *La céramique gallo-romaine de Genève*. Geneva 1981.
Peacock, D. P. S. "Amphorae and the Baetican Fish Industry." *The Antiquaries Journal* 54 (1974): 232–43.
———. "Amphorae in Iron Age Britain: A Reassessment." in *Cross-Channel Trade Between Gaul and Britain in the Pre-Roman Iron Age*. Sarah Macready and F. H. Thompson, eds. London 1984, pp. 37–42.
———. "Roman Amphorae in Pre-Roman Britain." in *The Iron Age and Its Hill Forts*. David Hill and Margaret Jesson, eds. Southampton 1971, pp. 161–88.
———. and D. F. Williams. *Amphorae and the Roman Economy. An Introductory Guide*. London 1986.
Pedrosa-Menabrito, Alberto and Joe M. Regenstein. "Shelf-life Extension of Fresh Fish—a Review. Part I—Spoilage of Fish." *Journal of Food Quality* 1,2 (1988): 117–27.
Pellati, Francesco. "I monumenti del Portogallo romano." *Historia* 5 (1931): 196–217.
Pilar G. Serrano, Maria. "Ánforas romanas en las costas de Mallorca." *Archivo español de arqueología* 36 (1963): 207–10.
Pirazzoli, Paolo Antonio. "Submerged Remains of Ancient Megisti in Castellorizo Island (Greece): a Preliminary survey." *International Journal of Nautical Archaeology and Underwater Exploration* 16,1 (1987): 57–66.
Ponsich, Michel. *Aceite de Oliva y Salazones de Pescado. Factores Geo-Economicos de Betica y Tingitania*. Madrid 1988.
———. "Pérennité des relations dans le circuit du Détroit de Gibraltar." in *Aufstieg und Niedergang der römischen Welt*. Hildegard Temporini and Wolfgang Haase, eds. Vol. II, Pt. 3. Berlin 1975, pp. 655–84.
———. "A propos d'une usine antique de salaisons à Belo (Bolonia-Cadix)." *Mélanges de la Casa de Velazquez* 12 (1976): 69–79.
———. *Recherches archéologiques à Tanger et dans sa région*. Paris 1970.
———. and Miguel Tarradell. *Garum et industries antiques de salaison dans la Méditerranée occidentale*. Preface by André Piganiol. Paris 1965.
Preisigke, Friedrich. *Wörterbuch der griechischen Papyrusurkunden*. 3 vols. Berlin 1925.
Purpura, Gianfranco. "Pesca e stabilimenti antichi per la lavorazione del pesce in Sicilia: 1. S. Vito (Trapani), Cala Minnola (Levanzo)." *Sicilia Archeologica* 48 (1982): 45–60.
———. "Pesca e stabilimenti antichi per la lavorazione del pesce in Sicilia: II. Isola delle Femmine (Palermo), Punta Molinazzo (Punta Rais), Tonnara del Cofano (Trapani), S. Nicola (Favignana)." *Sicilia Archeologica* 57–58 (1985): 59–86.
Radcliffe, William. *Fishing from the Earliest Times*. London 1921.
Rebuffat, René. *Thamusida III*. Supplement 2 of *Mélanges d'archéologie et d'histoire de l'École de Française de Rome*. Rome 1977.
Reil, Theodor. *Beiträge zur Kenntnis des Gewerbes im hellenistischen Ägypten*. Leipzig 1913.
Remark, Peter. *De Amphorarum Inscriptionibus Latinis Quaestiones Selectae*. Tübingen 1912.
Remondon, R. "Un nouveau document concernant Probus." *Revue de Philologie* 28 (1954): 199–210.
Rey-Coquais, Jean-Paul. *Inscriptions grecques et latines découvertes dans les fouilles de Tyr (1963–1974). I. Inscriptions de la nécropole*. Bulletin du Musée de Beyrouth, 19. Paris 1977.
Rhode, Paul. *Thynnorum Captura Quanti Fuerit apud Veteres Momenti*. Leipzig 1890.
Riley, J. A. "The Coarse Pottery from Berenice." in *Excavations at Sidi Khrebish Benghazi (Berenice)*. 2 Vols. Suppl. 5 to *Libya Antiqua*. Tripoli 1979, 2: 91–449.
Robert, Louis. "Épitaphes ex acclamations Byzantines à Corinthe." *Hellenica* 11–12 (1960): 21–52.
Roesch, Paul. "Sur le tarif des poissons d'Akraiphia." *Zeitschrift für Papyrologie und Epigraphik* 14 (1974): 5–9.
Rose, Valentine. "Aringus, der Hering." *Hermes* 8 (1874): 224–27.

Rostovtzeff, M. *The Social and Economic History of the Hellenistic World*. 3 vols. Oxford 1941.
———. *The Social and Economic History of the Roman World*. 2 vols. Rev. by P. M. Fraser. Oxford 1957.
Saisithi, Prasert, Bung-orn Kasemsarn, J. Liston, and Alexander M. Dollar. "Microbiology and Chemistry of Fermented Fish." *Journal of Food Science* 31 (1966): 105–10.
Salviat, F. and C. Vatin. "Le tarif des poissons d'Akraiphia." in *Inscriptions de Grèce centrale*. Paris 1971, pp. 95–109.
Salza Prina Ricotti, Eugenia. *L'arte del convito nella Roma antica*. Rome 1985.
Sanchez Leon, Maria Luisa. *Economía de la Hispania meridional durante la dinastia de los Antoninos*. Salamanca 1978.
Sanquer, René. "Les industriels des salaisons en Armorique romaine." *Caesarodonum* 10 (1975): 148–56.
———. "Informations archéologiques. Bretagne (Finistère): Douarnenez." *Gallia* 35 (1977): 355–60.
———. "Informations archéologiques. Bretagne (Finistère): Douarnenez." *Gallia* 41 (1983): 291–92.
———. "Informations archéologiques. Bretagne. Lanester." *Gallia* 41 (1983): 289–90.
———. "Informations archéologiques. Bretagne (Morbihan): Lanester." *Gallia* 39 (1981): 316–18.
———. "Informations archéologiques. Bretagne: Plonevez-Porzay." *Gallia* 37 (1979): 365.
———. "Une nouvelle lecture de l'inscription à Neptune trouvée à Douarnenez (Finistère) et l'industrie du garum armoricain." *Annales de Bretagne* (Rennes) 80 (1973): 215–36.
———. and Patrick Galliou. "Garum, sel et salaisons en Armorique gallo-romaine." Gallia 30 (1972): 199–223.
Sato, Tokuro, Tomitaro Fukuyama, Taedo Suzuki, Junko Takayanagi, Tadashige Murakami, Nobuya Shiotsuki, Ryozo Tanaka, and Ryo Tsuji. "Studies of the Causation of Gastric Cancer: 2. The Relation Between Gastric Cancer Mortality Rate and Salted Food Intake in Several Places in Japan." *Bulletin of the Institute of Public Health* (Tokyo,Japan) 8 (1959): 187–98.
Sazanov, A. V., "O xronologii Bospora rannevizantijskogo vremeni." *Sovetskaja Arxeologija*. No. 4 (1989): 41–60.
———. and Ju. F. Ivanščenko. "K voprosu o datirovkax pozdneantičnyx sloev gorodov Bospora." *Sovetskaja Arxeologija*. No. 1 (1989): 84–102.
Scarborough, John. "Adaptation of Folk Medicine in the Formal Materia Medica of Classical Antiquity." in *Folklore and Folk Medicines*. John Scarborough, ed. Madison, Wisconsin 1987, pp. 21–32.
———. "Diphilus of Siphnos and Hellenistic Medical Dietetics." *Journal of the History of Medicine and Allied Sciences* 25,2 (April 1970): 194–201.
———. *Roman Medicine*. Ithaca, N.Y. 1969.
———. "Roman Pharmacy and the Eastern Drug Trade: Some Problems as Illustrated by the Example of Aloe." *Pharmacy in History* 24,4 (1982): 135–43.
Schleiermacher, Wilhelm. "Tipasa." *Germania* 43 (1965): 165–68.
Schmeling, Gareth. "Trimalchio's Menu and Wine List." *Classical Philology* 65 (1970): 248–51.
Schuring, Josine M. "Studies on Roman Amphorae, I-II." *Bulletin Antieke Beschaving* 59,2 (1984): 137–95.
Sealey, Paul R. *Amphoras from the 1970 Excavations at Colchester Sheepen*. BAR British Series, 142. Oxford 1985.
Semenov-Zuser, S. "Rybnyj rynok v Xersonese." *Vestnik Drevnej Istorii* 2 (1947): 237–46.
Shelton, John. "Garum rouge Sang." *Zeitschrift für Papyrologie und Epigraphik* 17 (1975): 156.
Sherwin-White, Susan. *Ancient Cos*. Hypomnemata, 51. Göttingen 1978.
Siebert, Gunther. "Enzymes of Marine Fish Muscle and Their Role in Fish Spoilage." in *Fish in Nutrition*. Eirik Heen and Rudolf Kreuzer, eds. London 1962, pp. 80–82.
Sijpesteijn, P. J. *Customs Duties in Graeco-Roman Egypt*. Studia Amstelodamensia ad Epigraphicam Ius Antiquum et Papyrologicam Pertinentia, XVII. Zutphen, Holland 1987.
———. "Vierzehn Wiener Papyri." *Aegyptus* 61 (1981): 69–92.
Smidth, J. K. "Historical Observations on the Condition of the Fisheries Among the Ancient Greeks and Romans, and on Their Mode of Salting and Pickling Fish." U.S. Congress, Senate, 43rd Congress, 2nd session, *Miscellaneous Documents*, No. 108. Washington 1875, pp. 3–20.

Smith, W. D. "The Development of Classical Dietetic Theory." in *Hippocratica Actes du Colloque hippocratique de Paris (4–9 septembre 1978)*. M. D. Grmek, ed. Paris 1980, pp. 439–48.

Solier, Y. "Dépôt d'huîtres au Boulevard de 1848." *Bulletin de la Commission archéologique de Narbonne* 38 (1964–1965): 73–76.

———. "Les épaves de Gruissan." *Archaeonautica* 3 (1981): 8–264.

Solin, Heikki. "Tabelle plumbee di Concordia." *Aquileia Nostra* 48 (1977): 145–64.

Sotomayor, M. "Nueva factoría de salazones de pescado en Almuñécar (Granada)." *Noticiario arqueológico hispánico* 15 (1971): 147–78.

Sperber, Daniel. "Objects of Trade Between Palestine and Egypt in Roman Times." *Journal of the Economic and Social History of the Orient* 19 (1976): 113–47.

———. "On Social and Economic Conditions in Third Century Palestine." *Archiv orientální* 38 (1970): 1–25.

———. *Roman Palestine 200–400: Money and Prices*. Ramat-Gan 1974.

———. "Some Observations of Fish and Fisheries in Roman Palestine." *Zeitschrift der deutschen morgenländischen Gesellschaft* 118 (1968): 265–69.

Stannard, Jerry. "Hippocratic Pharmacology." *Bulletin of the History of Medicine* 34 (1961): 497–518.

Steinkraus, Keith H., Roger E. Culler, Carl S. Pederson, Lois F. Nellis, and Ben K. Gavitt, eds. *Handbook of Indigenous Fermented Foods*. New York 1983.

Stuart, Piet. "Nehalennia: Goddess from the Sea." *Delta* 14 (Aug., 1971): 5–23.

———. "130 römische Steindenkmäler aus dem Meer." *Archäologisches Korrespondenzblatt* 2 (1972): 299–302.

———. and J. E. Bogaers. "Catalogus van de monumentem." in *Deae Nehalenniae*. Leiden 1971, pp. 59–80.

Taffanel, Odette and Jean Taffanel. "Marques d'amphores trouvées au Cayla de Mailhac (Aude)." *Gallia* 5 (1947): 143–46.

Tailliez, Philippe. "Travaux de l'été 1958 sur l'épave du 'Titan' à l'île du Lévant (Toulon)." in *Atti del II Congresso Internazionale di Archeologia Sottomarina, Albenga 1958*. Bordighera 1961, pp. 173–98.

Tanzer, Helen H. *The Common People of Pompeii: A Study of the Graffiti*. Baltimore 1939.

Tarradell, Miguel. "Marruecos antiquo: neuvas perspectivas." *Zephyrus* 5 (1954): 105–39.

Tavares da Silva, Carlos and Mateus Gonçalves Cabrita. "O problema da destruição da povoação romana de Tróia de Setúbal." *Revista de Guimarães* 76 (1966): 147–55.

Tchernia, André. "Les amphores romaines et l'histoire économique." *Journal des savantes* 65 (1967): 216–34.

———. "Direction des recherches archéologiques sous-marines." *Gallia* 27 (1969): 465–99.

Testaguzza, Otello. *Portus*. Rome 1970.

Théodoridès, Jean. "Considerations on the Medical Use of Marine Invertebrates." in *Oceanography: the Past*. M. Sears and D. Merriman, eds. New York 1980, pp. 734–49.

Thompson, D'Arcy W. "Byzantios olent lacertos (Stat. *S*. 4, 9, 13)." *Classical Review* 46 (1932): 246–48.

———. *A Glossary of Greek Fishes*. London 1947.

Thouvenot, Raymond. *Essai sur le province romaine de Bétique*. Paris 1940.

Tomašević, Theodora. *Die Keramik der XIII Legion aus Vindonissa*. Veröffentlichungen der Gesellschaft pro Vindonissa, no. 7. Vindonissa 1970.

Tsirkin, Yu. B. "Economy of the Phoenician Settlements in Spain." in *State and Temple Economy in the Ancient Near East, II*. Orientalia Lovaniensia Analecta, 6. Leuven 1979, pp. 547–64.

Vaggi, Giuseppina. "Siria e Siri nei documenti dell'Egitto greco-romano." *Aegyptus* 37 (1937): 29–51.

Van Veen, A. G. "Fermented and Dried Seafood Products in Southeast Asia." in *Fish as Food*. Georg Borgström, ed. 4 vols. New York 1965, 3: 227–50.

Veiga Ferreira, O. Da. "Algumas considerações sobre as fábricas de conservas de peixe da antiquidade encontradas em Portugal." *Arquivo de Beja* 23–24 (1966–1967): 123–34.

———. "Algumas notas acera da pesca na antiguidade." *O Arqueologo português*. 3rd ser. 2 (1968): 113–33.

Vieillefond, Jean-René. *Les 'Cestes' de Julius Africanus*. Florence 1970.

Vivenza, Gloria. "Gli 'Hedyphagetica' di Ennio e il commercio del pesce in età repubblicana." *Economia e Storia* 1 (1981): 5–44.

Voskresensky, N. A. "Salting of Herring." in *Fish as Food*. Georg Borgström, ed. 4 vols. New York 1965, 3: 107–31.

Vrsalović, Dasen. *Istraživanja i Zaštita Podmorskih Arheoloških Spomenika u SR Hrvatskoj*. Zagreb 1974.

Wang, H. L. and C. W. Hesseltine. *Indigenous Fermented Food of Non-western Origin*. Mycologia Memoirs, No. 11. Berlin 1986.

Wąsowicz, Aleksandra. *Olbia pontique et son territoire. L'aménagement de l'espace*. Centre de Recherches d'Histoire Ancienne, vol. 13. Paris 1975.

Wheeler, Alwyne and Alison Locker. "The Estimation of Size in Sardines (Sardina pilchardus) from Amphorae in a Wreck at Randello, Sicily." *Journal of Archaeological Science* 12 (1985): 97–100.

White, Jonathan W. Jr. "Relative Significance of Dietary Sources of Nitrate and Nitrite." *Journal of Agricultural and Food Chemistry* 23 (1975): 886–91.

Wilcken, Ulrich. *Griechische Ostraka aus Aegypten und Nubien*. 2 vols. Leipzig-Berlin 1899.

———. "Zusätze zu dem Aufsatz: Zur Topographie der Ruinenstätte des alten Schet (Krokodilopolis-Arsinoë)." *Zeitschrift der Gesellschaft für Erdkunde zu Berlin* 22 (1887): 79–88.

Wilkes, W. G. St. J. "Underwater Exploration of the Ancient Port of Nora, Sardinia." *Papers of the British School at Rome* 35 (1967): 4–11.

Will, Elizabeth Lyding. "Ähnlichkeiten zwischen Stempeln auf Amphoren und auf arretinischen Gefässen." *Rei Cretariae Romanae Fautores Acta* 23–24 (1984): 9–11.

———. "Amphoras and Trade in Roman Sardinia." in *Studies in Sardinian Archaeology*. Vol. II: *Sardinia in the Mediterranean*. Miriam S. Balmuth, ed. Ann Arbor 1986, pp. 211–28.

Williams, D. F. "The Roman Amphora Trade with Late Iron Age Britain." in *Production and Distribution: a Ceramic Viewpoint*. Hilary Howard and Elaine L. Morris, eds. BAR International Series, 120. Oxford 1981, pp. 123–32.

Williams, Charles K., II. "Corinth, 1977: Forum Southwest." *Hesperia* 47 (1978): 1–39.

———. "Corinth, 1978: Forum Southwest." *Hesperia* 48 (1979): 105–44.

———. "Corinth Excavations, 1979." *Hesperia* 49,2 (1980): 107–34.

Wölfflin, Eduard von. "Salsamentarius." *Archiv für lateinische Lexikografie und Grammatik* 12 (1902): 366.

Worp, K. A. "Deux papyrus byzantins d'Amsterdam." *Chronique d'Égypt* 49 (1974): 130–34.

Wright, R. P. and M. W. C. Hassall. "Roman Britain in 1973: II. Inscriptions." *Britannia* 5 (1974): 467, no. 44.

Yu, S. I., C. L. Siaw, and A. Z. Idrus. "The Application of Technology to the Processing of Dry-Salted Fish in Peninsular Malaysia: comparison of Sun-dried and oven-dried Fish." *Journal of Food Technology* 17,2 (April 1982): 211–18.

Zahn, R. "Garum," in *Real-encyclopädie der classischen Altertumswissenschaft*. A. Pauly, G. Wissowa, and W. Kroll, eds. Stuttgart 1912, vol. 7, cols. 841–49.

Zaninović, Marin, "The Economy of Roman Dalmatia." *Aufstieg und Niedergang der römischen Welt*. Hildagard Temporini and Wolfgang Haase, eds. II,6 (Berlin 1977), pp. 767–809.

Zemer, Avshalom. *Storage Jars in Ancient Sea Trade*. Haifa 1977.

Zevi, Fausto. "Appunti sulle anfore romane." *Archeologia classica* 18 (1966): 208–47.

———. [Review of *Roman Amphorae* by M. H. Callender]. *Journal of Roman Studies* 57 (1967): 234–38.

———. and André Tchernia. "Amphores de Byzacène au Bas-Empire." *Antiquités africaines* 3 (1969): 173–214.

INDEX

I. Ancient Sources

The index of ancient sources must of necessity be a selective one, although I have included a few important citations properly Byzantine, Medieval and later. No attempt has been made to list every occurrence of an ancient citation. I have included those instances where the text has been quoted, where the passage has been discussed at length, where the source has been spotlighted in the text or footnotes, or where the citation has been considered worthy of inclusion for other reasons, such as the relative obscurity of the author or work. These criteria have also been followed for epigraphical and papyrological sources as well.

A. LITERATURE

B. EPIGRAPHY

C. PAPYRI

II. General

This index is of necessity selective. No effort has been made to be exhaustive, nor has every occurrence of each entry been listed. With few exceptions names and works cited in Part I–A of the Index have been omitted from this section. Roman names appear under their *nomen*.

STUDIES IN ANCIENT MEDICINE

1. F. Kudlien and Richard Durling (eds.). *Galen's Method of Healing*. Proceedings of the 2nd International Galen Symposium. 1991. ISBN 90 04 09272 2
2. Hippocrates. *Pseudepigraphic Writings*. Letters — Embassy — Speech from the Altar — Decree. Edited and translated by Wesley D. Smith. 1990. ISBN 90 04 09290 0
3. Robert I. Curtis. *Garum and Salsamenta*. Production and Commerce in Materia Medica. 1991. ISBN 90 04 09423 7

In preparation:

Jody Rubin Pinault. *Hippocratic Lives and Legends.*